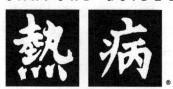

SANFORD GUIDE®

W9-CHT-654

THE SANFORD GUIDE TO HIV/AIDS THERAPY 2006-2007

15th Edition

THE SANFORD GUIDE TO HIV/AIDS THERAPY 2006–2007
15TH EDITION

Jay P. Sanford, M.D.
1928–1996

EDITORS

Merle A. Sande, M.D.
Professor of Medicine
University of Washington
Seattle, Washington

George M. Eliopoulos, M.D.
Chief, James L. Tullis Firm,
Beth Israel Deaconess Hospital
Professor of Medicine
Harvard Medical School
Boston, Massachusetts

Robert C. Moellering, Jr., M.D.
Shields Warren-Malinckrodt Professor of Medicine
Harvard Medical School
Boston, Massachusetts

David N. Gilbert, M.D.
Director of Medical Education & Earl A. Chiles Research Institute
Providence Portland Medical Center
Professor of Medicine

CONTRIBUTING EDITOR
Andrew T. Pavia, M.D.
George and Esther Gross Presidential Professor
Chief, Division of Pediatric Infectious Diseases
University of Utah
Salt Lake City, Utah

The Sanford Guides are published annually by

ANTIMICROBIAL THERAPY, INC.
P.O. Box 276, 11771 Lee Highway
Sperryville, VA 22740 USA
Tel 540-987-9480 Fax 540-987-9486
Email: info@sanfordguide.com   www.sanfordguide.com

Printed in the United States of America
ISBN 1-930808-34-8
Pocket Edition

The Sanford Guide is available from a variety of sources. You may have purchased your copy at
a bookstore or directly from us. You may also have received your copy from a pharmaceutical
company representative. Regardless of the source, you can be assured that the Sanford Guide
has been, and continues to be, independently prepared and published since its inception in
1969. Decisions regarding the content of the Sanford Guide are solely those of the editors and the
publisher. We welcome your questions, comments and feedback concerning the Sanford Guide.
All of your feedback is reviewed and taken into account in preparing the next edition. Content-
related notices are posted on the Sanford Guide website at **www.sanfordguide.com**

You may notice that this edition is longer than last year's book. In addition to new material added,
we have re-designed the manuscript to reduce density in an effort to make the text easier to
read. Our thanks to Gerette Braunsdorf for her efforts in updating the design of this complex
manuscript.

IMPORTANT NOTE TO READER

Every effort is made to ensure the accuracy of the content of this guide. However, current full
prescribing information available in the package insert for each drug should be consulted before
prescribing any product. The editors and publisher are not responsible for errors or omissions
or for any consequences from application of the information in this book and make no warranty,
express or implied, with respect to the currency, accuracy, or completeness of the contents of
the publication. Application of this information in a particular situation remains the professional
responsibility of the practitioner.

— TABLE OF CONTENTS —

TABLE 1	Assessment of **HIV Risks** & Recommendations for **Testing**.	*Page 1*
TABLE 2	**Initial Evaluation & Follow-Up** of HIV-Infected Adults.	*Page 3*
TABLE 3	**Diagnostic Tests**: HIV-1, HIV-2, HTLV-1, HTLV-2.	*Page 5*
TABLE 4	**HIV Classification**: CDC (1993 Revision), Karnofsky Scale, WHO Clinical Staging System.	*Page 15*
TABLE 5	**TMP/SMX Desensitization**.	*Page 16*
FIGURE 1	**Course** of HIV Infection/Disease in Adults, Clinical Decision Points.	*Page 17*
TABLE 6	**Antiretroviral Therapy** in Adults. Antiretroviral Drugs, Dosage, Adverse Effects. Drug Adverse Effects By Clinical Presentation. Drugs in the Anti-HIV Pipeline. Antiretroviral Approved or Tentatively Approved by FDA	*Page 18* *Page 28* *Page 30* *Page 33* *Page 34*
TABLE 7	**Penicillin Desensitization**.	*Page 34*
TABLE 8	HIV/AIDS in **Women/Newborn/Children**.	*Page 35*
TABLE 9	Management of **Occupational Exposure**.	*Page 50*
TABLE 10	Primary **Prophylaxis** Against Opportunistic Pathogens.	*Page 53*
TABLE 11	Diagnosis & Differential Diagnosis of **Opportunistic Infections**. **Immune Reconstitution & Novel Clinical Syndromes** Associated with **HAART**.	*Page 55* *Page 103*
TABLE 12	Treatment of **Specific Infections**. Dosages.	*Page 106*
TABLE 13	**Adverse Effects**, Comments on Drugs for Specific Infections.	*Page 137*
TABLE 14	**Pharmacokinetics** of Drugs Used in HIV Patients.	*Page 147*
TABLE 15	Drug Dosage Adjustments in **Renal & Hepatic Dysfunction**. Dosage of **Antiretroviral Drugs** in **Impaired Hepatic Function**.	*Page 149*
TABLE 16	**Drug-Drug Interactions**.	*Page 156*
TABLE 17	Antimicrobics in **Pregnancy**.	*Page 164*
TABLE 18	Treatment of HIV-Associated **Malignancies**.	*Page 165*
TABLE 19	**Immunization** of HIV-Infected **Children**.	*Page 167*
TABLE 20	**Immunization** of HIV-Infected **Adults**.	*Page 168*
TABLE 21	Preparing Patients for **Overseas Travel**.	*Page 169*
TABLE 22	Drugs Used in Treatment of **Hematocytopenias**.	*Page 170*
TABLE 23	AIDS **Information** & **Referral Services**.	*Page 171*
TABLE 24	**Generic** & Common **Trade Names**.	*Page 172*
INDEX		*Page 173*

TABLE 1: ASSESSMENT OF HIV INFECTION RISKS & RECOMMENDATIONS FOR HIV TESTING

I. General

HIV risk assessment is an essential component of primary care for all patients. In talking to patients, avoid medical jargon (e.g., "intercourse"), vague terms ("sexually active"), group designations ("homosexual"), or judgmental terms ("promiscuous"). Learn the language & terminology understood & used by patients. Question responses to the depth necessary to elicit risky behavior & define extent of risk of acquisition & transmission. Eliciting risk is particularly difficult but equally important in resource-limited areas of the world, esp. when working through translators. It is essential that the clinician be knowledgeable about cultural sensitivities, customs & traditions relative to HIV risk behavior.

Risk-reduction counseling works to reduce high-risk behavior in North America, Europe, Africa, & SE Asia. *(Cochrane Database Syst Rev 1: CD001230, 2003; AIDS 16:953 & 2209, 2002; J AIDS 29:284 & 409, 2002; J AIDS 30:S118, 2002; J AIDS 31:2002, 2002; Sex Trans Dis 29:520, 2002; CID 36:1577, 2003; MMWR 152:329, 2003).* Revised CDC Guidelines: *MMWR 50(RR-19):1, 2001.* It is time to include HIV counseling & testing as a critical component of health care maintenance *[MMWR 51(RR-12), 2003].*

II. Specific Behaviors Associated With HIV Transmission

A. Sexual Behaviors. The CDC now recommends ART post-exposure prophylaxis within 72 hrs after sexual, injection-drug use, or other non-occupational exposure to HIV *(MMWR Recomm Rep 54:1, 2005) (See Table 9).* Not 100% effective; seroconversion still detected in 1% of 702 exposed individuals *(CID 41:1507, 2005).*

1. **High-Risk Sexual Partner(s)**
   - HIV-infected partners [especially those with ↑ HIV-RNA *(NEJM 342:921,2000, Sex Trans Dis 29:38, 2002)]*
   - Partners who are at risk but have not been HIV tested [risk of HIV often underappreciated by partners; example, 15.7% crack cocaine smokers HIV+ vs 5.2% in non-smokers in one series, women > men (sex for money or drugs) *(NEJM 331:1422, 1994)* or do not disclose their HIV status to their partners *(MMWR 52:81, 2003)]*
   - Multiple partners: Unsafe sexual activity appears to be ↑ with MSM in American & European cities *(AIDS 16:1537 & 2329, 2002; J AIDS 30:522, 2002; J AIDS 31:63, 2002).*
   - Presence of mucosal ulceration or other STD in either partner *(JID 178:1060, 1998)*

2. **Sexual Practices**
   a. **High infection risk**
      - Unprotected anal receptive intercourse: on the rise in young gay males
      - Unprotected vaginal receptive intercourse
   b. **Infection risk documented**
      - Unprotected anal insertive intercourse
      - Unprotected vaginal insertive intercourse (risk may be higher during menses)
      - Unprotected oral receptive intercourse [HIV RNA levels in rectal secretions > serum with & without ART use *(JID 190:156, 2004)]*
      - Unprotected oral insertive intercourse rare *(ArIM 159:303, 1999)*
   c. **Lower infection risk**
      - Any of the above with latex/vinyl condom (vaginal or penile) protection. In 343 HIV-neg. women partners of HIV+ men, seroconversion for those who used condoms with every encounter was 1.1/100 person years while for those who used condoms intermittently or not at all, rate was 7.2/100 person years. In Thailand, aggressive condom campaign reduced seroprevalence from 7.2 to 3.8% in military conscripts. In 1995, rate was 0.55/100 person years *(AIDS 12:F29, 1998).* In U.S., condom use estimated to reduce risk 20-fold *(Sex Trans Dis 29:38, 2002).* However, among female sex workers, 12.5% still became HIV infected during the 100% condom program *(J AIDS 21:373, 1999).* Male condoms are 80–95% effective in ↓ risk of HIV infection *(AmFAR Issue Brief #1, Jan. 2005);* female condoms 94–97% effective.
      - Cunnilingus, esp. with rubber dam, microwaveable plastic food wrap or other water-impervious barrier
      - Circumcision reduced HIV infection by 60% in a prospective randomized study in 3,274 men in South Africa RR, 0.40 (p<.001) *(PLoS Med e298, 2005)* Other studies in progress.
      - Microbicides currently in development but data on effectiveness lacking *(JID 193; 36, 2006).* Nonoxynol-9 actually facilitated transmission *(JAMA 287:1171,2002)*
   d. **Safer**
      - Deep kissing
      - Protected sex with HIV test negative partner
      - Mutual monogamy
      - Mutual masturbation
      - Masturbation or massage
   e. **Safest**
      - Abstinence

3. **Conditions That Facilitate HIV Sexual Transmission** *(J AIDS 30:73, 2002; JID 191:333, 2005)*

Male-to-Female Transmission — Relative Risk Reported

(a) Oral contraceptives	2.5–4.5
(b) Gonococcal cervicitis	1.8–4.5
(c) Candida vaginitis	3.3–3.6
(d) Genital ulcers	2.0–4.0
(e) Bacterial vaginosis	2.4 *(J AIDS 29:409, 2002)*
(f) HSV-2	2.5
(g) Vitamin A deficiency	2.6–12.9
(h) CD4 count <200	6.1–17.6
(i) Depomedroxyprogesterone acetate (DMPA) subdermal implant use as contraceptive	2.2 *(JID 178:1053, 1998)*
(j) Sharing of HLA-B alleles in discordant couples	2.23 *(Ln 363:2137, 2004)*

Female-to-Male Transmission

(a) Lack of circumcision (but not male to female)	5.4–8.2 risk/coital act ↓ from 1/80 to 1/200 *(Ln 1: 223, 2001; Ln 363:1039, 2004; JID, Feb. 15, 2005)*
(b) Genital ulcers	2.6–4.7
(c) Sex during menses	3.4
(d) Herpes simplex type 2 (genital herpes)	6–16.8 *(JID 187:1513, 2003 & 189;1209, 2004))*

↑ Titers of viral DNA in vaginal secretions *(JID 175:57, 1997)*

(a) With low CD4 count	9.6 (<200 vs >500)
(b) Vitamin A deficiency	2.6
(c) Presence of cervical mucopus	2.1
(d) Acute primary HIV infection	↑
(e) With ↑ plasma HIV-RNA	↑ *(JID 177:1100, 1998)*
(f) Cervicitis	↑ *(AIDS 15:105, 2001)*
(g) Peak titer just prior to onset of menses	↑ *(JID 189:2192, 2004)*

TABLE 1 (2)

↑ Titers of viral DNA in semen (ejaculate) (*JID 172:1469, 1995; J AIDS & HR 18:277, 1998*)
   (a) Gonococcal urethritis   3.2
   (b) Acute primary HIV infection   ↑ (*AIDS 16:1529, 2002*)
Not protective:
   (a) Nonoxynol-9 intravaginally (*Ln 360:971, 2002; AIDS 18:2191, 2004*)
   (b) IUD use

4. Programs Aimed at Reducing Sexual Transmission
The major route of HIV spread worldwide is via heterosexual vaginal intercourse. Efforts to change sexual behavior by reducing number of sexual partners & using safe sex techniques (condoms) have met with varying degrees of success. These are summarized here:

   a. Voluntary counseling & testing (VCT): Prevention based on identifying infected persons & counseling them to prevent transmission to sexual partner(s). Variable success (*AIDS 15:1045, 2001; J AIDS 31:106, 2002; ArIM 162:1818, 2002*)
      (1) In >10,000 pregnant women in Tanzania, 3/4 agreed to be tested. 2/3 of those returned for results but only 1/6 of positives disclosed result to sexual partner because of fear of stigma & divorce (*J AIDS 28:458, 2001*).
      (2) Others reported VCT associated with ↓ risk behaviors & ↓ HIV transmission among discordant couples (*Soc Sc Med 53:1397, 2001*) & both men & women in Thailand (*J AIDS 29:284, 2002; J AIDS 15:493, 2002*).
      (3) Acceptance ↑ if test results available same day (*Ann NY Acad Sci 918:64, 2000*).
   b. Counseling & controlling STD in female sex workers: ↓ seroincidence of HIV from 16.3 to 6.5/100 person yrs in 500 subjects in Cote d'Ivoire (*AIDS 15:1421, 2000*) & Benin (*AIDS 16:463, 2002; J AIDS 30:69, 2002*), & U.S. (*JAMA 292:171, 2004*)
   c. Condom distribution campaigns: Successfully ↓ HIV prevalence in Thailand from 17% in 1992 to 2% in 1999. In South Africa <10% of distributed condoms discarded (*AIDS 15:789, 2001*).
   d. Prevention campaign focused on education about AIDS & promotion of safer sexual behavior: Appears to have been effective in Uganda, Senegal, Zambia (*J AIDS 25:77, 2000*), Mexico (among CSWs) (*AIDS 16:1445, 2002*), & U.S. (*JAMA 292:171, 2004*).
   e. Delivery of message complex. Examples of communication methods used:
      (1) Radio soap opera (Tanzania, *J Health Comm 5(Suppl):81, 2000*)
      (2) Combination of drama or video reached >85% in Uganda (*Health Educ Res 16:411, 2001*)
      (3) Traditional healers or theater in Sierra Leone (*J Assoc Nurs AIDS Care 12:48, 2001*)
      (4) Folk media in rural Ghana (*Am J Publ Health 91:1559, 2001*)
      (5) Religion has been shown to reduce protective behaviors toward AIDS & suggest a critical need to work with clergy to embrace the prevention message (*AIDS 14:2027, 2000*)
   f. HAART ↓ VL in genital secretions & transmission of HIV (by 53%) in Taiwan (*JID 190:879, 2004*). Studies have not demonstrated ↑ in high-risk heterosexual activity on HAART (*JAMA 292:224, 2004*), but remains a concern.

B. Injection (intravenous or "skin popping") Drug Use (IDU) or Smoking Crack Cocaine. Assess injectable anabolic steroid use! Assess sexual behaviors in all drug users! In one study, infection rates in crack cocaine-smoking women are as high as in men who had sex with men (41% vs 43%). Risk-reduction intervention can ↓ high risk sexual activity in crack cocaine users (*AIDS Educ Prev 15:15, 2003*) & IVDUs (*J AIDS 30:573, 2002*). IVDU is currently driving explosive spread of syphilis & HIV in Russian cities (*Int J STD AIDS 13:618, 2002; AIDS 16:F25, 2002*). Interestingly, transmission of drug-resistant HIV ↓ in Amsterdam (*AIDS 18:1571, 2004*). Buprenorphine, shows promise in reducing opioid-dependence, thus reducing HIV transmission (*CID 41:891, 2005*).
   Drug Use Practices: (Drug abuse treatment & methadone use programs reduce HIV transmission: *AIDS 13:2151 & 1807, 1999*)
   1. Riskiest
      • **Sharing uncleaned needles,** syringes, other paraphernalia & works, especially in "shooting galleries." HIV DNA found on 85% of needles/syringes & 1/3–2/3 cottons, cookers, wash waters from shooting galleries.
      • Practicing "registering," "booting," or "back loading"
   2. Less risky
      • Sharing cleaned needles, syringes, works. (Household bleach is effective, especially after washing & when contact time is greater than 5 minutes. It is important to rinse with water after bleach use)
      • Drug paraphernalia used repeatedly but by single user
   3. Least risky
      • Single use needles, syringes, works (needle exchange programs reduce HIV transmission, (see MMWR 54:673,2005 for update of US programs))
      • Sterile needles, syringes, works (needle/syringe exchange appears effective & has not ↑drug use)

C. Blood Product Infusion Recipient
   Blood Product Risks:
   1. Riskiest
      • Receipt of multiple units of blood products between **1978–1985**
      • Receipt of blood products obtained from donors in countries where screening is unreliable or not done
   2. Less risky
      • Receipt of heterologous blood products in U.S. after 1985 (risk per unit 1:450,000 to 1:660,000 units or 1:28,000 after an average of 5.4 units).[This is because of a window period (18–20 days) between infection & seroconversion (18–27 donations/yr are in this window).] HIV p24 antigen testing of all blood products (instituted 3/96) reduces the "window" by 6 days & ↓ infectious donations by 25%/yr to 1:600,000 – 1:800,000 units (*MMWR 45(RR2):1, 1996*). RhoGAM & hepatitis B vaccine (serum-derived) have never been reported to transmit HIV-1.
      • Receipt of donor-selected blood products in U.S. after 1985 (but no safer than random donors)
   3.   Safest
      • Receipt of autologous blood products
      • Receipt of genetically engineered blood product substitutes

D. Perinatal Infection: See Table 8

E. Occupational Exposure (*See Table 9*) (*CDC Guidelines, MMWR 50 (RR-11):1, 2001; AIDS 16:397, 2001*)
   Relative Risk Determinants
   1. Riskiest [risk may be decreased by glove use, which removes >50% blood from exposure site in some studies but HIV-size microbes can pass through 1/3 of latex gloves tested (*J All Clin Imm 97:575, 1996*). With double-glove use, blood-hand contacts ↓ from 71 to 32/100 procedures.
      • Deep parenteral inoculation (RR 16.8) via hollow needle of blood from source with high-titer viremia; seroconversion or advanced HIV disease (RR 7.8)
      • Parenteral inoculation of materials containing high titer virus in research laboratory setting
      • Failure to use ZDV after inoculation (RR 0.1 when used)

TABLE 1 (3)

2. **Less risky**
   - **Small volume exposure via non-hollow needle**
   - Mucosal exposure/non-intact skin exposure [risk is too low to be quantified in prospective studies; not zero but estimated to be at least a log (90%) lower than needlestick risk. Risk may be increased if large volume or prolonged contact occurs]
3. **Risk not identified**
   - **Cutaneous contact** (intact skin)
   - Exposure to urine, saliva, sweat, tears

F. **Donor Organ or Tissue Transplantation**
   1. Test potential donors for HIV (note window between infection & seroconversion *(C.2 above)*
   2. Assess donors for risk factors
   3. Evaluate risk/benefits
      - Risk following artificial insemination with semen from HIV+ donor is 3.5% *(Ln 351: 728, 1998)*. HIV testing recommended but **not legally required**

III. Recommendations for HIV Testing

A. HIV pre-test counseling should be provided to **all persons at risk** & HIV testing recommended. Use of HIV testing as "routine" medical care ↑ from 11 to 25% from 1998 to 2002 in U.S. *(AIDS Reader 15:35, 2005)*. Use pre-test counseling to encourage reduction of risk for acquisition &/or transmission *(Examples: "What do you expect your test results to be? Why? What will you do if you are HIV+? Is there anything different you will do if you are HIV–?")* *(ArIM 159:1994, 1999)*.

B. **"At Risk" Persons May Include:**
   1. All persons (men & women) with identified risk behaviors
   2. All persons with sexually transmitted diseases
   3. All persons with conditions associated with HIV infection *(see above)*
   4. All persons with tuberculosis [among patients seen in TB clinics in 1988–1989, 3.4% (range 0–46%) were HIV+]. Much higher association in 3ʳᵈ World.
   5. Pregnant women in areas of high prevalence. Some authorities recommend testing all pregnant women. Modeling suggests universal antenatal testing would be cost effective even in low-prevalence populations *(JID 190:166, 2004)*.
   6. Women of childbearing age in areas of high prevalence
   7. All patients, age 15–54yrs, in-patient or out-patient, receiving care in institutions where HIV prevalence is ≥1% or AIDS diagnosis rate is ≥1.0 per 1000 discharges *[MMWR 42:(RR-2), 1993 (Jan. 15)]*. Such screening would involve only 593 of the 5558 U.S. Acute Care Hospitals & 12% of all patients but would detect 68% of HIV+ patients hospitalized for conditions other than symptomatic HIV disease. Studies in high-prevalence areas have questions about the 54-year upper age cutoff. For guidelines regarding the conduct of blinded HIV serosurveys in hospitals, contact Seroepidemiology Branch, Mail Stop E-46, CDC, Atlanta, GA 30333.
   8. Patients with unexplained lymphadenopathy, fever, weight loss, other STDs such (syphilis, gonorrhea, chlamydia or genital herpes), signs of subtle immunodeficiency (herpes zoster, oral candidiasis, or oral hairy leukoplakia), those with unexplained pneumococcal bacteremia as well as the well defined AIDS associated OIs & malignancies.

C. **Post-test Counseling:**
   Rapid HIV antibody tests, which can provide results within 20 minutes has improved the efficiency of point of care testing. However a confirmatory test such as Western Blot is still required. It is critically important to offer counseling to those who test positive. Issues to be discussed should include:
   1. Emphasize that HIV infection can now be can be managed successfully as a complicated disease like diabetes
   2. Stigma & the fear of disclosure HIV status
   3. Need to inform previous/current sexual partner
   4. Testing of children & partners at potential risk
   5. Strict adherence to safe-sex practices (especially consistent use of condoms)
   6. Avoidance of drugs that may cause disinhibition (amphetamines, etc)

TABLE 2A: INITIAL EVALUATION OF HIV-INFECTED ADULT PATIENT
(See NEJM 353:16, 2005 for excellent review)

I. **Insist on documentation of a positive HIV antibody test: confirm with a 2ⁿᵈ antibody test, a Western blot, or positive plasma viral quantitation**

II. **History, Review of Systems, & Past Medical History**
   A. **General health status**
      1. General well-being: constitutional symptoms
      2. Infectious disease (TB, leishmaniasis, cocci, histo, etc.): childhood infections, infections in adult life, previous physician visits, hospitalizations (where, when)
      3. Immunization history, e.g., hepatitis A, B, BCG, pneumococcal
   B. **Drug history**
      1. Medications & dosages
         a. Prescription; non-prescription
         b. Alternative therapies
      2. "Recreational" drug use *(see Table 1, above)*
         a. Intravenous/injection; crack cocaine
         b. Other
            c. Identify partners at risk
      3. Smoking & alcohol history
   C. **Sexual history**
      1. Sexual practices *(see Table 1, pg1)*
      2. Past sexually transmitted diseases
      3. Obstetrical/gynecologic history
      4. Contraceptive use
      5. Identify partners at risk

D. **Past or present HIV-related illness, e.g., candidiasis**
E. **Risks for opportunistic infections**
   1. Travel history
   2. Geographic location of current/prior residence, e.g., southwest, midwest of USA
   3. Occupational history, e.g., poultry worker
   4. Avocational activities
   5. Tuberculosis status: history of BCG vaccination, family members with &/or treated for tuberculosis, contacts (close) with patients with known tuberculosis, results of previous tuberculin tests &/or chest x-rays if known
   6. Pets, e.g., cats—Bartonella henselae; fish—M. marinum. Cat ownership not associated with toxoplasma antibody seroconversion
F. **Past history of viral hepatitis, to include type if known, past history of herpes zoster**

III. **Comprehensive Physical Examination**
   A. Document weight & height
   B. Careful funduscopic & oral examination
   C. Dermatologic examination, to include back, buttocks, & extremities, hands, feet
   D. Exam of all lymph node areas: postoccipital, preauricular, cervical, submental, supraclavicular, axillary, epitrochlear, inguinal (measure & record size if palpable, record as negative if not palpable)

TABLE 2A (2)

E. Rectal/genital examination, to include pelvic exam with Pap smear in women, inspection for perianal/genital Herpes simplex. Pap smears should be repeated every 12 months.

F. Assess mental status for evidence of dementia.

IV. Laboratory Evaluation

A. Baseline
1. Complete blood count with differential (anemia may complicate zidovudine rx)
2. Electrolytes, blood sugar (diabetes may complicate use of PIs which cause insulin resistance), renal function tests: BUN, creatinine (abn renal function may complicate use of tenofovir or adjustment in NRTI/NNRTI dosages)
3. Liver function tests: serum bilirubin, aspartate aminotransferase (AST, SGOT), alanine aminotransferase (ALT, SGPT), alkaline phosphatase (Indinavir & atazanavir can elevate indirect bilirubin levels.
4. Creatine kinase (inc level may indicate HIV myopathy & baseline to monitor zidovudine which may cause drug-induced myopathy)
5. Lipid profile (elevated levels may indicate need for dietary/drug therapy or avoidance of certain PIs)

B. HIV staging (important for all future care decisions including when to initiate HAART & prophylaxis)
1. CD4 & CD8 T-lymphocyte count
2. Quantitative measurement of plasma HIV (Table 3)—"viral load" or plasma "viral burden"
3. Possibly baseline genotyping (in areas of ↑ prevalence of drug resistance)

C. Additional studies
1. PPD intermediate (5TU,) or blood assay for M. tbc infection (QuantiFERON-TB GOLD), MMWR 54 (RR-15), 2005 see Table 12, pg109
2. Chest x-ray (baseline important for future care)
3. VDRL or RPR (tests for syphilis) (evidence of past or recent exposure requires treatment unless there is documentation of adequate course of treatment)

4. IgG antibody to toxoplasmosis (if + primary prophylaxis indicated when CD4 <100
5. Hepatitis B surface antigen (HBsAg), antibody to Hep B surface Ag (anti-HBsAg), antibody to Hep C (important in consideration of treatment decisions for chronic active infection & HAART)
6. CMV antibody, IgG
7. G6PD assay (African-Americans)
8. Urine nucleic acid amplification test for N. gonorrhoeae & C. trachomatis

V. Initial Health Care Maintenance
A. HIV risk reduction education (see Table 1)
B. Drug rehabilitation/safer needle use/needle exchange
C. Smoking cessation (smoking ↑ risk of thrush, hairy leukoplakia, bacterial pneumonia)
D. Partner notification
E. Reproductive counseling
F. Psychosocial support
G. Immunizations (see Table 20). Immunizations transiently ↑ HIV viral load, clinical significance uncertain
1. Pneumococcal vaccine
2. Influenza vaccine (annually)
3. Hepatitis B vaccine, if sexually active or sharing needles; hepatitis A vaccine
H. Preventive dentistry
I. If CD4 count <100 cells/mm³, baseline ophthalmologic evaluation
J. Cervical Pap smear females; anal Pap smear males

VI. Primary Care of Patients Infected With HIV
Multiple studies demonstrate that physicians & other health care givers who care for large numbers of HIV-infected persons & who make delivery of this care a major focus of their practice, training & continuing education have better outcomes (see IDSA position statement, CID 26:275, 1998). A team approach with coordination of services around patients' needs & integration of acute & long-term care is emerging as the most effective management. 3rd-party payment with private insurance & Medicaid to pay for services remains a challenge

TABLE 2B: INFORMATION NEEDED FOR MAKING DECISIONS ON WHEN TO START ANTIRETROVIRAL TREATMENT & WHAT TO START WITH: Treatment Plan for ART-Naive Patients

Age & weight (Tables 6 & 8)
Clinical stage of HIV infection (Tables 4A & B)
• CD4 count (Tables 3 & 6)
• Viral load (Tables 3 & 6)
Underlying medical conditions:
• HIV-associated opportunistic infections & malignancies (Tables 11 & 18)
• Tuberculosis (Tables 11 & 12)
• Hepatitis B & C (Tables 11 & 12) & hepatic function (Table 15B)
• Diabetes & other causes of cardiovascular disease (Table 11)

• Renal diseases & renal function (Tables 11 & 15A)
• Pregnancy (Tables 8 & 17)
• Dementia & other CNS conditions (Table 11)
Other medications: drug-drug interactions (Table 16) & allergies
Psychosocial conditions that could influence adherence:
• Depression or other psychiatric conditions
• Illicit drug use, alcoholism, or other addiction
• Stability of living conditions, employment, insurance, finances

TABLE 2C: FOLLOW-UP OF THE HIV-INFECTED PATIENT

Follow-up visits: every 3–6mos/earlier if symptoms dictate or after starting HAART
• Discuss new symptoms, sexual activity & safe sex practices, pregnancy planning, nutrition, mental health, substance abuse, including smoking cessation, adherence to medication, side effects of medications, & any questions brought by patient
• Complete initial assessment (immunizations, lab work)
• Perform focused physical exam
• Labs: CD4 count/viral load, CBC with differential, comprehensive metabolic panel, fasting lipid profiles on HAART, consider HIV genotype/phenotype if patient failing HAART: VL ↑ & CD4 ↓, chest x-ray if indicated (+ PPD)
• Follow-up call or early return if significant abnormalities are found & requiring action (initiation of or change of HAART, initiation of prophylaxis of opportunistic infections, etc.)

Annual exam:
• History as above—review immunization status (influenza vaccine, hepatitis, Pneumovax, Td)
• Complete physical exam including vision test (ophthalmologic referral if CD4 count <100 or abnormalities are found), dental exam
• Labs: PPD, RPR, chlamydia & gonorrhea urinary tests (if indicated by risk activity or signs/symptoms), pelvic exam & Pap smear (q6 mos initially & then annually if normal), testosterone level (if indicated by evidence of wasting), health maintenance appropriate for age & sex (screening for cancer, hypercholesterolemia, etc.). Consider repeat hepatitis serologies if non-immune & repeat toxoplasma serology if initially seronegative & CD4 count <100.

TABLE 3: LABORATORY TESTS COMMONLY USED IN THE DIAGNOSIS & MANAGEMENT OF INFECTION WITH HIV-1, HIV-2, HTLV-1, & HTLV-2

1. **Classification of HIV-1 genetic forms**

2. **HIV-1 & HIV-2 antibody tests**
   A. Serum antibody detection
      (1) EIA ± Western blot
      (2) Rapid detection methods
      (3) Home test kits
   B. Detection of HIV-1 antibody in other body fluids
      (1) Antibody in saliva
      (2) Antibody in urine

3. **HIV-2 antibody tests**

4. **HTLV-1 antibody tests**

5. **HTLV-2 antibody tests**

6. **Detection/quantitation of HIV**
   A. HIV p24 antigen
   B. Qualitative PCR: Circulating cells or plasma
   C. Quantitative plasma viral "burdens"

7. **Guide to logarithmic change**

8. **CD4/CD8 T-lymphocyte counts**
   A. CD4 T-lymphocytes
   B. CD8 T-lymphocytes

9. **Resistance of HIV to antiretroviral medications**
   A. Genotypic resistance testing
   B. Phenotypic resistance testing

1. **Classification of HIV-1—genetic forms.** Ref.: *Ln ID* 2-461, 2002
   A. **Three phylogenetic groups:**
      M = Main   O = Outlier—Central Africa. Rare   N = Novel: Non-M & Non-O—Central Africa. Rare

      9 subtypes (clades)

      A B C D F G H J K

   B. **Circulating recombinant forms (CRFs)** = Intersubtype recombinant viruses identified in 3 or more epidemiologically unlinked people with full-length genome sequencing. CRFs identified by number (in order of discovery) & letters of parental subtypes (CPX = complex: recombinant virus from 3 or more subtypes).
      Examples: CRF01_AE; CRF06 CPX; CRF14_BG—currently 13 CRFs reported (2/2003).
   C. **Geographic distribution of HIV genetic forms**

Area	Circulating Genetic Forms	Area	Circulating Genetic Forms
North & Central America	B	Central Africa	A, (CRF02_AG), C, D, F1, F2, G, H, J, (CRF01_AE), O, N
South America	B, F1, (CRF12 BF)	South Africa	C
Western Europe	B, G, (CRF14 BG)	South Asia	C, B, A
Eastern Europe	A, B, C, F1, (CRF03_AB)	Southeast Asia	B, (CRF01_AE)
Australia	B	China	B, (CRF07_BC), (CRF08_BC), (CRF01_AE)

TABLE 3 (2)

Test	Primary Purpose(s)	Sensitivity %	Specificity %	Comment
2. HIV-1 antibody tests (http://hivinsite.ucsf.edu)				
A. **Detection of antibody in serum or plasma**				
(1) **Enzyme Immunoassay (EIA) followed by Western blot** for confirmation. All detect antibodies to HIV-1 & HIV-2 (see **Comment**)	For all high-risk groups (Table 1); antibody becomes positive approx. 3 wks. post-disease acquisition in majority, 6 mos. after infection. 95% pts antibody-positive.	99.9	99.9	EIA detects IgG, IgA, & IgM antibody to HIV-1, Group B subtype. **Most U.S. HIV infections are due to M group, subtype B.** Current EIAs detect nearly all Group M subtypes. Increasing concern, worldwide, regarding circulating recombinant forms (CRFs) of HIV (*Ln ID 2:461, 2002*)—see section 1.B. above. **False-positive** EIA rare, e.g., autoimmune diseases, pregnancy, post-immunization (influenza, HIV vaccine, hepatitis B, rabies) (*ArM 160:2386, 2000).* **False-negative** in 1/500,000 units donated blood due to (1) 1–2wk window between infection & antibody response (*JAMA 284:210, 2000*), (2) agammaglobulinemia, (3) Gp O or N genetic variants. Only 2 pts in U.S. with Gp O as of 7/2000 (*AIDS 18:269, 2002*). So far no N group in U.S. EIA negative in 20–30% HIV-2 pts.
Western blot confirms HIV-1 antibody. No confirmatory test for HIV-2. Interpretation: 1. No antibodies (bands) detected = **negative** 2. Antibody (bands) to Gp41 & Gp120/160 or either of latter plus p24 = **positive**. 3. Any other pattern of positive = **indeterminate**. Proceed to plasma viral load testing.				
(2) **Rapid detection methods:** Results available within 30 minutes. Large number available—see websites: www.cdc.gov/hiv/testing.htm & www.rapid-diagnostics.org/rti-hiv-com.htm				
Need confirmation of pos. results with EIA & Western blot; for protocol, see *MMWR 53:221, 2004.*				
Clinical uses for all: (a) In labor, no prenatal HIV test (*JAMA 292:219, 2004);* (b) Patient who is source of needlestick injury to health care provider (*JCM 41:3868, 2003);* (c) Evaluation of acutely ill patient with possible PCP; (d) Patients who are unlikely to return for test results.				
Examples of Available Tests:				
(a) Single use diagnostic system (SUDS) (FDA-approved)		99.6	99.6	Need serum/plasma; refrigeration of reagents
(b) Merlin		95	100	Whole blood. Ref.: *CID 34:653, 2002*
(c) Uni-Gold Recombigen (FDA-approved); results in 10 min.		100	99.7	Whole blood, serum, or plasma; no refrigeration; detects HIV 1 & 2 antibody; CLIA waived
(d) Determine HIV-1/2 (www.abbottdiagnostics.com)		> 90	> 90	Whole blood; no refrigeration; no instruments; **not available in USA**
(e) Oraquick (FDA-approved); results in 20min., read by provider		99.6	100	Whole blood; oral fluid; no refrigeration needed. Ref.: *MMWR 51:1051, 2002.* **DOES NOT REQUIRE CLIA-APPROVED LAB.** Detects antibody to HIV-1 & -2.
(f) Reveal G2 (FDA-approved); results in 3min., read by provider		99.8	99.1	Serum or plasma; no refrigeration; needs CLIA lab; need centrifuge
(3) **Home sample collection test,** e.g., Home Access Express (*LnID 4:640, 2004*). **NOTE: Other kits sold on Internet unreliable.**	Encourage individuals at risk to determine their antibody status. Convenient. Anonymity maintained.	100	99.95	Patient pricks fingertip & blood spotted on filter paper. Positives confirmed with standard antibody. Counseling included. Takes 3–7 days. Cost: **$44–66** online.

TABLE 3 (3)

Test	Primary Purpose(s)	Sensitivity %	Specificity %	Comment
B. Detection of HIV-1 antibody in other body fluids				
(1) **Antibody in oral mucosal transudate** (OraQuick Advance Rapid HIV-1/2) (Ref: *JAMA* 277:254, 1997)	FDA approved for point of care diagnosis of HIV infection.	99.3	99.8	Absorbent pad swabs between teeth & gums. Results in 20 minutes Detects HIV-1 IgG antibody. Confirmatory test with OraSure HIV-1 Western blot is necessary.
(2) **Antibody in urine** (Sentinel or Calypte): HIV-1 Urine EIA	Rapid—results in 2.5 hrs. Like rapid tests, could be used on source blood if occupational exposure or in ERs, STD clinics	99.7	94	Non-invasive & rapid turnaround time attractive. Positives confirmed with serum Western blot. Rare pt. urine antibody neg. & urine antibody pos. (*Ln* 342:1458, 1993). Cost: individual test $4
(3) **Vaginal secretions** IgG EIA (Wellozyme HIV-1 & 2)	HIV IgG antibodies in semen. Suggested for victims of rape.	97.7	97.6	
3. **HIV 2 antibody tests**—HIV-1 antibody tests neg. in 20-30% pts with HIV 2 infections. Suspect in patient from West Africa. Suspect HIV 2 infection in patient from West Africa. HIV 2 specific antibody tests available at CDC (used to screen all blood donors)				
4. **HTLV-1: Detection of antibody** Human T-lymphocyte virus-1 (Review: *Ln* 353:1951, 1999). ELISA followed by confirmatory Western blot	Screen all donated blood & blood components. Test pts with compatible illness: **Adult T-cell lymphoma** **Tropical spastic hemiparesis (myelopathy)**	>98	>98 (see Comment)	HTLV-1/2 infection in 7-12% IVDUs & 2-10% commercial sex workers; 80-90% of positives are HTLV-2. **HTLV-1 infection results in an increase in CD4 lymphocyte counts.** Specificity good but transient false-positives in 2-5% of blood donors who had received influenza vaccine in last 4 months (*MMWR* 42:173, 1993).
5. **HTLV-2: Detection of antibody** Human T-lymphocyte virus-2				Thus far an investigative tool in that there is no definite association of HTLV-2 infection with any disease process. Donated blood is NOT screened. Based on antibody studies, infection with HTLV-2 is endemic in Native Americans & injection drug users.

Test	Current Use	% Positive	Advantages	Disadvantages	Comment
6. Detection/quantitation of HIV					
A. **HIV p24 antigen** (Assumes acid pretreatment to dissociate immune complexes)	Diagnosis of acute HIV syndrome (antibody may not be detectable for 2-6mos)	% positive depends on method/stage of disease, e.g. in acute retroviral syn.: 100%, if CD4 200-500, 45-70%; if CD4 <200, 75-100%	Detection of infection before antibody appears	Not as good as quant. nucleic acid methods as a measure of effectiveness of therapy	In newborns at risk, HIV DNA PCR (if available) preferable to p24 antigen
B. **Qualitative HIV nucleic acid by PCR:** circulating cells or plasma	**Use to diagnose primary HIV instead of p24 antigen; also to resolve indeterminate Western blots.** Can use circulating cells or plasma	>99% for HIV variants from U.S. & Europe (subtype B). May fail to detect novel African HIV-1 variants	In meta-analysis, 97% sensitivity & 98% specificity with 1.9% false-pos. & 3.0% false-neg. (*AnM* 114:803, 1996).	Qualitative not quantitative	Trend is to use quantitative PCR methods.

TABLE 3 (4)

Test	Current Use	% Positive	Advantages	Disadvantages	Comment
C. **Quantitative measurement of plasma HIV "viral burdens"** Ref. *JID 190:2047, 2004*	• Clinical uses: (1) While decision to initiate antiretroviral rx is no longer based primarily on viral load measurements, high levels (>50,000/ml) may signal rapid decline in CD4 counts & poor prognosis. (2) Monitor response to anti-retroviral rx. (3) Predict likelihood of transmission of HIV from mother to fetus. (4) Diagnosis of infection in newborn.	Depending on stage of disease & sensitivity & specificity of method: 86 – >98%	At least 3 competing methods. Test availability varies with locale. Ability to accurately quantitate low levels of viremia (<40–50 viral RNA equivalents/ml). Changes in viral burden of ≥0.3 log (2-fold) may be just technical variation: changes ≥0.5 log (3-fold) reflect real changes in viral burden (see section 7, next page). Recommend repeat use of same test method for individual patients because of discrepancies between the different techniques. Roche Amplicor & Organon Teknika test kits may underdetect/underestimate Group M non-B subtypes. All assays have problems amplifying HIV-1 Gp O & **do not** amplify HIV-2 (*MMWR 50:RR-20, 2001*). In developing countries, samples can collect dried whole blood on filter paper, rather than plasma, for HIV viral loads (*Ln 362:2067, 2003*).		
(1) Due to assay differences, use same assay repeatedly for a given patient. Results with RT-PCR & NASBA consistently greater than bDNA (*MMWR 50:RR-20, 2001*). (2) For given assay, need change of ≥0.5 $\log_{10}$ (3-fold) for significant change. (3) **NOTE**: Use standard EDTA tubes; use of "plasma separation tubes" resulted in fictitious low-level viremia (*CID 41:1671, 2005*)	• Current methods: (1) Couples **RNA** reverse transcription (RT) to a **DNA PCR amplification (RT-PCR)** (Roche Amplicor HIV-1 Monitor, Version 1.5). NOTE: Ideally collect with EDTA & separate plasma within 6hrs. Freeze plasma until assayed. (2) Amplification of RNA of HIV, a **nucleic acid sequence-based amplification** (NASBA) (bioMerieux NucliSens, HIV-1 QT). Freeze plasma until assayed. (3) Identification of HIV-1 RNA, then **signal amplification by DNA branched-chain technique** (referred to as bDNA) (Bayer Versant HIV-1 RNA Quantiplex 3.0 Assay). Freeze plasma until assayed.	>98 >98 >98		**Preferred anticoagulant**: ACD/EDTA ACD/EDTA/HEP EDTA	Version 1.5 better at detection of subtypes other than B as well as genetic variants of subtype B. **Values roughly 2x higher than bDNA.** RT-PCR is less efficient than bDNA at quantitation of subtypes (*J AIDS 29:330, 2002*). For information, call bioMerieux (800-682-2666). May underestimate viral burden if subtype C (*Abst. 666, CROI, 2003*)[2] For information, call Bayer (800-434-2447). Detects subtypes A to G.

Reportable ranges (copies/ml)

Standard 400–750,000
Ultrasensitive assay 50–100,000

NucliSens: 50–5,390,000. Can quantify HIV in CSF, seminal fluid, breast milk, saliva, vaginal fluid.

Version 3.0: 50–500,000

D. **Interpretation**: Changes of ≥50% (2-fold or 0.3 $\log_{10}$) copies/ml are considered significant.
(1) **A guide to logarithmic changes**; for a person **starting with 100,000 copies of HIV-RNA**:

$\log_{10}$	n-Fold Change	Copies of HIV RNA Remaining
0.3	2-fold	50,000
0.5	3-fold	33,000
1.0	10-fold	10,000
1.5	30-fold	3,300
2.0	100-fold	1,000

---

[1] **ACD** = acid citrate dextran; **EDTA** = ethylenediaminetetraacetic acid; **HEP** = heparin   [2] **CROI** = Conference on Retroviruses & Opportunistic Infections

TABLE 3 (5)

(2) **Factors that increase viral load:**
   a. Progressive uncontrolled HIV infection due to non-compliance or ineffective regimen
   b. Active non-HIV infection, e.g., tuberculosis (5–160 fold ↑), pneumococcal pneumonia (3–5 fold ↑)
   c. Immunization, e.g., influenza, pneumococcal

(3) **Falsely low viral loads:**
   a. Non-B subtype not detected with Amplicor assay
   b. HIV-2 infection

7 **CD4/CD8 antigen T-lymphocyte counts (CD=cluster differentiation)**—CDC Guidelines for absolute CD4 T cell counts: MMWR 52(RR-2);1-13, 2003

Test	Current Use	% Positive	Advantages	Disadvantages	Comment
A. **CD4 T-lymphocyte count (T-helper lymphocyte)** Principles of flow cytometry: Crit. Care Med. 33 (Suppl)/S426, 2005	(1) Decision to initiate antiretroviral rx (200–350/mm³ (Table 6); (2) Assess magnitude of injury to host immune system; (3) Changes used to monitor effectiveness of antiretroviral rx. **Normals: CD4 500–1400/mm³. CD8 180–805/mm³ CD4/CD8 ratio 1.1–3.5;** (4) Initiation of prophylaxis vs opportunistic infections (Table 10)	Not applicable	Generally available. Rate of ↓ in CD4 count correlates with HIV disease progression. **New method (reference above): flow cytometry with 3 different monoclonal antibodies measures absolute CD4 count in single step.**	Test must be done within ≤18 hrs after blood collection. **CD4 counts may ↓ due to:** time of day, time of year, lab doing test, intercurrent infection, & corticosteroids (CID 21;1121, 1995) **CD4 levels may ↑ due to:** HTLV-1 co-infection, splenectomy. Cost varies from $80-$150.	Fluorescinated monoclonal antibodies are added to pt blood & the % fluorescent cells counted in cell sorter. CD4 count calculated as: WBC × % lymphocytes × % CD4 cells. **To avoid influence of change in WBC, can use % CD4s (≥29% = CD4 count of >500; 14–28% = CD4 200–499; <14% = CD4 <200/mm³. Try not to use this method. See reference above for single-step measurement.**
B. **Total lymphocyte count (TLC)** CD4 surrogate in resource-poor areas	TLC <1200/mm³ = approx. CD4 count of 200 cells/mm³ (J AIDS 31;378, 2002) For review & meta-analysis: Ln 366;1868, 2005.				
C. **CD8 T-lymphocyte count (T-suppressor/ cytotoxic lymphocyte)**	Often measured in parallel with CD4, even though role in disease process less well defined—see Comment	Not applicable	3–4 wks following infection, both CD4 & CD8 counts ↑ but CD8 is greater with inversion of normal CD4/CD8 ratio. CD8 cells believed to play a role in control of viral replication in many cells including CD4 cells.		

8 Discordant virologic (HIV viral burden, copies per ml) & immunologic responses (CD4 T-lymphocyte count) to antiretroviral therapy (ART).

	CD4 Count	Viral Burdens	Possible Explanation
A.	Increases	Decreases	Expected response to ART
B.	Fails to ↑ or decreases	Decreases	Drug toxicity: e.g. combination of tenofovir & didanosine (AIDS 19;1107, 2005); Deficiency in CD4 cell regeneration &/or increased apoptosis (JID 191;1670, 2005).
C.	Remains elevated		Drug-induced defective virus with reduced replicative capacity (JID 187;1027, 2003; JID 191;1670, 2005; Pediatrics 114; 604, 2004)
D.	Fails to increase	Increases	Non-adherence to therapy, drug-resistant HIV

TABLE 3 (6)

9. Drug Resistance Testing in the Treatment of HIV Infection *(NEJM 350:1023, 2004)*
A. Mechanism of action & resistance of drugs used to treat HIV infection

Drugs	Mechanism of Action	Mechanism of Resistance
Nucleoside analogues (NRTIs):	Analogues of nucleosides; Active when triphosphorylated; Incorporated into new viral DNA; & Prematurely terminate synthesis of HIV DNA	a. Thymidine analogue (stavudine & zidovudine) mutations promote ATP- & pyrophosphate- mediated **excision** of incorporated chain terminator into new HIV DNA
Abacavir		
Didanosine		
Emtricitabine/lamivudine		
Stavudine		
Zalcitabine		
Zidovudine		b. Other mutations **impair incorporation** of nucleoside analogues into new HIV DNA
Nucleotide analogue (Nucleotide RTI):	Same as nucleosides	Specific mutation impairs incorporation into HIV DNA
Tenofovir		
Non-nucleoside reverse-transcriptase inhibitors (NNRTIs)	Binds to hydrophobic pocket of HIV, type 1 reverse transcriptase; HIV, type 2 resistant	Mutations decrease affinity for the enzyme; & Single mutation can lead to high level of resistance
Delavirdine		
Efavirenz		
Nevirapine		
Protease inhibitors (PIs)	Binds to, & interferes with, the active site of the protease	Mutations reduce affinity of inhibitors for the protease; & High level resistance usually requires multiple mutations
Atazanavir		
Fosamprenavir		
Indinavir		
Lopinavir		
Nelfinavir		
Ritonavir		
Saquinavir		
Tipranavir		
Fusion Inhibitor	Interferes with glycoprotein 41-dependent membrane fusion	Mutations in a portion of glycoprotein 41
Enfuvirtide		

B. **When & why to test for resistance?**
   (1) **Always test while on therapy except acute HIV.** Off therapy ≥2 wks, wild type virus "emerges." Once resistant, always resistant.
   (2) Results identify drugs to avoid.
   (3) Past history of clinical resistance better predictor than lab evidence of resistance

C. **Who should have HIV resistance testing?**
   (1) All pts with primary (acute) HIV infection. *(JAMA 288:181, 2002; NEJM 347:385 & 438, 2002)*
   (2) Chronic HIV infection & no prior therapy. Pretreatment resistance to one drug class is 14.5% (CROI 2005)
   (3) Treatment failure: Recommend testing. See definition of treatment failure below.[a]
   (4) Pregnancy: Recommend testing

D. **How to test? Genotype or phenotype?**
   (1) Genotype identifies specific mutations. Can use genotype to predict a "virtual" phenotype
   (2) Phenotype exposes virus to drugs in tissue culture system.
   (3) Prefer genotyping during failure of 1st or 2nd regimen; many prefer phenotyping of highly-treated pts with many PI mutations; some data support genotyping in these pts also *(CID 188:194, 2003)*.

[a] **Definition of rx failure:** (1) Failure to ↓ viral load (VL) >0.5–0.7 $\log_{10}$ copies/ml (≥3-fold) by 4 wks of rx OR (2) failure to ↓ VL > 1 $\log_{10}$ copies/ml (10-fold) by 8 wks of rx

TABLE 3 (7)

E. **Does resistance testing predict virologic response?** *(CID 37:113, 2003)*
  (1) Using genotypic & phenotypic testing to guide treatment results in:
    • **EXTRA 0.5–0.6 log₁₀ copies/ml** (approx. 30,000 copies/ml or 3-fold) ↓ in viral load
    • **EXTRA 10–20% of patients with viral loads below 200–500 copies/ml**
  (2) Improved longterm virologic outcome in treatment-experienced pts *(CID 41:92, 2005)*.

F. **Genotype resistance testing**
  (1) **DETECTS MUTATIONS IN TARGET PROTEINS THAT ARE ASSOCIATED WITH DRUG RESISTANCE. EXPERT ADVICE ON INTERPRETATION IMPROVES VIROLOGIC RESPONSE** *(CID 37:708, 2003)*
    a. Use PCR to amplify HIV protease & reverse transcriptase genes
    b. Sequence genes. Report mutations found. Pattern of mutations used to predict response to antiretrovirals
    c. **Mutation pattern updates on the internet: www.iasusa.org or http://hivdb.stanford.edu**
    d. Selected mutations, or combinations of mutations, may ↓ the **replication capacity** of HIV clinical isolates. **Definitions: Replication capacity** = number of progeny produced per round of infection per unit time. **Fitness** = relative reproductive success of various subtypes of HIV. **Virulence** = ability to destroy CD4 lymphocytes.

  (2) **Commercial assays**
    a. Approx. cost $300–500; results in approx. 2wks
    b. Companies:

Test Name	Manufacturer	Website	Phone	Minimum Viral Load
Trugene	Bayer Diagnostics	www.trugene.com	510-705-5700	1000
ViroSeq	Celera Diagnostics	www.celeradiagnostics.com	800-422-2688	1000–2000
GeneSeq	Monogram Biosciences	www.monogrambio.com	650-635-1100	500
Virco Type HIV-1	Virco	www.vircolab.com	800-325-7504	200–400; combines genotype & phenotype

  (3) **Nucleoside analog derivation of drugs:**

Drug	Analog of:	Drug	Analog of:	Drug	Analog of:
Abacavir	Guanosine	Lamivudine	Cytidine	Zalcitabine	Cytidine
Didanosine	Deoxyadenosine	Stavudine	Thymidine	Zidovudine	Thymidine
				Tenofovir	Adenosine
				Emtricitabine	Cytidine

  (4) **Description of resistant mutations**
    a. In addition to above gene numbers, the resulting change in amino acid may be indicated by:
      i. A prefix letter code indicating amino acid encoded in wild-type virus
      ii. A suffix letter code after the codon number indicating amino acid encoded in the mutant virus, e.g., M46i = at codon 46, isoleucine has replaced methionine
    b. Amino acid codes

Code Letter	Amino Acid	Code Letter	Amino Acid	Code Letter	Amino Acid	Code Letter	Amino Acid
A (Ala)	Alanine	G (Gly)	Glycine	M (Met)	Methionine	S (Ser)	Serine
C (Cys)	Cytosine	H (His)	Histidine	N (Asn)	Asparagine	T (Thr)	Threonine
D (Asp)	Aspartic acid	I (Ile)	Isoleucine	P (Pro)	Proline	V (Val)	Valine
E (Glu)	Glutamic acid	K (Lys)	Lysine	Q (Glu)	Glutamine	W (Trp)	Tryptophan
F (Phe)	Phenylalanine	L (Leu)	Leucine	R (Arg)	Arginine	Y (Tyr)	Tyrosine

c. To save space, specifics of amino acid substitutions deleted in some of the tables below. For full data, see www.iasusa.org.

(5) Selected Genotype Mutations that Result in Resistance to NRTIs (www.iasusa.org; AAC 49:1671, 2005)

Mutation	Selected By	Mechanism	Effects On Other NRTIs	Comment
M184V	Lamivudine, Emtricitabine	Impairs drug incorporation	Decreased suscept. To lamivudine & emtricitabine; increased suscept to zidovudine, stavudine & tenofovir	Presence delays appearance of thymidine analogue mutations (TAMs)
Thymidine analogue mutations (TAMs): M41L, D67N, K70R, L210W, T215Y/F, K219 Q/E/N/R	Zidovudine, stavudine	Mutation leads to excision of drug from DNA chain terminus	Decreased suscept to all NRTIs; the more TAMs, the more resistance.	TAM acquisition slowed by presence of M184V
Q151M complex, T69 insertion	(Zidovudine/didanosine) or (Stavudine/didanosine)	Impairs drug incorporation	Q151M complex: resistance to all NRTIs except tenofovir; T69 insertion: resistance to all NRTIs	
K65R	Tenofovir, abacavir, didanosine		Variable decreased suscept. To abacavir, didanosine, lamivudine/emtricitabine & especially tenofovir	Increases suscept to zidovudine & stavudine
L74V	Abacavir, didanosine		Decreased suscept to abacavir, didanosine & tenofovir	
E44D, V118I	Zidovudine, tenofovir, stavudine		Decreased suscept to all NRTIs	Prevented by presence of zidovudine in treatment regimen

(6) Mutations in Non-Nucleoside Reverse Transcriptase Inhibitors (NNRTIs). Cross-resistance is the rule. Amino acid substitutions shown only once per codon numer.

Multi-NNRTI resistance[1]:

Multi-NNRTI resistance mutations[2]	L100I	K103N	V106M / V106A	V108I	Y181C/I	Y188L	G190S/A	P225H	M230L	P236L
Delavirdine	100	103	106		181	188	190			236
Efavirenz[a]	100	103	106	108	181	188	190	225	230	
Nevirapine	100	103	106 106	108	181	188	190			

[1] K103N most common & usually occurs first
[2] Expect cross-resistance among all NNRTIs
[3] New NNRTIs in development

(7) Mutations in the Protease Gene Associated with Resistance to Protease Inhibitors (PIs)—major mutations in bold print; others "minor"

a. In general, multiple mutations needed for high level resistance
b. Cross-resistance common: e.g. mutations at codons 82, 84, 90. EXCEPTIONS-no cross-resistance: D30N nelfinavir, I50L atazanavir mutations
c. Specific amino acid substitutions shown only once to avoid cluter

Multi-PI resistance mutations:

Drug	10	13	16	20	24	D30N	V32I	33	35	36	43	**M46L**	**I47V/A**	**G48V**	**I50L/V**	53	54	58	60	62	63	69	71	73	74	77	**V82A**	83	**I84V**	88	**L90M**	93	96
Atazanavir	10		16		24		32	33		36		**46**		**48**			54		60	62			71	73			**82**		**84**	88	**90**	93	
Fosamprenavir	10			20	24		32					**46**	**47**		**50V**		54							73			**82**		**84**		**90**		
Indinavir	10			20	24		32			36		**46**					54						71	73		77	**82**		**84**		**90**		
Lopinavir/Ritonavir	10			20	24		**V32I**	33				**46**	**47**		**50**	53	54				63		71	73			**82**		**84**		**90**		
Nelfinavir	10					**D30N**				36		**46**											71			77	**82**		**84**	88	**90**		
Ritonavir	10			20			32	33		36		**46**					54						71			77	**82**		**84**		**90**		
Saquinavir	10													**G48V**			54			62			71	73		77	**82**		**84**		**90**		
Tipranavir/Ritonavir	10	13		20				33	35	36	43	**46**	**47**				54	58				69			74		**82**	83	**84**		**90**		96

TABLE 3 (9)

(8) Mutations in Gp41 Envelope Gene Associated with Resistance to Entry Inhibitors

	36	37	38	39	42	43	HR1 Region
Enfuvirtide							

(9) Virtual Phenotype: Genotype used to project a phenotype based on a large library of compared genotypic & phenotypic test results.

See next section for phenotypic drug resistance testing.

G. Phenotypic drug resistance testing: Measures susceptibility of recombinant viruses to an individual drug in cell culture

(1) Indications for phenotypic testing
   a. After multiple treatment failures
   b. Genotype shows many & complex mutation patterns
   c. Evaluate suscept to a new drug
   d. Patient infected with nonsubtype-B HIV

(2) General Comments
   a. Methods & interpretation evolving
   b. Results reflect combination of:
      i. Accumulated genetic mutations
      ii. Variables in assay system
      iii. End-point (cutoff) used—see below
   c. Compared to genotyping, phenotypic resistance assays:
      i. Take longer (2–8wks); easier to interpret; quantitative degree of resistance
      ii. Cost more ($800–1000)
      iii. Need viral burden of 500–1000 RNA HIV equivalents/ml of plasma
      iv. If circulating drug-resistant virus represents less than 10% of plasma virus burden, resistant virus probably not detected.
      v. Only detect resistance to single drug, not combinations

(3) Method Comments
   a. Overview of laboratory procedure:
      Genes for reverse transcriptase & protease from patients circulating HIV are inserted into laboratory clone of HIV → HIV replication in various drug concentrations measured by expression of a reporter gene → results compared to replication of laboratory strain of HIV.
   b. **Results expressed as fold increase (or fold resistance)**
      IC_{50} = drug concentration that inhibits viral replication by 50%
      IC_{50} patient virus/IC_{50} reference virus = fold increase (or fold resistance)
   c. **Definition of phenotypic resistance**
      i. Phenotypic resistance definition varies with cutoff value used; "cutoff" is separation of sensitive from resistant virus—3 levels of cutoffs in use:
      ii. **3 resistance cutoffs.** Ref. *J AIDS 31:128, 2002*
         (a) **Technical or reproducibility cutoffs:** Based on variability of repeated testing of pt samples
            (1) Definition: lowest fold difference for which susceptible isolates reliably separated from reference laboratory HIV strains
            (2) Sensitive <4-fold increase IC_{50} patient/IC_{50} patient/IC_{50} lab HIV in presence of test drug
               Intermediate 4–10-fold increase
               Resistant >10-fold increase
            (3) Technical cutoffs now rarely used
         (b) **Biologic cutoffs:** Based on variability of wild-type virus from pts
            (1) Determined by study of IC_{50} concentration of test drug vs HIV from wild type (treatment-naïve) patients. Cutoff defined as IC_{50} above mean +2SD (99% percentile).
            (2) More relevant but still arbitrary—see *Clinical cutoffs*
            (3) Cutoffs vary from one commercial assay to another

TABLE 3 (10)

(c) **Clinical cutoffs: Outcome data from clinical trials**
   (1)   Determined by correlation of in vitro IC_{50} with virologic response in clinical trial
   (2)   **Best definition of phenotypic resistance but most difficult to obtain** Examples:
         Abacavir: 4.5 "fold increase" = resistance (0.5-6.5, some pts may have at least 0.5 log ↓ in viral load)
         Didanosine & stavudine: 1.7 "fold increase = reduced susceptibility
         Lopinavir: 10 fold increase = reduced susceptibility
         Tenofovir: 1.4 fold increase = reduced susceptibility (JID 189:837, 2004)
         Indinavir & ritonavir: 10 fold increase = reduced susceptibility
   (3)   Difficult to determine—need large-scale trials
   (4)   With multi-drug regimen, individual drug response influenced by other drugs used

(3) Commercial labs

Test Name	Manufacturer	Website	Phone	Minimum Viral Load
Virco Type HIV-1	Virco (Belgium)	www.vircolab.com	800-325-7504	1000 copies/ml; combines genotype & phenotype
PhenoSense	Monogram Biosciences (USA)	www.monogrambio.com	650-635-1100	500 copies/ml; also offers combined genotypic/phenotypic testing
Phenoscript	Specialty Labs & Viralliance (France)	www.specialtylabs.com	800-421-7110	500 copies/ml

H. Interpretation of discordance in drug susceptibility by genotype & phenotype

Genotype	Phenotype	Cause	Interpretation
Resistant	Susceptible	Mixture HIV subtypes	Resistant
Resistant	Susceptible	Hypersusceptibility	Partial resistance mutation, e.g., 184
Not available	Susceptible or resistant	New drug	Phenotype result
Susceptible	Resistant	Novel drug	Resistant

I. In summary, failure to respond to treatment depends on:
   (1) % of viral population that is drug-resistant   (4) Low drug potency
   (2) Plasma viral load   (5) Poor pharmacokinetics
   (3) Compliance with prescribed treatment regimen (6) High plasma protein binding

TABLE 4A: 1993 REVISED CDC HIV CLASSIFICATION SYSTEM & EXPANDED AIDS SURVEILLANCE DEFINITION FOR ADOLESCENTS & ADULTS
(MMWR 41:RR-17, Dec. 18, 1992)

The revised system emphasizes the importance of CD4 lymphocyte testing in clinical management of HIV infected persons. The system is based on 3 ranges of CD4 counts & 3 clinical categories giving a matrix of 9 exclusive categories. This system is less valuable in clinical decision analysis in 1997 because of availability of measures of viral RNA.

CRITERIA FOR HIV INFECTION: Persons 13 years or older with repeatedly (2 or more) reactive screening tests (ELISA) + specific antibodies identified by a supplemental test, e.g., Western blot ["reactive" pattern = + vs any two of p24, gp41, gp120/160 *(MMWR 40:681, 1991)*]. Other specific methods of diagnosis of HIV-1 include virus isolation, antigen detection, & detection of HIV genetic material by PCR or branched DNA assay (bDNA).

CLASSIFICATION SYSTEM				Clinical Category A	Clinical Category B	Clinical Category C
	Clinical Category			Asymptomatic HIV infection	Symptomatic, not A or C	Candidiasis: esophageal, trachea, bronchi
CD4 Cell* Category	A	B	C	Persistent generalized lymphadenopathy (PGL) †	conditions.	Coccidioidomycosis, extrapulmonary
(1) ≥500/mm³	A1	B1	C1	Acute (primary) HIV illness	Examples include but not limited to:	Cryptococcosis, extrapulmonary
					Bacillary angiomatosis	Cervical cancer, invasive
(2) 200–499/mm³	A2	B2	C2		Candidiasis, vulvovaginal; persistent >1 month, poorly responsive to rx.	Cryptosporidiosis, chronic intestinal (>1 month)
						CMV retinitis, or CMV in other than liver, spleen, nodes
(3) <200/mm³	A3	B3	C3		Candidiasis, oropharyngeal	Herpes simplex with mucocutaneous ulcer >1 month, bronchitis, pneumonia
					Cervical dysplasia, severe, or carcinoma in situ	Histoplasmosis: disseminated, extrapulmonary
* See table for clinical definitions. Shaded area indicates expansion of AIDS surveillance definition. Cats. A3, B3 & C3 require reporting as AIDS.					Constitutional sx, e.g., fever (38.5°) or diarrhea >1 month	Isosporiasis, chronic, >1 month
						Kaposi's sarcoma
† There is a diurnal variation in CD4 counts averaging 60/mm³ higher in the afternoon in HIV+ individuals. Blood for sequential CD4 counts should be drawn at about the same time of day each time *(J AIDS 3:144, 1990)*. The equivalence between CD4 counts and CD4 % of total lymphocytes is ≥500 = ≥29%, 200–499 = 14–28%, <200 = <14%.				‡ Nodes in 2 or more extrainguinal sites, at least 1 cm in diameter for ≥3 mos	The above must be attributed to HIV infection or have a clinical course or management complicated by HIV.	Lymphoma: Burkitt's, immunoblastic, primary in brain
						M. avium or M. kansasii, extrapulmonary
						M. tuberculosis, pulmonary or extrapulmonary
						Pneumocystis carinii pneumonia
						‡ Pneumonia, recurrent (≥2 episodes in 1 year)
						Progressive multifocal leukoencephalopathy
						Salmonella bacteremia, recurrent
						Toxoplasmosis, cerebral
						Wasting syndrome due to HIV

* These are the 1987 CDC case definitions *(MMWR 36:15, 1987)*. The 1993 *CDC Expanded Surveillance Case Definition* includes all conditions contained in the 1987 definition (above) plus persons with documented HIV infection & any of the following: (1) CD4 T-lymphocyte count <200/mm³ (or CD4 <14%); (2) pulmonary tuberculosis; (3) recurrent pneumonia (≥2 episodes within 1 year) or (4) invasive cervical carcinoma. There are no CDC definitions utilizing viral load available to date.

TABLE 4B: 'PERFORMANCE STATUS' (KARNOFSKY SCALE)/WHO CLINICAL STAGING SYSTEM

PERFORMANCE STATUS (Karnofsky Scale)		WHO CLINICAL STAGING SYSTEM
Able to carry on normal activity; no special care is needed	100	Normal; no complaints; no evidence of disease
	90	Able to carry on normal activity; minor signs or symptoms of disease
		WHO Clinical Stage 1
		No clinical symptoms
		May have persistent generalized lymphadenopathy (PGL)
		Performance scale 1
		* Normal activity
Unable to work; able to live at home & care for most personal needs; a varying amount of assistance is needed	80	Normal activity with effort; some signs or symptoms of disease
	70	Cares for self; unable to carry on normal activity or to do active work
		WHO Clinical Stage 2
		Weight loss <10%
		Minor skin rash
		Herpes zoster
		Recurrent upper respiratory infection
		Performance scale 2
		* Symptomatic but normal activity
	60	Requires occasional assistance but is able to care for most needs
Unable to care for self; requires equivalent of institutional or hospital care; disease may be progressing rapidly	50	Requires considerable assistance & frequent medical care
		WHO Clinical Stage 3
		Weight loss >10%
		Chronic diarrhea >1 month
		Recurrent fevers >1 month
		Oral thrush
		Pulmonary tuberculosis
		Performance scale 3
		* Bedridden <50% of the day during the last month
	40	Disabled; requires special care & assistance
	30	Severely disabled; hospitalization is indicated although death not imminent
	20	Very sick; hospitalization necessary; active supportive treatment necessary
		WHO Clinical Stage 4
		Cryptococcal meningitis
		Toxoplasmosis of the brain
		Kaposi sarcoma
		Dementia
		Performance scale 4
		* Bedridden >50% of the day during the last month
	10	Moribund; fatal processes progressing rapidly
	0	Dead

NOTE that patients may move from a later stage to an earlier stage if the presenting opportunistic infection is treated.
See HIV Infection. Ed. E. Katabira, M.R. Kamya, F.X. Mubiru, N.N. Bakyaita. Makerere Univ. Printery, 2000. 2nd Edition.

TABLE 5: RAPID ORAL TMP/SMX DESENSITIZATION

HOUR	DOSE TMP/SMX (mg)
0	0.004/0.02
1	0.04/0.2
2	0.4/2

HOUR	DOSE TMP/SMX (mg)
3	4/20
4	40/200
5	160/800

COMMENT
Perform in hospital or clinic. Use oral suspension [40 mg TMP/200 mg SMX/5 ml (tsp]. Take 6 oz. water after each dose. Corticosteroids, antihistamines NOT used. NOT used. Refs. *CID 20:849, 1995; AIDS 5:311, 1991*

FIGURE 1 *(see Table 10)*

Clinical Decision Points: course of HIV infection and disease in adults and following effective response to HAART.

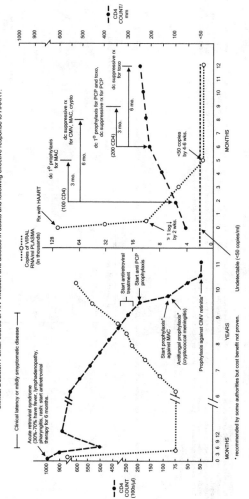

TABLE 6A: ANTIRETROVIRAL THERAPY IN TREATMENT-NAÏVE ADULTS

In late 2005, DHHS guidelines for treatment of infected adults & adolescents, guidelines for the use of antiretroviral therapy (ART) in pediatrics, recommendations for ART in pregnant women to prevent mother-to-child transmission, & use of antiretrovirals in pregnancy were updated. In addition, guidelines for management of occupational exposures of healthcare workers were updated & recommendations for post-exposure prophylaxis after non-occupational exposure to HIV [*MMWR 54(RR-2):1, 2005*] were introduced. These documents are available online at www.aidsinfo.nih.gov. Since the previous version of this HIV Guide, new antiretroviral agents or formulations have been introduced, & others have been discontinued (See Table 3 for tests of viral RNA).

The following concepts guide therapy:
- **The goal of rx is to inhibit maximally viral replication, allowing re-establishment & persistence of an effective immune response that will prevent or delay HIV-related morbidity.**
- **The lower the viral RNA can be driven, the lower the rate of accumulation of drug resistance mutations & the longer the therapeutic effect will last.**
- **To achieve maximal & durable suppression of viral RNA, combinations of potent antiretroviral agents are required, as is a high degree of adherence to the chosen regimens.**
- **Treatment regimens must be tailored to the individual as well as to the virus. Antiretroviral drug toxicities can compromise adherence in the short term & can cause significant negative health effects over time. Carefully check for specific risks to the individual, for interactions between the antiretrovirals selected & between those & concurrent drugs, & adjust doses as necessary for body weight, for renal or hepatic dysfunction, & for possible pharmacokinetic interactions.**

A. When to start therapy? (www.aidsinfo.nih.gov)

HIV Symptoms	CD4 cells/μl	Start Treatment	Comment
Yes	Any	Yes	
No	<200	Yes	* Risk for progression to AIDS also depends on viral load; consider on individual basis
No	≥200–≤350	Offer*	*Maybe if CD4 decreasing rapidly &/or viral load >100,000 copies/ml
No	>350	No*	

B. Suggested Initial Therapy Regimens for Untreated Chronic HIV Infection Doses & use assume normal renal & hepatic function unless otherwise stated. *See additional comments, section F.*

(For pregnancy, see next page & Table 8; for additional explanation & alternatives, see www.aidsinfo.nih.gov)

1. **Preferred Regimens**

	Regimen	Pill strength (mg)	Usual Daily Regimen (oral)	No. pills/day	Cost/mo (Avg. Whole-sale Price)	Comment (See also individual agents & Table 6B)
a.	(Zidovudine + Lamivudine) + Efavirenz	(300 + 150) + 600	(Combination—Combivir 1 tab bid) + 1 tab q24h at bedtime, empty stomach (see Comment)	3	$1198	Good efficacy, low pill burden, low AE profile. If rx stopped, dc efavirenz 1–2wks before Combivir (for explanation, see section E.2 below). Avoid efavirenz in pregnancy or in women who might become pregnant (**Pregnancy Category D**). Food may ↑ serum efavirenz concentration, which can lead to ↑ adverse events.
b.	(Tenofovir + Emtricitabine) + Efavirenz	(300 + 200) + 600	(Combination—Truvada 1 tab q24h) + 1 tab q24h at bedtime, empty stomach	2	$1207	Analysis at 48-wks of ongoing trial reported superior virus suppression, CD4 ↑ & AEs of ZDV/3TC/efavirenz (NEJM 354:251, 2006). Tenofovir: reports of renal toxicity (CID 42:283, 2006). Avoid efavirenz in pregnancy or in women who might become pregnant (**Pregnancy Category D**). Food may ↑ serum efavirenz concentration, which can lead to ↑ adverse events.

TABLE 6A (2)

	Regimen	Pill strength (mg)	Usual Daily Regimen (oral)	No. pills/ day	Cost/mo (Avg. Wholesale Price)	Comment (See also Individual agents & Table 6B)
c.	(Zidovudine + Lamivudine) + Lopinavir/ Ritonavir	(300 + 150) + 200/50	(Combination—Combivir 1 tab bid) + 2 tabs bid without regard to food	6	$1341	Good virologic efficacy & durable effect. Tolerable AEs. ↓ accumulation of resistance mutations than nelfinavir regimen (NEJM 346:2039, 2002). Lopinavir/ritonavir can be given as 4 tabs once daily in rx-naive pts.
2.	**Alternative Regimens**					
a.	Didanosine EC + Lamivudine + Efavirenz	400 + 300 + 600	1 cap q24h at bedtime, fasting + 1 tab q24h + 1 tab q24h at bedtime, empty stomach **Didanosine dosage shown for ≥60 kg**	3	$1142	Low pill burden. Efficacy & durability under study(AHFE). Potential didanosine AEs (pancreatitis, peripheral neuritis). Avoid efavirenz in pregnancy or in women who might become pregnant (**Pregnancy Category D**). Food may ↑ serum efavirenz concentration, which can lead to ↑ adverse events. Can substitute emtricitabine 200 mg po q24h for lamivudine 300 mg po q24h.
b.	(Abacavir + Lamivudine) + Efavirenz	(600 + 300) + 600	(Combination–Epzicom 1 tab q24h) without regard to food + 1 tab q24h at bedtime, empty stomach	2	$1260	Low pill burden. **However, note risk of abacavir hypersensitivity reaction.** Comparison of abacavir/lamivudine with tenofovir/emtricitabine as backbone in rx-naive pts under study(AHFE). Avoid efavirenz in pregnancy or in women who might become pregnant (**Pregnancy Category D**). Food may ↑ serum efavirenz concentration, which can lead to ↑ adverse events.
c.	(Zidovudine + Lamivudine) + Fosamprenavir + Ritonavir	(300 + 150) + 700 + 100	(Combination—Combivir 1 tab bid) + 1 tab bid fed or fasting + 1 cap q24h fed or fasting	6	$1890	Can take without regard to meals. Skin rash, GI symptoms. Fosamprenavir contains sulfa moiety. Alternative fosamprenavir regimens available for rx-naive pts, including fosamprenavir without ritonavir & once-daily fosamprenavir/ritonavir regimens (see label for use & doses).
d.	(Zidovudine + Lamivudine) + Nelfinavir	(300 + 150) + 625	(Combination—Combivir 1 tab bid) + 2 tabs bid, with food	6	$1445	Nelfinavir-associated diarrhea in 20%. Nelfinavir contraindicated with drugs highly dependent on CYP3A4 elimination where ↑ levels may cause life-threatening toxicity.
e.	(Zidovudine + Lamivudine) + Atazanavir	(300 + 150) + 200	(Combination—Combivir 1 tab bid) + 2 caps q24h, with food	4	$1576	Lower potential for lipid derangement by atazanavir than other PIs. Many experts prefer ritonavir-boosted atazanavir regimens when possible (see label). Acid-lowering agents can markedly ↓ absorption of atazanavir. Avoid with PPIs. Give atazanavir 2hr before or 10hr after H2-blockers, or boost with ritonavir (see 2006 drug label changes). May ↑ PR interval & bilirubin (jaundice especially likely in Gilbert's syndrome (JID 192:1381, 2005)).

TABLE 6A (3)

Regimen	Pill strength (mg)	Usual Daily Regimen (oral)	No. pills/day	Cost/month (Avg. Whole-sale Price)	Comment (See also individual agents & Table 6B)
† (Zidovudine + Lamivudine) + Indinavir + Ritonavir	(300 + 150) + 400 + 100	(Combination—Combivir 1 tab bid) + 2 caps bid + 1 cap bid, without regard to food	8	$1556	Nephrolithiasis—hydrate! GI symptoms. Metabolic effects of PI. May ↑ bilirubin, with jaundice more likely in Gilbert's syndrome (JID 192: 1381, 2005).
3. Triple nucleoside regimen: Due to inferior virologic activity, use only when preferred or alternative regimen not possible. Seek expert advice about alternatives.					
a. (Zidovudine + Lamivudine + Abacavir)	(300 + 150 + 300)	(Combination-Trizivir 1 tab bid)	2	$1164	Reduced activity as compared with preferred or alternative regimens. Potentially serious abacavir AEs (see comments for individual agents.)
4. During pregnancy. Expert consultation mandatory. Timing of rx initiation & drug choice must be individualized. Viral resistance testing should be strongly considered. Long-term effects of agents unknown. Certain drugs hazardous or contraindicated. For additional information & alternative options, see www.aidsinfo.nih.gov. For regimens to prevent perinatal transmission, see Table 8A					
a. (Zidovudine + Lamivudine) + Nevirapine	(300 + 150) + 200	(Combination-Combivir 1 tab bid) + 1 tab bid fed or fasting [after 14-day lead-in period of 1 tab q24h]	4	$1144	See especially nevirapine **Black Box warnings**—among others ↑ risk of **potentially fatal hepatotoxicity** in women with CD4 >250. Avoid in this group unless benefits clearly outweigh risks; monitor intensively if drug must be used.
b. (Zidovudine + Lamivudine) + Nelfinavir	(300 + 150) + 625	(Combination-Combivir 1 tab bid) + 2 tabs bid with food	6	$1445	See section 2.d above.
c. (Zidovudine + Lamivudine + Saquinavir + Ritonavir)	(300 + 150 + 500 + 100)	(Combination-Combivir 1 tab bid) + 2 tabs bid + 1 cap bid	8	$1980	Use saquinavir tabs only in combination with ritonavir. Certain drugs metabolized by CYP3A4 are contra-indicated with saquinavir/ritonavir. (Original DHHS recommendations were based on saquinavir soft gel caps, which are no longer available, plus ritonavir.)
C. Suggested Regimen for Acute HIV Infection (see Comments)					
(Zidovudine + Lamivudine) + Efavirenz	(300 + 150) + 600	(Combination-Combivir 1 tab bid) + 1 tab q24h at bedtime, empty stomach	3	$1198	Benefits of rx acute HIV infection uncertain, so treatment is considered optional, & best undertaken in clinical research setting. Perform resistance testing. Optimal duration of rx unknown. (See www.aidsinfo.nih.gov). Avoid efavirenz in pregnancy or in women who might become pregnant (**Pregnancy Category D**). Food may ↑ serum efavirenz concentration, which can lead to ↑ adverse advents.

D. Antiretroviral Therapies That Should NOT Be Offered (Modified from www.aidsinfo.nih.gov)
1. Regimens not recommended

Regimen	Logic	Exception
a. Monotherapy	Rapid development of resistance & inferior antiretroviral activity	Perhaps pregnancy for mother with HIV RNA <1000 copies/ml to prevent mother-child transmission. See Table 8

Regimens not recommended (continued)

TABLE 6A (4)

b. Two-drug combinations	Inferior antiretroviral activity compared to 3- or 4- drug combinations	Pts who have been on such regimens with sustained virological response could continue with careful monitoring
c. Triple-NRTI combinations	Triple-NRTI regimens have shown inferior virologic efficacy in clinical trials: (tenofovir + lamivudine + abacavir) & (didanosine + lamivudine + tenofovir) & others	(Zidovudine + lamivudine + abacavir) could be used if no alternative (see section B.3.)

2. Drug, or drugs, not recommended as part of antiretroviral regimen

a. Saquinavir hard gel cap or tab (Invirase) as single (unboosted) PI	Bioavailability only 4%, inferior antiretroviral activity	No exceptions
b. Stavudine + didanosine	High frequency of toxicity: peripheral neuropathy, pancreatitis & mitochondrial toxicity (lactic acidosis). In pregnancy lactic acid acidosis, hepatic steatosis, ± pancreatitis	Toxicity partially offset by potent antiretroviral activity of the combination. Use only when potential benefits outweigh the sizeable risks.
c. Efavirenz in pregnancy or in women who might become pregnant	Teratogenic in non-human primates **Pregnancy Category D—may cause fetal harm**	Only if no other option available. Note that oral contraceptives alone may not be reliable for prevention of pregnancy in women on ART or other medications (see Safety & Toxicity of Individual Agents in Pregnancy at www.aidsinfo.nih.gov).
d. Amprenavir oral solution in pregnancy, children <4 y/o, presence of renal &/or hepatic failure, with metronidazole or disulfiram, or with ritonavir oral solution	Oral solution contains large amounts of propylene glycol, which can cause toxicities in pts indicated	
e. Stavudine + zidovudine	Antagonistic	
f. Stavudine + zalcitabine	Additive risk of peripheral neuropathy	
g. Didanosine + zalcitabine	Additive risk of peripheral neuropathy	
h. Atazanavir + indinavir	Additive risk of hyperbilirubinemia	
i. Emtricitabine + lamivudine	Same target. Same resistance profile	
j. Fosamprenavir + amprenavir	Fosamprenavir is pro-drug of amprenavir	
k. Lamivudine + zalcitabine	Inhibition of intracellular phosphorylation	

E. Selected Characteristics of Antiretroviral Drugs

1. Selected Characteristics of Nucleoside or Nucleotide Reverse Transcriptase Inhibitors (NRTIs)

All agents have Black Box warning: Risk of lactic acidosis/hepatic steatosis. Also, labels note risk of fat redistribution/accumulation with ARV rx. For combinations, see warnings for component agents.

Generic/Trade Name	Pharmaceutical Prep. (Avg. Wholesale Price)	Usual Adult Dosage & Food Effect	% Absorbed, po	Serum T½, hrs	Intracellular T½, hrs	Elimination	Major Adverse Events/Comments (See Table 6B)
Abacavir (ABC; Ziagen)	300 mg tabs or 20 mg/ml oral solution ($446/month)	300 mg po bid or 600 mg po q24h. Food OK	83	1.5	20	Liver metab., renal excretion of metabolites, 82%	**Hypersensitivity reaction:** fever, rash, N/V, malaise, diarrhea, abdominal pain, respiratory symptoms. (Severe reactions may be ↑ with 600 mg dose.) Do not rechallenge! Report to 800-270-0425
Abacavir/lamivudine/zidovudine (Trizivir)	Film-coated tabs: ABC 300 mg + 3TC 150 mg + ZDV 300 mg ($1164/month)	1 tab bid (not recommended for wt <40 kg or CrCl <50 ml/min or impaired hepatic function)	(See individual components)				(See Comments for individual components) Note Black Box warnings for ABC: hypersensitivity reaction & others. Should only be used for regimens intended to include these 3 agents. Black Box warning for VL >100,000 copies/ml.

TABLE 6A (5)

Generic/Trade Name	Pharmaceutical Prep. (Avg. Wholesale Price)	Usual Adult Dosage & Food Effect	% Absorbed, po	Serum T½, hrs	Intracellular T½, hrs	Elimination	Major Adverse Events/Comments (See Table 6B)
Didanosine (ddi; Videx or Videx EC)	25, 50, 100, 150, 200mg chewable tabs; 100, 167, 250mg powder for oral solution; 125, 200, 250, 400 enteric-coated caps $332/month Videx EC). (Tablets discontinued in US in 2006 pkgs.)	≥60kg. Usually 400mg enteric-coated po q24h hr before or 2hrs after meal. Do not crush. <60kg: 250mg EC po q24h. See Comment	30-40	1.6	25-40	Renal excretion, 50%	**Pancreatitis**, peripheral neuropathy, lactic acidosis & hepatic steatosis (rare but life-threatening, esp. combined with stavudine in pregnancy). Retinal, optic n. changes. **ddI + TDF is used: reduce dose of ddI-EC from 400mg to 250mg EC q24h (or from 250mg EC to 200mg EC for adults <60kg). Monitor for ↑ toxicity & possible in ↓ efficacy of this combination pkgs; may result in ↓ CD4.**
Emtricitabine (FTC, Emtriva)	200mg caps; 10mg/mL oral solution.	200mg po q24h. Food OK.	93	Approx. 10	39	Renal excretion 86%, minor biotransformation. 14% excretion in feces	Well tolerated; headache, nausea, vomiting & diarrhea occasionally, skin rash rarely. Skin hyperpigmentation. Differs only slightly in structure from lamivudine (5-fluoro substitution). **Exacerbation of Hep B reported in pts after stopping FTC**
Emtricitabine/tenofovir disoproxil fumarate (Truvada)	Film-coated tabs: FTC 200mg + TDF 300mg ($728/month)	1 tab po q24h for CrCl ≥50 ml/min. Food OK	92/25	10/17	—	Primarily renal/renal	See Comments for individual agents **Black Box warning**—not indicated for treatment of chronic Hep B. **Exacerbation of HepB after stopping FTC.**
Lamivudine (3TC; Epivir)	150, 300mg tabs; 10mg/mL oral solution	150mg po bid or 300mg po q24h. Food OK	86	5-7	18	Renal excretion, minimal metabolism	**Use HIV dose, not Hep B dose.** Usually well-tolerated. **Risk of exacerbation of Hep B after stopping 3TC.**
Lamivudine/abacavir (Epzicom)	Film-coated tabs: 3TC 300mg + abacavir 600mg ($781/month)	1 tab po q24h. Food OK. Not recommended for CrCl <50ml/min or impaired hepatic function	86/86	5-7/1.5	16/20	Primarily renal/ metabolism	See Comments for individual agents. **Note abacavir hypersensitivity Black Box warnings** (severe reactions may be somewhat more frequent with 600 mg dose).
Lamivudine/ zidovudine (Combivir)	Film-coated tabs: 3TC 150mg + ZDV 300mg ($719/month)	1 tab po bid. Not recommended for CrCl <50 ml/min or impaired hepatic function	86/64	5-7/0.5 ~3	—	Primarily renal/ metabolism with renal excretion of glucuronide	See Comments for individual agents See **Black Box warning**—exacerbation of Hep B in pts stopping 3TC
Stavudine (d4T, Zerit)	15, 20, 30, 40 mg capsules; 1 mg/mL oral solution ($370/month 40 mg caps)	≥60 kg: 40 mg bid <60 kg: 30 mg po bid Food OK	86	1.2-1.6	3.5	Renal excretion, 40%	**Highest incidence of lipoatrophy, hyperlipidemia, & lactic acidosis of all NRTIs.** Pancreatitis. Peripheral neuropathy. (See didanosine comments.)

TABLE 6A (6)

Generic/Trade Name	Pharmaceutical Prep. (Avg. Wholesale Price)	Usual Adult Dosage & Food Effect	% Absorbed, po	Serum $T_\frac{1}{2}$, hrs	Intracellular $T_\frac{1}{2}$, hrs	Elimination	Major Adverse Events/Comments (See Table 6B)
Tenofovir disoproxil fumarate (TDF, Viread)—a nucleotide	300 mg tabs ($478/month)	CrCl ≥50 ml/min: 300 mg po q24h. Food OK; high-fat meal ↑ absorption	39 (with food) 25 (fasted)	17	>60	Renal excretion	Headache, N/V. **Cases of renal dysfunction, reported;** avoid concomitant nephrotoxic agents. Must adjust dose of ddI (↓) if used concomitantly but best to avoid this combination (see ddI Comments). Atazanavir & lopinavir/ritonavir ↑ tenofovir concentrations; monitor for adverse effects. **Black Box warning**—Not indicated for treatment of Hep B; **exacerbations of Hep B reported after stopping tenofovir.**
Zalcitabine (ddC, Hivid)	0.375, 0.75 tabs	0.75 mg po q8h. Food OK	85	2	3	Renal excretion, 70%	**Peripheral neuropathy,** stomatitis, rarely life-threatening lactic acidosis, pancreatitis. To ↓ discontinued in 2006 (GRS)
Zidovudine (ZDV, AZT, Retrovir)	100 mg caps, 300 mg tabs; 10 mg/mL oral solution; 10 mg/mL syrup ($387/month)	300 mg po q12h. Food OK	60	1.1	11	Metabolized to glucuronide & excreted in urine	**Bone marrow suppression.** GI intolerance, headache, insomnia, malaise, myopathy.

2.

Selected Characteristics of Non-Nucleoside Reverse Transcriptase Inhibitors (NNRTIs)

Generic/Trade Name	Pharmaceutical Prep. (Avg. Wholesale Price)	Usual Adult Dosage & Food Effect	% Absorbed, po	Serum $T_\frac{1}{2}$, hrs	Elimination	Major Adverse Events/Comments
Delavirdine (Rescriptor)	100, 200 mg tabs ($325/month)	400 mg po TID. Food OK	85	5.8	Cytochrome P450 (3A inhibitor), 51% excreted in urine (<5% unchanged), 44% in feces	Rash severe enough to stop drug in 4.3%. ↑ AST/ALT, headaches. Not recommended.
Efavirenz (Sustiva) **(Pregnancy Category D)**	50, 100, 200 mg capsules; 600 mg tablet ($479/month)	600 mg po q24h at bedtime, without food. Food may ↑ serum conc., which can lead to ↑ in risk of adverse events	42	40-55 See Comment	Cytochrome P450 (3A mixed inducer/ inhibitor). 14-34% of dose excreted in urine as glucuronidated metabolites, 16-61% in feces	Rash severe enough to dc use of drug in 1.7%. High frequency of diverse CNS AEs: somnolence, dreams; confusion, agitation. Serious psychiatric symptoms. False-pos. cannabinoid screen. **Pregnancy Category D—may cause fetal harm—avoid in pregnant women or those who might become pregnant.** (Note: No single method of contraception is 100% reliable). Very long tissue T1/2. **If rx to be discontinued, stop efavirenz 1-2 wks before stopping companion drugs.** Otherwise, risk of developing efavirenz resistance, as after 1-2 days only efavirenz in blood &/or tissue. Some authorities bridge this gap by adding a PI to the NRTI backbone if feasible. (CID 42:401, 2006; 11th CROI, 2004, abstr. 131)(GME6)

TABLE 6A (7)

Selected Characteristics of Non-Nucleoside Reverse Transcriptase Inhibitors (NNRTIs) *(continued)*

Generic/Trade Name	Pharmaceutical Prep. (Avg. Wholesale Price)	Usual Adult Dosage & Food Effect	% Absorbed, po	Serum T½, hrs	Elimination	Major Adverse Events/Comments
Nevirapine (Viramune)	200 mg tablet, 50 mg/5 mL oral suspension ($425/month)	200 mg po q24h x14 days & then 200 mg po bid (see *Comments & Black Boxing*) Food OK	> 90	25–30	Cytochrome P450 (3A4, 2B6) inducer; 80% of dose excreted in urine as glucuronidated metabolites, 10% in feces	**Black Box warning—fatal hepatotoxicity.** Women with CD4 >250 esp. vulnerable, inc. pregnant women, but men in this group unless benefits clearly > risks (www.fda.gov/cder/drug/advisory/nevirapine.htm). If used, intensive monitoring required. Men with CD4 >400 also at ↑ risk. Rash severe enough to stop drug in 7%, **severe or life-threatening skin reactions** in 2%. Do not restart if any suspicion of such reactions. 2wk dose escalation period may ↓ skin reactions. As with efavirenz, because of long T1/2, consider continuing companion agents for several days if nevirapine is discontinued

Selected Characteristics of Protease Inhibitors (PIs).

All PIs: Glucose metabolism: new diabetes mellitus or deterioration of glucose control; fat redistribution; possible hemophilia bleeding; hypertriglyceridemia or hypercholesterolemia. Exercise caution re: potential drug interactions & contraindications. QTc prolongation has been reported in a few pts taking PIs; some PIs can block HERG channels in vitro (*Lancet* 365:682,2005).

Generic/Trade Name	Pharmaceutical Prep. (Avg. Wholesale Price)	Usual Adult Dosage & Food Effect	% Absorbed, po	Serum T½, hrs	Elimination	Major Adverse Events/Comments (See *Table 6B*)
Atazanavir (Reyataz)	100, 150, 200 mg capsules ($857/month)	400 mg q24h with food (exception is atazanavir 300 mg po q24h + ritonavir 100 mg po q24h when combined with either efavirenz 600 mg po q24h or TDF 300 mg po q24h). Take with food 2 hrs pre or 1 hr post buffered ddI. Ritonavir-boosted dose also recommended for ARV rx-experienced pts.	Good oral bioavailability; food enhances bioavailability & ↓ pharmacokinetic variability. Absorption ↓ by antacids, H₂-blockers, proton pump inhibitors. Avoid with PPIs. Give 2hr before or 10hr after H2-blockers or boost with ritonavir (see *2006 drug label changes*)	Approx. 7	Cytochrome P450 (3A4, 1A2 & 2C9 inhibitor) & UGT1A1 inhibitor, 13% excreted in urine (7% unchanged). 79% excreted in feces (20% unchanged)	No ↑ lipids in available studies. Asymptomatic unconjugated hyperbilirubinemia common;jaundice especially likely in Gilbert's syndrome (*JID* 192:1381, 2005). Headache, rash, GI symptoms. Prolongation of PR interval (1st degree AV block) reported; caution in pre-existing conduction system disease. Efavirenz & tenofovir ↓ atazanavir exposure; use atazanavir/ritonavir regimen; also, atazanavir ↑ tenofovir concentrations—watch for adverse events.
Fosamprenavir (Lexiva)	700 mg tablet ($629/month when used with ritonavir)	1400 mg (two 700 mg tabs) po bid **OR** with ritonavir: [1400 mg fosamprenavir (2 tabs) + ritonavir 200 mg] po q24h **OR** [700 mg fosamprenavir (1 tab) + ritonavir 100 mg] po bid	Bioavailability not established. Food OK		7.7	Hydrolyzed to amprenavir, then cytochrome P450 (3A4 substrate, inhibitor, inducer)	Amprenavir prodrug. Contains sulfa moiety. Potential for drug interactions (see label). Rash, inc. Stevens-Johnson syndrome. (See *amprenavir* adverse events; *Table 6B*.) Once daily regimen: (1) not recommended for PI-experienced pts, (2) additional ritonavir needed if given with efavirenz (see *label*). Boosted twice daily regimen is recommended for PI-experienced pts.

TABLE 6A (8)

Generic/Trade Name	Pharmaceutical Prep. (Avg. Wholesale Price)	Usual Adult Dosage & Food Effect	% Absorbed, po	Serum T_½ hrs	Elimination	Major Adverse Events/Comments (See Table 6B)
Indinavir (Crixivan)	100, 200, 333, 400 mg capsules ($300/month) Store in original container with desiccant	Two 400 mg caps (800 mg) po q8h without food or with light meal. Can take with enteric-coated Videx. [If taken with ritonavir (e.g., 800 mg indinavir + 100 mg ritonavir po q12h), no food restrictions]	65	1.2–2	Cytochrome P450 (3A4 inhibitor)	**Maintain hydration. Nephrolithiasis,** nausea, inconsequential ↑ of indirect bilirubin (jaundice in Gilbert's syndrome), ↑ AST/ALT, headache, asthenia, blurred vision, metallic taste, hemolysis. ↑ urine WBC (>100/hpf) has been assoc. with nephritis/medullary calcification, cortical atrophy.
Lopinavir + ritonavir (Kaletra)	(200 mg lopinavir + 50 mg ritonavir) tablets. Tabs do not need refrigeration. Oral solution: (80 mg lopinavir + 20 mg ritonavir) per mL. Refrigerate caps but can be kept at room temperature (≤77 °F) x2 mos. ($622/month)	(400 mg lopinavir + 100 mg ritonavir)—2 tabs po bid. Higher dose may be needed in non–tx-naive pts when used with efavirenz, nevirapine, amprenavir, or unboosted fosamprenavir. [Dose adjustment in concomitant drugs may be necessary: see Table 16B & C.]	No food effect with tablets. (Earlier capsule formulation required food.)	5–6	Cytochrome P450 (3A4 inhibitor)	Nausea/vomiting/diarrhea, ↑ AST/ALT, pancreatitis. Oral solution 42% alcohol. Lopinavir + ritonavir can be taken as a single daily dose of 4 tabs (total 800 mg lopinavir + 200 mg ritonavir), except in treatment-experienced pts or those taking concomitant efavirenz, nevirapine, amprenavir, or nelfinavir. (Note that drug content of tabs is not the same as previously available capsules.)
Nelfinavir (Viracept)	625, 250 mg tabs; 50 mg/gm oral powder ($726/month)	Two 625 mg tabs (1250 mg) po bid, with food	20–80 Food ↑ exposure & ↓ variability	3.5–5	Cytochrome P450 (3A4 inhibitor)	Diarrhea. Coadministration of drugs with life-threatening toxicities & which are cleared by CYP3A4 is contraindicated.
Ritonavir (Norvir)	100 mg capsules; 600 mg/7.5 mL solution. Refrigerate caps but solution. Room temperature for 1 mo. is OK. ($9.03/capsule)	Full dose: 6 caps (600 mg) po bid, with food. Escalate to full dose: 300 mg bid x2 days; 400 mg bid x3 days; 500 mg bid x7 days; then full dose. *"Booster drug"—see Comment	Food ↑ absorption	3–5	Cytochrome P450. Potent 3A4 & 2D6 inhibitor	Nausea/vomiting/diarrhea, paresthesias, hepatitis, pancreatitis, taste perversion, ↑ CPK & uric acid. **With few exceptions, used exclusively to enhance pharmacokinetics of other PIs, using lower ritonavir doses. Black Box warning**—potentially fatal drug interactions. Many drug interactions—see Table 16A–C.

TABLE 6A (9)

Generic/Trade Name	Pharmaceutical Prep. (Avg. Wholesale Price)	Usual Adult Dosage & Food Effect	% Absorbed, po	Serum $T_{1/2}$ hrs	Elimination	Major Adverse Events/Comments (See Table 6B)
Saquinavir (Invirase—hard gel caps or tabs) + **ritonavir**	Saquinavir 200 mg caps, 500 mg film-coated tabs; ritonavir 100 mg caps ($719/month)	[2 tabs saquinavir (1000 mg) + 1 cap ritonavir (100 mg)] po bid with food	Erratic; 4 (saquinavir alone)	1-2	Cytochrome P450 (3A4 inhibitor)	Nausea, diarrhea, headache. ↑ AST, ALT. Avoid rifampin with saquinavir + ritonavir. ↑ hepatitis risk. **Black Box warning**— Invirase to be used only with ritonavir
Tipranavir (Aptivus)	250 mg caps. Refrigerate unopened bottles. Use opened bottles within 2 mo. ($871/month)	[500 mg (two 250 mg caps) + ritonavir 200 mg] po bid with food.	Absorption low, ↑ with high fat meal. ↓ with Al⁺⁺⁺ & Mg⁺⁺ antacids.	5.5-6	Cytochrome 3A4 but with ritonavir, most of drug is eliminated in feces.	Contains sulfa moiety. **Black Box warning**—hepatitis, fatal hepatic failure. Use cautiously in liver disease, esp. hepB, hepC; contraindicated in Child-Pugh class B-C. Monitor LFTs. Coadministration of certain drugs contraindicated (see label). For highly ARI-experienced pts or for multiple-PI resistant virus.

4.

Selected Characteristics of Fusion Inhibitors

Generic/Trade Name	Pharmaceutical Prep. (Avg. Wholesale Price)	Usual Adult Dosage & Food Effect	% Absorbed, po	Serum $T_{1/2}$ hrs	Elimination	Major Adverse Events/Comments (See Table 6B)
Enfuvirtide (T20, Fuzeon)	Single-use vials of 90mg/mL when reconstituted. Vials should be stored at room temperature. Reconstituted vials can be refrigerated for 24 hrs only. ($25,400/year)	90 mg (1 ml) subcut. bid. Rotate injection sites, avoiding those currently inflamed.	84	3.8	Catabolism to its constituent amino acids with subsequent recycling of the amino acids in the body pool. Elimination pathway(s) have not been performed in humans. Does not alter the metabolism of CYP3A4, CYP2D6, CYP1A2, CYP2C19 or CYP2E1 substrates.	Local reaction site reactions 98%, 4% discontinue; erythema/induration – 80-90%, nodules/cysts – 80%. **Hypersensitivity reactions reported** (fever, rash, chills, N/V, ↓ BP &/or ↑ AST/ALT)—do not restart if occur, including background regimens, peripheral neuropathy 8.9%, insomnia 11.3%, ↓ appetite 6.3%, myalgia 5%, lymphadenopathy 2.3%, eosinophilia – 10%. ↑ incidence of bacterial pneumonias. Alone offers little benefit to a failing regimen [NEJM 348:2249, 2003].

TABLE 6A (10)

F. **Other Considerations in Selection of Therapy**
   Caution: Initiation of ARV therapy may result in immune reconstitution syndrome with significant clinical consequences. *(AIDS Reader 16:199, 2006).*

   1. Resistance testing: Given current rates of resistance, in a model of ART-naive individuals with chronic HIV infection, genotype resistance testing was cost effective over a wide range of assumptions *(CID 41:1316, 2005).*
   2. Repeated detection of genetic archival data on resistance *(see Table 6C)*
   3. Drug-induced disturbances of glucose & lipid metabolism *(see Table 6C)*
   4. Drug-induced lactic acidosis & other FDA "box warnings" *(see Table 6C)*
   5. Drug-drug interactions *(see Table 16)*
   6. Risk in pregnancy *(see Table 17)*
   7. Use in children & children *(see Table 8)*
   8. Dosing in patients with renal or hepatic dysfunction *(see Table 17)*
   9. Other special populations *(see www.aidsinfo.nih.gov)*

      a. **Injection drug users.** Active drug use may compromise adherence. Potentially co-existing neuropsychiatric symptoms & ↑ prevalence of Hep B & C add to risk of drug toxicities. Drug interactions may potentially cause ↑ or ↓ blood levels of ART drugs, & of methadone or drugs of abuse *(Mt Sinai J Med 67:429, 2000; see Table 16A)*.

      b. **Co-infection with Hep B &/or C.** Lamivudine, emtricitabine & tenofovir are active against HBV *(CID 39:1062, 2004),* but only 3TC currently has FDA indication for Hep B. Severe hepatitis flare (see Black Box warnings) may occur in pts with chronic Hep B after stopping any of these 3 drugs used for HIV therapy. In HCV/HIV co-infected pts, ↑ rate of progression to cirrhosis. Proper sequencing of rx for HIV/HCV important to avoid ↑ toxicities *(see Table 12, pg131–134)*. Avoid ddI/d4T (lactic acidosis/steatosis) & full-dose ritonavir (hepatotoxicity), *CID 38[Suppl.2]:S90, 2004)*. Some experts find that an NRTI backbone of [tenofovir + (emtricitabine or lamivudine)] is better tolerated in this population than one of [zidovudine + lamivudine]. Changes in ART drug elimination with hepatic dysfunction may necessitate dosing changes *(CID 40:174, 2005; see Table 15B)*. Therapeutic drug monitoring should be considered when there is significant liver dysfunction.

G. **Response to Antiviral Therapy**

   1. **Adequate response to antiviral therapy: Continue current regimen**
      a. 0.5–0.75 log$_{10}$ ↓ in plasma HIV RNA by 4 weeks but generally effective rx ↓ VL by 1.5–2.0 log (90%–99%) within 2 weeks
      b. Undetectable by 4–6 months
      c. A sustained ↑ in CD4 counts: counts typically ↑ ≥50 cells/ml at 4 to 8 weeks after rx initiated or changed followed by 50–100 cells/ml per year thereafter

2. **Virologic/clinical failure to antiretroviral therapy: Confirm adherence. If OK, suspect resistance. Check susceptibility & change current regimen.**
   a. <0.5–0.75 log$_{10}$ ↓ in plasma HIV RNA by 4 weeks
   b. <1 log$_{10}$ ↓ in plasma HIV RNA by 8 weeks
   c. Failure to suppress plasma HIV RNA to below 400 copies/ml by 24 weeks or 50 copies/ml by 48 weeks
   d. Repeated detection of virus in significant level of virus in plasma after initial suppression to undetectable levels, suggesting the development of resistance
   e. Persistent decline in CD4 counts, as measured on at least 2 separate occasions
   f. Clinical deterioration

H. **Changing Treatment Regimens Due to Intolerance or Failure** *(Lancet 362:2002, 2003; www.aidsinfo.nih.gov)*

   1. For drug **intolerance** to a specific antiretroviral agent, it is acceptable to substitute a single alternative agent.
   2. For **failure** to achieve complete viral suppression or with sustained reappearance of virus after initial suppression, goal is to re-establish suppression to preserve immunologic function & minimize accumulation of drug resistance. This is easiest in less antiretroviral-experienced patients & with early intervention.
   3. Review history for potential impediments to maximal adherence. If adherence seems good & no other explanation, could consider therapeutic drug monitoring (PI or NRTI trough concentrations) if any concerns about absorption (e.g., GI disease) or too-rapid elimination (e.g., from drug interactions).
   4. Review history of antiretroviral use (or clue to archived mutant virus) & perform resistance testing (genotype &/or phenotype, see *Table 3*) while on failing regimen.
   5. Possible approaches to treatment for pts who are not extensively treatment-experienced:

      a. Most aggressive approach for relatively treatment-inexperienced patients is switch from NNRTI-based regimen to PI-based regimen, or vice versa. Select new NRTIs from resistance testing results & history. Pts on PI-based regimen could also be switched to an alternative PI (with appropriate NRTIs) based on resistance testing.

      b. For patients with partial suppression (low-detectable viral loads), consider intensification of regimen with additional agents (e.g., tenofovir if not on a TDF-based regimen) or boosting a PI-based regimen with ritonavir

      c. If possible, avoid adding only one active drug to a failing regimen

      d. In failing, adherent patient with no or minimal demonstrable genotypic or phenotypic resistance, consider measuring plasma drug levels (therapeutic drug monitoring)

      e. If resistant to multiple licensed drugs, investigate available clinical trials or agents available for compassionate use *(see Table 6D)*

TABLE 6B: ANTIRETROVIRAL DRUGS & ADVERSE EFFECTS (See also www.aidsinfo.nih.gov; for combinations, see individual components)

DRUG NAME(S); GENERIC (TRADE)	MOST COMMON ADVERSE EFFECTS	MOST SIGNIFICANT ADVERSE EFFECTS
Nucleoside Reverse Transcriptase Inhibitors (NRTI) (Black Box warning for all nucleoside/nucleotide RTIs: lactic acidosis/hepatic steatosis, potentially fatal. Also carry Warnings that fat redistribution has been observed)		
Abacavir (Ziagen)	Headache 7-13%, nausea 7-19%, diarrhea 7%, malaise 7-12%	**Hypersensitivity reaction** in 8% with malaise, fever, GI upset, rash, lethargy, & respiratory symptoms most commonly reported; myalgia, arthralgia, edema, paresthesia less commonly reported. Severe hypersensitivity reaction may be more common with once-daily dosing. **Rechallenge contraindicated; may be life-threatening.**
Didanosine (ddI) (Videx)	Diarrhea 28%, nausea 6%, rash 9%, headache 7%, fever 12%, hyperuricemia 2%	**Pancreatitis 1-9%. Black Box warning—Cases of fatal & nonfatal pancreatitis** have occurred in pts receiving ddI, especially when used in combination with d4T or d4T + hydroxyurea. Fatal lactic acidosis in pregnancy with ddI + d4T. Peripheral neuropathy in 20%, 12% required dose reduction. Rarely, retinal changes.
Emtricitabine (FTC) (Emtriva)	Well tolerated. Headache 20%, diarrhea, nausea, rash, skin hyperpigmentation	Potential for lactic acidosis (as with other NRTIs). Also in **Black Box—severe exacerbation of hepatitis B on stopping drug reported—monitor clinical/labs for several months after stopping in pts with hepB.** Anti-HBV rx may be warranted if FTC stopped.
Lamivudine (3TC) (Epivir)	Well tolerated. Headache 35%, nausea 33%, diarrhea 18%, abdominal pain 9%, insomnia 11% (all in combination with ZDV). Pancreatitis more common in pediatrics (15%).	**Black Box warning.** Make sure to use HIV dosage, not Hep B dosage. **Exacerbation of hepatitis B on stopping drug. Patients with hepB who stop lamivudine require close clinical/lab monitoring for several months.** Anti-HBV rx may be warranted if 3TC stopped.
Stavudine (d4T) (Zerit)	Diarrhea, nausea, vomiting, headache	**Peripheral neuropathy** 15-20%. Pancreatitis 1%. Appears to produce lactic acidosis more commonly than other NRTIs. **Black Box warning—Fatal & nonfatal pancreatitis with d4T + ddI + hydroxyurea. Fatal lactic acidosis/steatosis in pregnant women receiving d4T + ddI.** Motor weakness in the setting of lactic acidosis mimicking the clinical presentation of Guillain-Barré syndrome (including respiratory failure) (rare).
Zalcitabine (ddC) (Hivid)	Oral ulcers 13%, rash 8%	**Peripheral neuropathy** 22-35%. Severe continuous pain, slowly reversible when ddC is discontinued. ↑ risk with diabetes mellitus. **Hepatic failure in pts with Hep B.** Esophageal ulcers. Pancreatitis 1%.
Zidovudine (ZDV, AZT) (Retrovir)	Nausea 50%, anorexia 20%, vomiting 17%, **headache 62%.** Also reported: asthenia, insomnia, myalgias, nail pigmentation. Macrocytosis expected with all dosage regimens.	**Black Box warning—hematologic toxicity, myopathy. Anemia** (<8 gm, 1%), **granulocytopenia** (<750, 1.8%). Anemia may respond to epoitin alfa if endogenous serum erythropoietin levels are ≤500 milliU/mL.
Nucleotide Reverse Transcriptase Inhibitor (NRTI) (Black Box warning for all nucleoside/nucleotide RTIs: lactic acidosis/hepatic steatosis, potentially fatal. Also carry Warnings that fat redistribution has been observed)		
Tenofovir (TDF) (Viread)	Diarrhea 11%, nausea 8%, vomiting 5%, flatulence 4% (generally well tolerated)	**Severe exacerbations of hepatitis B** reported in pts who stop tenofovir. Not indicated to treat Hep B. Monitor carefully if drug is stopped; anti-HBV rx may be warranted if TDF stopped. Possible ↑ bone demineralization. Reports of Fanconi syndrome & **renal injury induced by tenofovir** (CID 37:e174, 2003; J AIDS 35:269, 2004; CID 42:283,2006). Modest decline in Ccr with TDF may be greater than with other NRTIs (CID 40:1194, 2005).
Non-Nucleoside Reverse Transcriptase Inhibitors (NNRTI)		
Delavirdine (Rescriptor)	Nausea, diarrhea, vomiting, headache	**Skin rash** has occurred in 18%, can continue or restart drug in most cases. Stevens-Johnson syndrome & erythema multiforme have been reported rarely. ↑ in liver enzymes in <5% of patients

TABLE 6B (2)

DRUG NAME(S): GENERIC (TRADE)	MOST COMMON ADVERSE EFFECTS	MOST SIGNIFICANT ADVERSE EFFECTS
Non-Nucleoside Reverse Transcriptase Inhibitors (NNRTI) (continued)		
Efavirenz (Sustiva)	**CNS side-effects 52%;** symptoms include dizziness, insomnia, somnolence, impaired concentration, psychiatric sx, & abnormal dreams; symptoms are worse after 1st or 2nd dose & improve over 2–4 weeks; discontinuation rate 2.6%. Rash 26% (vs. 17% in comparators); often improves with oral antihistamines; discontinuation rate 1.7%. Can cause false-positive urine test results for cannabinoid with CEDIA DAU multi-level THC assay.	Serious neuropsychiatric symptoms reported, including severe depression (2.4%) & suicidal ideation (0.7%). Elevation of liver enzymes. **Teratogenicity reported in primates; pregnancy category D—may cause fetal harm, avoid in pregnant women or those who might become pregnant** (see Table 8E). NOTE: No single method of contraception is 100% reliable. Contraindicated with certain drugs metabolized by CYP3A4.
Nevirapine (Viramune)	**Rash 37%;** occurs during 1st 6 wks of therapy. Follow recommendations for 14-day lead-in period to ↓ risk of rash (see Table 6A). Women experience 7-fold ↑ in risk of severe rash (CID 32:124, 2001). 50% resolve within 2 wks of dc drug & 80% by 1 month. 6.7% discontinuation rate.	**Black Box warning—Severe life-threatening skin reactions reported:** Stevens-Johnson syndrome, toxic epidermal necrolysis, & hypersensitivity reaction or drug rash with eosinophilia & systemic symptoms (DRESS) (AnIM 161:2501, 2001). For severe rashes, dc drug immediately & do not restart. In a clinical trial, the use of prednisone ↑ the risk of rash. **Black Box warning—Life-threatening hepatotoxicity reported,** 2/3 during the first 12 wks of rx. Overall 1% develop hepatitis. Pts with preexisting ↑ in ALT or AST &/or history of chronic Hep B or C ↑ susceptible (Hepatol 35:182, 2002). Women with CD4 >250, including pregnant women, at ↑ risk. Avoid in this group unless no other option. (Men with CD4 >400 also at ↑ risk. Monitor pts intensively (clinical & LFTs), esp. during the first 12 wks of rx. If clinical hepatotoxicity occurs, dc drug & never rechallenge.
Protease inhibitors (PI)		
Abnormalities in glucose metabolism, dyslipidemias, fat redistribution syndromes are potential problems. Pts taking PI may be at increased risk for developing osteopenia/osteoporosis. (See Table 6C). Spontaneous bleeding episodes have been reported in HIV+ pts with hemophilia being treated with PIs (An Rheum Dis 61:82, 2002). Potential of some PIs for QTc prolongation has been suggested (Lancet 365:682, 2005). **Caution for all PIs**—Coadministration with certain drugs dependent on CYP3A for elimination & for which ↑ levels can cause serious toxicity may be contraindicated.		
Amprenavir (Agenerase)	Nausea 43–74%, vomiting 24–34%, diarrhea 39–60%, paresthesias 26–31%	Skin rash 28%. Most maculopapular of mild–moderate intensity, some with pruritus. Severe or life-threatening rash, including Stevens-Johnson syndrome, in 1% of pts. Skin rash onset 7–73 days, median 11 days. **Black Box warning**—potential propylene glycol toxicity. Do not use in pregnancy, children <4 years old, renal/hepatic failure, or with disulfiram or metronidazole. Contains sulfa moiety.
Atazanavir (Reyataz)	Asymptomatic unconjugated hyperbilirubinemia in up to 60% of pts, jaundice in 7–9% (especially with Gilbert syndrome (JID 192: 1381, 2005)). Moderate to severe events: Diarrhea 1–3%, nausea 6–14%, abdominal pain 4%, headache 6%, rash 5–7%	Prolongation of PR interval (1st degree AV block) reported; rarely 2° AV block. One case acute interstitial nephritis (Am J Kid Dis 44:E81, 2004).
Fosamprenavir (Lexiva)	Skin rash ~ 20% (moderate or worse in 3–8%), nausea, headache, diarrhea.	Rarely Stevens-Johnson syndrome, hemolytic anemia. Pro-drug of amprenavir. Contains sulfa moiety.
Indinavir (Crixivan)	↑ in indirect bilirubin 10–15% (≥2.5 mg/dl), with overt jaundice especially likely in those with Gilbert syndrome (JID 192: 1381, 2005). Nausea 12%, vomiting 4%, diarrhea 5%. Paronychia of big toe reported (CID 32:140, 2001).	**Kidney stones.** Due to indinavir crystals in collecting system. Nephrolithiasis in 12% of adults, higher in pediatrics. Minimize risk with good hydration (at least 48 oz. water/day) (AAC 42:332, 1998). Tubulointerstitial nephritis/renal cortical atrophy reported in association with asymptomatic ↑ urine WBC. Severe hepatitis reported in 3 cases (Ln 349:924, 1997). Hemolytic anemia reported.

TABLE 6B (3)

DRUG NAME(S): GENERIC (TRADE)	MOST COMMON ADVERSE EFFECTS	MOST SIGNIFICANT ADVERSE EFFECTS
Protease Inhibitors (PI): (continued)		
Lopinavir/Ritonavir (Kaletra)	GI: **diarrhea** 14-24%, nausea 2-16%.	Lipid abnormalities in up to 20-40%. Pancreatitis. Inflammatory edema of legs (*AIDS* 16:673, 2002).
Nelfinavir (Viracept)	Mild to moderate **diarrhea** 20%. Oat bran tabs, calcium, or oral anti-diarrheal agents (e.g., loperamide, diphenoxylate/atropine sulfate) can be used to manage diarrhea.	
Ritonavir (Norvir) (With rare exceptions, used to enhance levels of other anti-retrovirals, because of toxicity; interactions with full-dose ritonavir)	GI: bitter aftertaste ↓ by taking with chocolate milk, Ensure, or Advera; nausea 23%, ↓ by initial dose esc (titration) regimen; vomiting 13%, diarrhea 15%; Circumoral paresthesias 5-6%; ↑ dose >100mg bid assoc. with ↑ GI side-effects & ↑ in lipid abnormalities.	Hepatic failure (*AnIM* 129:670, 1998). **Black Box warning** relates to many important drug-drug interactions—inhibits P450 CYP3A & CYP2D6 system—may be life-threatening (see Table 16). Rarely Stevens-Johnson syndrome, anaphylaxis.
Saquinavir (Invirase: hard cap, tablet)	**Diarrhea**, abdominal discomfort, nausea, headache	**Black Box Warning**—Invirase & Fortovase (which has been discontinued) are not bioequivalent. **Use Invirase only with ritonavir.**
Tipranavir (Aptivus)	Nausea & vomiting, diarrhea, abdominal pain. Rash in 8-14%, more common in women, & 33% in women taking ethinyl estradiol. Major lipid effects.	**Black Box Warning—associated with hepatitis & fatal hepatic failure.** Risk of hepatotoxicity in hepB or hepC co-infection. Potential for major drug interactions. Contains sulfa moiety.
Fusion Inhibitor		
Enfuvirtide (T20, Fuzeon)	Local injection site reactions (98%; at least 1 local ISR, 4%; dc because of ISR (pain & discomfort, induration, erythema, nodules & cysts, pruritus, & ecchymosis). Diarrhea 32%, nausea 23%, fatigue 20%.	↑ Rate of bacterial pneumonia (6.7 pneumonia events/100 pt yrs). **hypersensitivity reactions** ≤1% (rash, fever, nausea & vomiting, chills, rigors, hypotension, & ↑ serum liver transaminases).

TABLE 6C: DRUG ADVERSE EFFECTS BY CLINICAL PRESENTATION

Clinical Presentation	Implicated Drug Class or Drug(s) (in alphabetical order)	Onset; Clinical Signs & Symptoms (S&S)	Estimated Frequency	Risk Factors	Prevention/ Monitoring	Clinical Management
LIFE THREATENING ADVERSE EFFECTS (in alphabetical order)						
Drug-induced hepatitis	Nevirapine (Viramune)	Onset: Any time 1st wks. S&S: nausea/vomiting/icterus. Skin rash in 50%	2.5-11% in clinical trials	Females; CD4 >250. Chronic Hep B or C. Alcoholism	Monitor ALT/AST q2wks x1mo, then q mo x3, then q3mos.	DC all antiretrovirals + other potential hepatotoxic drugs
Lactic acidosis/ hepatic steatosis ± pancreatitis	Nucleoside reverse transcriptase inhibitors: stavudine (Zerit), didanosine (Videx), zidovudine (Retrovir)	Onset: Months after starting therapy. S&S: Nausea, vomiting, fatigue, dyspnea, icterus. Lab: Metabolic acidosis with anion gap & elevated lactate	Rare: 0.85 cases/1000 pt yrs, mortality up to 50%	Didanosine + stavudine. Female, pregnancy, obesity	Lactic acid levels if suggestive symptoms; routine lactate levels **not** recommended	DC all antiretrovirals. IV thiamine &/or riboflavin reported helpful. If needed, use NRTIs with low potential for mitochondrial toxicity: abacavir, tenofovir, lamivudine, emtricitabine

1 NRTI = nucleoside reverse transcriptase inhibitor

TABLE 6C (2)

Clinical Presentation	Implicated Drug Class or Drug(s)	Onset; Clinical Signs & Symptoms (S&S)	Estimated Frequency	Risk Factors	Prevention/ Monitoring	Clinical Management
LIFE THREATENING ADVERSE EFFECTS (in alphabetical order) (continued)						
Lactic acidosis/rapid progressive ascending neuromuscular weakness	Stavudine (Zerit)	Onset: After months S&S: Rapid progressive ascending polyneuropathy that mimics Guillain-Barre. Lab: Metabolic acidosis with anion gap, ↑ elevated lactate + high CPK	Rare	Prolonged stavudine use	Early recognition	DC all antiretrovirals, mechanical ventilation. Unclear benefit from plasmapheresis, IVIG, corticosteroids, carnitine
Stevens-Johnson syndrome/toxic epidermal necrosis (see drug-induced hepatitis above)	Non-nucleoside reverse transcriptase inhibitors. Rare case reports other classes	Onset: ↑ few days to weeks S&S: Skin eruption with mucosal ulcers ± epidermal detachment	Nevirapine (Viramune) 0.3–1% Efavirenz (Sustiva) & delavirdine (Rescriptor) 0.1%	Nevirapine—female, black, Asian, Hispanic	Educate pts for early recognition	DC all antiretrovirals + other possible drug etiology; e.g., TMP/SMX. Usually requires ICU.
Systemic hyper-sensitivity reaction	Abacavir (Ziagen)	Onset: Median 11 days; 90% within 1 6wks S&S: Fever, diffuse rash, nausea/ vomiting/diarrhea/arthralgia, dyspenia, cough, or pharyngitis	8% in clinical trials (range 2–9%)	HLA-B 5701, HLA-DR7. Risk less with 600mg q24h rather than 300mg q12h	Educate pts for early recognition	DC all antiretrovirals. Should resolve within 48 hrs after stopping abacavir. **DO NOT rechallenge with abacavir.**
SERIOUS ADVERSE EFFECTS (in alphabetical order)						
Bleeding increase in hemophiliac pts	Protease inhibitors	Onset: Few weeks S&S: Spontaneous bleeding	Unknown	Protease inhibitor use	Use non-protease inhibitor regimen	
Bone marrow suppression	Zidovudine (Retrovir)	Onset: Weeks to months S&S: Fatigue Lab: Anemia &/or neutropenia	Anemia 1.1–4% Neutropenia 1.8–8%	AIDS; high dose concomitant marrow suppressive drug(s)	Avoid marrow suppressive drugs. CBC & differential at least q3 mos	If severe, could use G-CSF &/or erythropoetin
Nephrolithiasis/ urolithiasis/crystalluria	Indinavir (Crixivan)	Onset: Any time S&S: Flank pain & dysuria Lab: Hematuria, crystalluria, pyuria	Range in clinical trials: 4.7–34.4%	Dehydration, history of nephrolithiasis	Intake of 1.5–2 liters water/day	Hydration
Nephrotoxicity– tenofovir (CID 42:283, 2006)	Indinavir (Crixivan) crystalluria (see above) & tenofovir (Viread) tubular injury	Onset: Tenofovir—weeks to months S&S: Tenofovir—nephrogenic diabetes insipidus. **Fanconi syndrome** Lab: Non-anion gap metabolic acidosis, glycosuria, hypokalemia, hypophosphatemia	Unknown	Other nephrotoxic drugs; other anti-HIV drugs handled by proximal tubular cells—see prevention	Monitor serum K⁺ & serum phosphorus. Theoretic drug-drug interactions with ritonavir, didanosine & atazanavir	Stop tenofovir
Pancreatitis	Didanosine (Videx); didanosine + stavudine (Zerit); lamivudine (Epivir) in children	Onset: Weeks to months S&S: Abd /back pain, nausea/vomiting Lab: ↑ amylase/lipase	Didanosine alone 1–7%; Lamivudine in children—range in clinical trials <1–15%	High serum/cell didanosine levels; alcoholism; hypertriglyceridemia. Failure to ↓ dose of didanosine if given with tenofovir	No didanosine if history of pancreatitis. Adjust dose of didanosine if tenofovir used	DC antiretrovirals

TABLE 6C (3)

ADVERSE EFFECTS WITH LONG-TERM COMPLICATIONS (in alphabetical order)

Clinical Presentation	Implicated Drug Class or Drug(s)	Onset; Clinical Signs & Symptoms (S&S)	Estimated Frequency	Risk Factors	Prevention/ Monitoring	Clinical Management
Atherosclerotic cardiovascular disease potential. Ref: NEJM 352:48, 2005	All protease inhibitors except atazanavir (Reyataz)	Onset: Months to years. S&S: Premature or accelerated atherosclerotic vascular disease (e.g., MI, stroke)	Incidence of MI: 3-6/1000 pts yrs on protease inhibitor.	Tobacco use, age, hyperlipidemia (see below), hypertension, diabetes	Address risk factors	Manage risk factors; may have to avoid protease inhibitors
Hyperlipidemia Ref: NEJM 352:48, 2005	All protease inhibitors (PIs) except atazanavir (Reyataz); stavudine (Zerit); efavirenz (Sustiva)	Onset: Weeks to months. Lab: ↑ LDL & total cholesterol & triglycerides; ↓ HDL.	Range in pts taking PIs: 47-57%.	Varies with PI: lopinavir > nelfinavir & amprenavir > indinavir & saquinavir > atazanavir	Use non-PI, non-stavudine regimen. Lipid profile baseline & then at 3-6 months of therapy	Lifestyle modification. For ↑ total cholesterol, LDL, triglycerides 200-500, Pravastatin or atorvastatin. For triglycerides >500 mg/dl, gemfibrozil
Insulin resistance/ diabetes mellitus Ref: NEJM 352:52, 2005	All protease inhibitors (PIs) inc. low dose ritonavir	Onset: Weeks to months. S&S: Polydipsia, polyuria, polyphagia	3-5% of pts	Underlying hyperglycemia, family history	Non-PI regimen. Ideally, monitor fasting insulin level.	Diet & exercise, metformin, "glitazones," sulfonylureas
Osteonecrosis Ref: NEJM 352:52, 2005	All protease inhibitors (PIs)	Onset: Insidious. S&S: Periarticular pain. 85% involve femoral head	Symptomatic 0.08-1.3%. Asymptomatic by MRI 4%	Diabetes; prior steroid use; alcohol use; hyperlipidemia	No steroids. Periodic MRIs to assess disease progression.	Remove risk factors; less weight-bearing; some total joint arthroplasty

ADVERSE EFFECTS THAT INFLUENCE QUALITY OF LIFE

Clinical Presentation	Implicated Drug Class or Drug(s)	Onset; Clinical Signs & Symptoms (S&S)	Estimated Frequency	Risk Factors	Prevention/ Monitoring	Clinical Management
Fat maldistribution Refs: NEJM 352:48, 2005; Antiviral Therapy 10 (Supp2):M117, 2005.	Protease inhibitors (PIs) & stavudine (Zerit)—esp. in combination with didanosine (Videx). Atazanavir ok. CID 42:273 & 281, 2006.	Onset: Months after treatment starts. S&S: • Lipoatrophy—fat loss with facial thinning, loss of subcutaneous fat of buttocks & extremities • ↑ in abdominal girth, breast size & development of "buffalo hump"	High (40-60% ambulatory pts; precise frequency unknown)	Low baseline body mass index	Avoid: (zidovudine plus stavudine) plus didanosine)	• DC thymidine analogues • Uridine (Nucleomax) 36gm tid 10 days per month, expensive • Pravastatin 40mg daily • Pioglitazone 30mg daily (CROI 40.745, 2005)
Gastrointestinal— Diarrhea	All protease inhibitors (PIs), didanosine (Videx)	Onset: Weeks to months. Symptoms: Perhaps worst with lopinavir/ritonavir, nelfinavir, & buffered didanosine	Varies	All patients	Antidiarrheals	(For diarrhea, consider: loperamide, diphenoxylate/atropine, calcium tabs, psyllium products, pancreatic enzymes
Peripheral neuropathy	Didanosine (Videx), stavudine (Zerit), zalcitabine (HIVID)	Onset: Weeks to months. S&S: Usually legs. Numbness & paresthesias. Often irreversible even if drug(s) stopped	Didanosine 12-34%. Stavudine 52%. Zalcitabine 22-35%	Pre-existing neuropathy; advanced HIV; concomitant drugs that ↑ intracellular didanosine, e.g., ribavirin, hydroxyurea	Avoid use, esp. in combination	If symptomatic, gabapentin or tricyclic antidepressants; high concentration capsaicin dermal patch (Conference on Retroviruses & Opportunistic Infections (CROI), 2006)

TABLE 6D: SELECTIVE LIST OF DRUGS IN THE ANTI-HIV PIPELINE (www.aidsinfo.nih.gov: 800-448-0440)

Class of Drug	Drug Name(s), Number(s), Manufacturer	Anti-HIV Activity/Comments	Development Status
Non-Nucleoside Reverse Transcriptase Inhibitors (NNRTI)			
	Etravirine, TMC-125 (Tibotec)	Over 1 log decrease in viral load even if 2 NNRTI resistance mutations present. Diarrhea & rash in 15%.	Phase II-III. Possible new formulation dose is 200 mg bid. Under study in combination with darunavir (TMC-114)
Protease Inhibitors (PI)			
	Brecanavir, GW640385 (GlaxoSmithKline)	Brecanavir 300mg + ritonavir 100mg bid + NRTIs resulted in viral load of <50 copies per ml in 77% of pts who failed other PIs.	Phase III in 2006. No serious adverse events.
	Darunavir, TMC-114 (Tibotec)	Dose: 600mg + 100mg ritonavir once a day. In treatment experienced pts, 62% with 1 log decrease in viral load at 24hrs.	Phase III. NDA filed with FDA. For expanded access: 1-866-889-2074 (USA) or TMC114-C266@i3research.com or www.tibotec.com
Maturation Inhibitor			
	PA-457 (Panacos Pharm.)	Oral dose not determined. Over 1 log decrease in viral load after 10 days.	Phase II. Little known about adverse reactions.
Entry Inhibitors			
Attachment Inhibitor			
	PRO-140 (Progenics Pharm. Co.)	Humanized monoclonal antibody that binds CCR5. Very active in animal models.	Phase I. At 5 mg per kg achieved therapeutic effect for over 60 days with no adverse events.
CCR5 Chemokine Inhibitors: All po; active vs. R5 monocytic tropic virus			
	Maraviroc, UK-427, 857 (Pfizer)	Possible dose: 300mg bid. Over 1.4 log decrease in viral load.	Phase II-III
	Vicriviroc, Sch-417690 (Sch-D)	Possible dose: 50mg bid. Likely active vs. T-20 resistant HIV.	Phase III. Responds to ritonavir boosting.
Integrase Inhibitors			
	GS9137 (JTK-303)(Gilead)	Possible dose: 50mg + 100mg ritonavir once daily. 2 log decrease in viral load in 10 days reported.	Phase II in progress. Well-tolerated.
	MK-0518 (Merck)	In dose ranging study, over 2 log decrease in viral load in 10 days in treatment-experienced pts.	Phase III soon.

TABLE 6E. ANTIRETROVIRALS APPROVED OR TENTATIVELY APPROVED BY FDA FOR INTERNATIONAL AIDS RELIEF (from www.fda.gov/oia/pepfar.htm)

As a requirement of the President's Emergency Plan for AIDS Relief (PEPFAR), the US FDA reviews international marketing applications for individual antiretroviral agents, fixed dose combinations & co-packaged ARVs, & grants approval (A) or tentative (T) approval (when products continue to have marketing protection) status to products that meet efficacy, safety & manufacturing standards for marketing in the US.

Generic name	Pharmaceutical Prep.	Supplier	Status	Generic name	Pharmaceutical Prep.	Supplier	Status
Single agents				**Single agents**			
Didanosine	200 mg, 250 mg, 400 mg delayed release caps	Bar Laboratories, Inc.	A	Nevirapine	200 mg tabs	Ranbaxy Laboratories, Ltd	T
Zidovudine (ZDV)	300 mg tabs	Ranbaxy Laboratories, Ltd	A		200 mg tabs 50 mg/mL oral suspension	Aurobindo Pharma, Ltd	T
	300 mg tabs, 50 mg/5 mL oral solution	Aurobindo Pharma, Ltd	A	Efavirenz	600 mg tabs	Aurobindo Pharma, Ltd	T
Lamivudine (3TC)	150 mg tabs	Ranbaxy Laboratories, Ltd	T	**Combinations &/or co-packaged products**			
	150 mg, 300 mg tabs 10 mg/mL oral solution	Aurobindo Pharma, Ltd	T	Lamivudine/ Zidovudine	Tabs (150 mg 3TC + 300 mg ZDV)	Aurobindo Pharma, Ltd	T
Stavudine	30 mg, 40 mg caps 1 mg/mL oral solution	Aurobindo Pharma, Ltd	T	Lamivudine/ Zidovudine co-packaged with nevirapine	Tabs (150 mg 3TC + 300 mg ZDV) with Tabs 200 mg nevirapine	Aspen Pharmacare, Ltd	T

TABLE 7: METHODS FOR PENICILLIN DESENSITIZATION

Perform in ICU setting. Discontinue all β-adrenergic antagonists. Have IV line. ECG & spirometer (Curr Clin Topics Int Dis 13:131, 1993). Once desensitized, rx must not lapse or risk of allergic reactions ↑. A history of Stevens-Johnson syndrome, exfoliative dermatitis, erythroderma are nearly absolute contraindications to desensitization (use only as an approach to IgE sensitivity).
Oral Route: If oral prep available & pt has functional GI tract, oral route is preferred. 1/3 pts will develop transient reaction during desensitization or treatment, usually mild.

Step*	1	2	3	4	5	6	7	8	9	10	11	12	13	14	15	16	17
Drug (mg/mL)	0.5	0.5	0.5	0.5	0.5	0.5	0.5	5	5	5	50	50	50	50	1000	1000	1000
Amount (mL)	0.1	0.2	0.4	0.8	1.6	3.2	6.4	1.2	2.4	4.8	1.0	2.0	4.0	8.0	0.16	0.32	0.64

* Interval between doses: 15 min. After Step 14, observe for 30 minutes; then 1 gm IV.

Parenteral Route:

Step**	1	2	3	4	5	6	7	8	9	10	11	12	13	14	15	16	17
Drug (mg/mL)	0.1	0.1	0.1	0.1	0.1	1	1	10	10	10	100	100	100	100	1000	1000	1000
Amount (mL)	0.1	0.2	0.4	0.8	0.16	0.32	0.64	0.12	0.24	0.48	0.1	0.2	0.4	0.8	0.16	0.32	0.64

** Interval between doses: 15 min. After Step 17, observe for 30 minutes, then 1 gm IV.

[Adapted from Sullivan, TJ, in Allergy: Principles & Practice, Middleton, E., et al. Eds. C.V. Mosby, 1993, p. 1726, with permission]

TABLE 8A: HIV/AIDS IN WOMEN/PREGNANCY

I. General Aspects

- A. Women represent half of persons with HIV/AIDS in the world. Among young people (15–24yrs) in developing countries with HIV/AIDS, 64% are women.
- B. Heterosexual transmission is dominant mode of transmission worldwide. Among new HIV/AIDS diagnoses among women in the U.S. in 2004: 79% heterosexual contact, 19% IDU.
- C. Transmission of HIV from men to women occurs more readily than from women to men. Risk factors for male-to-female transmission: genital ulcers, partner with advanced disease, other STDs, trauma.
- D. Risk after several years of unprotected sex with same infected partner is 10–45%.
- E. Despite these aspects, relatively less is written about women's issues. Only small numbers of women have been included in therapy trials.

II. Initial Assessment: See Table 2

III. Clinical Manifestations *(Adapted from Newman, MD, in Medical Mgmt of AIDS, 6th ed.; 1999; J AIDS 9:361, 1995)*

- A. **AIDS-defining diagnoses:**
  - Disease progression similar in women & men *(NEJM 333:751, 1995)*
  - Survival is related to access to care, which may be worse for women
  - Viral load at high CD4 counts tends to be lower in women *(CID 35:313, 2002)*
  - Gender difference narrows as CD4 drops
- B. **Human papillomavirus:**
  - HPV disease incidence increased! Cervical intraepithelial neoplasia (CIN) more prevalent in multiple studies. Prevalence increases with decreasing CD4 *(CID 38:737, 2004)*
  - Aggressive course, with high rate of progression to cancer if immunosuppressed
  - Pap smear recommended for HIV+ women. If initial Pap smear is neg, repeat in 6mos. If both are negative, annual Pap smears adequate (CDC Guidelines). We recommend q6mos for those with CD4 <200. Colposcopy recommended for any suspicious lesions. There are no contraindications to standard treatment modalities for CIN.
- C. **Recurrent/refractory vaginal candidiasis**
  - May be early manifestation (CD4 may be >500)
  - HIV diagnosis often missed because testing not offered
- D. **Other conditions**
  - PID may be more severe, 7–17% require hospitalization
  - Menstrual disorders (41% HIV+ women had menstrual abnormalities vs 24% in case controls) include irregular periods, heavier or scantier periods, early menopausal symptoms, ↑ in premenstrual symptoms

IV. Family Planning. 85% of women with AIDS are in child-bearing years. Certain contraceptives may pose health hazards for HIV+ women *(Zeeman B, Hirschhorn LR, p. 616, in HIV Infection, Libman H, Witzburg RA. 3rd Ed., Little Brown & Co.)*

Method of Contraception	Failure Rate	Risks
Sterilization	0.4	No HIV protection
Oral contraceptive	3	May ↑ disease progression; drug-drug interactions common
IUD	3	↑ risk of PID, not higher for HIV+ vs HIV–
Latex condom	12	—
Diaphragm cervical cap	18	Potential vaginal abrasions
Sponge	18–28	Potential vaginal abrasions
Nonoxynol-9	21	Irritation of vaginal mucosa with freq. use; may ↑ HIV transmission

V. Treatment Issues

- A. Inadequate gender-specific data!
- B. Theoretical issues
  - Baseline anemia (iron deficiency)
  - Low mean body weight, higher body fat, different hepatic metabolism compared to men
- C. Menstrual dysfunction
  - Amenorrhea should be evaluated; start with pregnancy test
  - Premature menopause occurs frequently; consider hormone replacement therapy
- D. Recommended treatment regimens currently identical for men & women
  - Rates of some side effects different in women (↑ rash on nevirapine, ↑ GI side-effects on lopinavir/ritonavir)
  - **Efavirenz should be avoided in women who may become pregnant**
  - Lactic acidosis may be more common in women, associated with d4T & ddI

VI. HIV in Pregnancy: Care of the Mother

- A. **Antepartum Care**
  - **All** pregnant women should be offered HIV testing & counseling **regardless** of risk factors. Inclusion in routine testing with opt-out preferred to opt-in
  - Quantitative measure of **HIV RNA**
  - Obtain CD4 count at outset & each trimester (some ↓ in normal pregnancy)
  - **Screening tests** (HBsAg, RPR, chlamydia) as in any pregnancy
  - Discourage illicit drug use, unprotected sex with multiple partners (↑ transmission)
- B. **Use of antiviral therapy in pregnancy** (www.aidsinfo.nih.gov). Treatment of HIV in pregnancy requires attention to 2 separate but equal goals:
  - Provide optimal treatment to the woman that does not limit future options
  - Prevent transmission to the infant without drug toxicity
  1. Risk factors for mother-to-child transmission (MTCT)
     - Maternal viral load (outset & at delivery are independent predictors *(JID 183:539, 2001)*
     - Maternal CD4 count (risk of transmission ↑ if CD4 <400)
     - Lack of antiviral therapy (independent of other factors) *(JID 183:539, 2001)*
     - Prolonged rupture of membranes (rate doubled if >4 hours) *(NEJM 334:1617, 1996)*
     - Mode of delivery *(see next page)*
     - Breastfeeding (additional 10–14% transmission) *(JAMA 282:744, 1999)*
  2. General principles
     - Preventing MTCT should be integrated with obstetrical & HIV medical care for the mother. The mother should be informed & involved in decisions.

TABLE 8A (2)

- Antiretroviral therapy ↓ risk of MTCT regardless of viral load
- ARV is generally safe for the mother (avoid use of ddl with d4T—↑ risk of lactic acidosis)
- Maximal viral suppression with combination therapy ↓ risk of resistance in mother & loss of future options, & appears more effective than 1- or 2-drug regimens
- Resistance testing recommended before beginning ARV if it is available
- Longterm safety of ARV for infant exposed in utero is not fully known. Generally safe, although conflicting data on mitochondrial toxicity
- Some data suggest ↑ rate of prematurity, low birth weight with PI use during pregnancy
- Optimal dosing in pregnancy has not been fully adequately studied
- PI levels fall in third trimester (nelfinavir, indinavir, lopinavir/ritonavir)

3. Combination therapy with ZDV, 1 other NRTI, & either nevirapine or potent protease inhibitor recommended:
   a. **For all women for whom ARV therapy is otherwise appropriate**
   b. **For all women with >1000 copies of HIV RNA**
   c. **Should be considered for all pregnant woman**
      - **Transmission in cohorts 0.7–2.0% with 3-drug HAART**
      - **d4T & 3TC are probably a reasonable choice of nucleosides if they are more readily available through national formulary, although data are limited**
      - **WHO recommends ZDV, 3TC & nevirapine or d4T, 3TC & nevirapine for pregnant women who will receive HAART**
4. Many trials have demonstrated significant efficacy of more limited regimens. Some may be more affordable or practical in specific settings. (For detailed overview, see http://womenchildrenhiv.org/wchi/?page=pi-10-02)
5. Single dose nevirapine should be considered for women without prenatal care. However, emergence of nevirapine resistance can occur in up to 50%. Use of additional drugs, such as ZDV & lamivudine, continued for 3–7 days after delivery has been shown to to ↓ the emergence of resistance.
6. **Efavirenz is contraindicated in pregnancy due to risk of teratogenicity.**
7. **Stavudine & didanosine combination should not be used in pregnancy due to risk of lactic acidosis.**
8. **Severe skin rash, ↑ transaminases & rarely fulminant hepatitis can occur after starting nevirapine. Rates higher in non-pregnant women than in men, esp. with higher CD4 count. Monitor LFTs, instruct mother to seek care for nausea, abdominal pain. Check transaminases in any woman who develops rash. Consider non-nevirapine containing regimens if CD4 count >250 unless benefits clearly outweigh risks.**

C. Specific situations
   1. **For pregnant women not on therapy:** Evaluate clinical, virologic, social factors, & previous therapy. Discuss options, risks, & benefits. Begin therapy after 10–14wks gestation & after nausea has resolved, when adherence can be assured.
   2. **For women on antiretroviral therapy when pregnancy is diagnosed:** If pregnancy dx after 1st tri, continue therapy, modify as necessary. Efavirenz & combination stavudine/didanosine must be avoided. If pregnancy dx in 1st tri, many experts would continue therapy to avoid viral rebound. Consideration can be given to stopping therapy until the 2nd tri, but all drugs should be stopped at once, with attention to 1/2 lives.
   3. **For women in labor with no prior therapy:** Several options may be considered:
      - Intrapartum IV ZDV & 4–6wks of po ZDV for the infant
      - Intrapartum ZDV & 3TC, followed by 1wk of ZDV & 3TC for the infant
      - 2-part nevirapine regimen with intrapartum po nevirapine (200mg) followed by single dose for the infant (2mg/kg). High risk of nevirapine resistance. Consider following option
      - Intrapartum nevirapine combined with ZDV & 3TC, followed by po nevirapine for the infant & 4–6wks po ZDV. Strongly consider 1wk of ZDV & 3TC for mother to reduce nevirapine resistance.
   4. **For infants born to HIV-infected women who did not receive therapy:**
      - Offer po ZDV to the infant begun as soon as possible & continue for 6wks
      - Some experts would use additional agents, e.g., ZDV & 3TC, or ZDV, 3TC & single dose nevirapine

D. **Elective C-section before the onset of labor** ↓ transmission by 50% for women on no therapy or ZDV monotherapy (NEJM 340:977, 1999). However, in recent cohorts on effective therapy, no apparent additional benefit of C-section was observed.
   - This should be discussed with the woman & she should be involved in the decision.
   - Elective C-section (before 38 weeks) should be considered if:
      - Maternal viral load >1000 at delivery despite HAART
      - Mother received less than 3-drug therapy
      - Mother presents late in pregnancy
      - Obstetrical indications or maternal preference
   - Elective C-section is not cost-effective in resource-poor settings

E. **PCP prophylaxis:** Recommended for women with CD4 count <200 or on prophylaxis. PCP during pregnancy can be more severe.
   - **TMP/SMX** may be used, although use in last trimester may be associated with ↑ bilirubin. Risk of kernicterus unknown but very small. TMP/SXZ reduced maternal & infant mortality among mothers with CD4 < 200 in resource poor settings.
   - **Dapsone:** no known adverse effects, although experience limited.
   - **Aerosolized pentamidine.** Little systemic absorption, although less effective in advanced disease. Effect of ventilation changes due to pregnancy on distribution is unknown.

TABLE 8B: HIV IN THE FETUS & NEWBORN

GENERAL:
- In 2004, only an est 48 children in the U.S. were diagnosed with AIDS, compared to an est 800,000 children newly infected with HIV worldwide. In the U.S., 1695 children were living with an AIDS diagnosis in 2004 & an additional 3000–3500 are living with HIV. Worldwide, an estimated 2.7 million children are living with HIV.
- In 1995, over 7,000 HIV-infected women gave birth. This number has ↑substantially, but accurate est. aren't available
- Thus, the success of HIV testing of pregnant women & intrapartum treatment in Western countries dramatically ↓ HIV infection in children. Universal testing & counseling **must be offered to all pregnant women** to improve this.
- At the same time, millions of children are infected in resource-poor settings.

TABLE 8B (2)

- In the U.S., 63% of children living with AIDS in 2004 were black, 22% Hispanic, & 14% white. Injection drug use identified as a risk factor for a minority of mothers; most due to demonstrated or presumed heterosexual transmission.

TRANSMISSION:[1]

- **Over 90% of HIV+ children in U.S. acquired infection from their mothers perinatally:** in utero, during delivery, or postpartum through breastfeeding. Risk of transmission 13–40% (http://aidsinfo.nih.gov/guidelines).
- **Time of transmission:**
  - **In utero:** HIV has been identified in fetal tissues as early as 8 weeks. Probably in the majority, in utero transmission occurs late in pregnancy *(Lancet 345:518, 1995)*.
  - **Intrapartum:** 50–70% of transmissions believed to occur through exposure to mother's blood, cervical secretions or amniotic fluid during delivery.
  - **Postpartum** acquisition rare in developed countries, important in developing countries. Breast-fed infants have a 10-14% add'l risk of becoming infected. In mothers seroconverting during lactation, risk is 1/3 *(Lancet 342:1437, 1993)*.

DIAGNOSIS: (See Table 8C, below)

- HIV can be diagnosed in most infants by 1mo & all infants by 6mos of age by demonstration of virus by viral culture, viral DNA PCR, or viral RNA PCR.
- DNA PCR is currently considered the preferred method because of more supportive data (http://aidsinfo.nih.gov/guidelines), but RNA PCR (e.g., Roche Amplicor) may be more sensitive *(JID 175:707, 1997; J AIDS 32:192, 2003)*. Some experts perform both assays.
- Maternal anti-HIV IgG crosses the placenta & persists until 9–15mos, so infants born to HIV-infected mothers may test positive for up to 15mos regardless of infection. Assays for p24 antigen are less sensitive & less specific than PCR.
- PCR should be performed:
  - By age 48hrs (not on cord blood)
  - At 2–8wks
  - Repeat at 3–6mos if initial tests negative
- Any pos test should be repeated immediately along with quantitative HIV RNA PCR (viral load) before treatment begun.
- Presumptive evidence of in utero infection is PCR positive in 1st 48 hours of life. Intrapartum infection defined by negative test in 1st 48 hours followed by positive test *(NEJM 275:606, 1995)*.
- If PCR is not available, HIV can be diagnosed by persistence of HIV antibody after 18 months of age.

NATURAL HISTORY:

Bimodal distribution. Approximately 20% will be rapid progressors with onset of symptoms by median 8 months & median survival of <2yrs. Median survival, untreated, for non-rapid progressors was 66mos. Survival has greatly ↑ in the era of HAART, & many perinatally infected children are reaching adolescence & young adulthood.

TABLE 8C: HIV INFECTION IN CHILDREN

1. HIV-Infected
   - Child <18mos known to be HIV+ or born to HIV+ mother & has positive results on 2 separate determinations from one or more: HIV culture, HIV PCR, HIV 24 antigen.
   - Child ≥18mos born to HIV+ mother or infected by blood products, sexual contact who is HIV antibody + by ELISA & Western blot or HIV culture, PCR or p24 antigen.
2. Perinatally Exposed: A child who does not meet criteria above but
   - is HIV seropositive & <18mos of age   • unknown antibody status but born to HIV+ mother
3. Seroreverter: (CDC definition) A child <18mos w/ mother: Documented HIV negative (2 or more neg. EIA at 6–18mos, or 1 neg. EIA at ≥18mos) & no other lab evidence of infection & not had an AIDS-defining condition
4. HIV-uninfected: Child w/2 or more HIV PCR assays which are neg after 1mo of age & 1 assay negative after 4mos

1994 CDC PEDIATRIC HIV CLASSIFICATION2

Immunologic Categories	Clinical Categories (Level of Signs/Symptoms)			
	N: None	A: Mild	B: Moderate	C: Severe
1: No evidence of suppression	N1	A1	B1	C1
2: Evidence of moderate suppression	N2	A2	B2	C2
3: Severe suppression	N3	A3	B3	C3

Immunologic Categories (CD4 counts change with age)						
	Age of Child					
	<12mos		1–5yrs		6–12yrs	
Immunologic Category	CD4 L	(%)	CD4 L	(%)	CD4 L	(%)
1: No evidence of suppression	≥1,500	(≥25)	≥1,000	(≥25)	≥500	(≥25)
2: Evidence of moderate suppression	750–1,499	(15–24)	500–999	(15–24)	200–499	(15–24)
3: Severe suppression	<750	(<15)	<500	(<15)	<200	(<15)

WHO STAGING SYSTEM FOR HIV INFECTION & DISEASE IN CHILDREN

Clinical Stage I:
1. Asymptomatic
2. Generalized lymphadenopathy

Clinical Stage II:
3. Chronic diarrhea >30 days duration in absence of known etiology
4. Severe persistent or recurrent candidiasis outside of the neonatal period
5. Weight loss or failure to thrive in absence of known etiology

6. Persistent fever >30 days duration in absence of known etiology
7. Recurrent severe bacterial infections other than septicemia or meningitis, e.g., osteomyelitis, bacterial (non-TB pneumonia, abscesses)

Clinical Stage III:
8. AIDS-defining opportunistic infection
9. Severe failure to thrive in absence of known etiology
10. Progressive encephalopathy
11. Malignancy
12. Recurrent septicemia or meningitis

---

[1] From Pediatric AIDS, A. Pavia, Medical Mgmt of AIDS, 6th Ed., Eds. M.A. Sande, P.A. Volberding, W.B. Saunders & Co., 1999.

[2] 1994 revised classification system for HIV infection in children less than 13yrs of age *[MMWR 43(RR-12):1–10, 1994]*

TABLE 8D: INITIATION OF ANTIRETROVIRAL THERAPY, P. CARINII PROPHYLAXIS, &
SUPPORTIVE THERAPY *[MMWR 47(RR-8):1, 2002. http://aidsinfo.nih.gov/guidelines]*

A. P. carinii Prophylaxis—1999 Revised Guidelines

1. In infants with perinatally acquired HIV, PCP occurs most frequently at 3–6mos, often acute in onset with poor prognosis. HIV+ infants <1yr of age at risk even with CD4 ≥1500.
   - Identify infants born to HIV+ mothers promptly (screen mothers during pregnancy), obtain PCR or viral culture at birth, 2–8wks, & 2–4mos.
   - Begin PCP prophylaxis at 4–6wks of age in all infants born to HIV-infected mothers.
   - Stop prophylaxis in children found to be HIV-negative (e.g., 2 negative PCRs obtained after 1mo of age)
   - Continued PCP prophylaxis in HIV-infected children depends on immunologic stage *(see previous page)*. Recommended for all children Immunologic Category 3. If CD4 not available, use for WHO Clinical Stages II & III. Some would give to all HIV+ children in resource-poor country.
2. Drug Regimens for PCP Prophylaxis in Children ≥4wks of age
   - **TMP/SMX (150mg TMP/M² /day)** po divided twice daily 3x/wk on consecutive days (i.e., Mon., Tues., Wed.) Alternatives: same daily dose 1x/day, divided q12h 7 days/wk or q12h on alternate days. Once-daily regimen may be best for adherence.
   - If TMP/SMX not tolerated:
     - **Dapsone 2mg/kg po 1x/day** (not to exceed 100mg) or 4mg/kg po q wk
     - **Aerosolized pentamidine (children ≥5yrs) 300mg** via Respirgard II inhaler monthly
     - **Atovaquone 30mg/kg po q24h** for children 1–3mos old. Atovaquone 45mg/kg po q24h for children 4–24mos.
     - **IV pentamidine 4mg/kg q2 or 4wks** when other options are not available

B. Antiviral Therapy

1. **When to start:** This decision is much more complex in children than in adults. Data specific to outcomes in children are limited, & clinical trial data do not adequately define when to start. Natural history studies in children & extrapolation from adult studies are used to derive guidelines. Some factors argue for **early** treatment in children:
   - 25–35% of HIV-infected children will be rapid progressors
   - Viral load & CD4 are associated with rapid progression but cannot accurately identify all rapid progressors in first year of life
   - Immune control of virus limited in first year of life
   - HIV encephalopathy, other neurological disease & cardiac involvement may occur at young age
   - Some trials of early therapy have shown promising results

   Some factors favor **delayed** institution of therapy.
   - Slow progressors may maintain good immune function for many years without treatment
   - Limited number of drugs with liquid formulation
   - Highly variable & inadequately understood pharmacokinetics of ARVs in children may lead to inadequate levels & drug failure
   - Metabolic complications, including abnormal lipids, glucose intolerance, fat redistribution & possibly bone mineral abnormalities can occur in children
   - Children may have excellent immune reconstitution even with advanced disease
   - Difficulties with adherence are common & lead to drug failure
   - Children may rapidly run out of treatment options

   Three sets of guidelines have been developed. They share several features. In infants who are known to be HIV-infected, they favor starting therapy at an early stage & consideration of treating all infants, due to the inability to identify rapid progressors. In older children, the guidelines favor treatment when the child reaches a more advanced disease stage. All emphasize the need for education to ensure adherence, & routine monitoring for efficacy & safety:

RECOMMENDATIONS FOR BEGINNING TREATMENT IN INFANTS & CHILDREN

	DHHS	PENTA	WHO
Infants	<1yr with CDC Category A, B, or C disease or CD4 <25% **(Recommended)**	<1yr with CDC Category B or C disease or CD4% < 25-35% **(Recommended)**	<18mos, virologically confirmed infection with WHO Pediatric Stage III **(Recommended)**
	All infants regardless of symptoms or CD4 % **(Consider)**	Younger than 1yr regardless of symptoms or CD4 % **(Consider)**	<18mos, virologically confirmed infection with WHO Pediatric Stage II (consider using CD4 <20%) **(Recommended)**
			<18mos, virologically confirmed infection with WHO Pediatric Stage I & CD4 <20% **(Recommended)**
			<18mos, HIV seropositive but virologic confirmation not available, WHO Pediatric Stage II & CD4 <20% **(Recommended)**
Children	CDC Category C disease **or** CD4 <15% **(Recommended)**	CDC Category C disease **or** CD4 <20% if 1-3 or <15% if >4 **(Recommended)**	WHO Pediatric Stage III disease **or** CD4 <15% **(Recommended)**
	CDC Category A or B disease **or** CD4 15–25% or viral load >5 log **(Consider)**	CDC Category B disease **or** CD4 <20% or viral load >5.3 log **(Consider)**	WHO Pediatric Stage II disease **(Recommended)**. Consider using CD4 <15% as a criterion

DHHS = Department of Health & Human Services (U.S.) Working Group (**www.aidsinfo.nih.gov**)
PENTA = Paediatric European Network for the Treatment of AIDS 2003 (www.pentatrials.com)
WHO = World Health Organization: Scaling up antiretroviral therapy in resource-limited settings (Draft: 2003 revision http://www.who.int/3by5/publications/documents/arv_guidelines/en/

2. **Recommended therapy**
   Combination therapy with at least 3 antiretroviral drugs is recommended for all children started on therapy. Choice of drugs depends on supporting data, age of the patient, local availability, & need for liquid formulation. WHO guidelines emphasize initial use of NNRTI-based regimens because of costs, local availability, & to

TABLE 8D (2)

complement adult guidelines. U.S. & European guidelines recommend either PI-based or NNRTI-based initial regimens, but recognize the risk of NNRTI-resistant virus being transmitted from mother to child *(see below)*.

If available, resistance testing should be considered for children before starting HAART, especially if an NNRTI is being considered. If the local prevalence of resistance is known, it may influence the need for resistance testing.

RECOMMENDED FIRST-LINE THERAPY FOR HIV-INFECTED INFANTS & CHILDREN

	DHHS	PENTA	WHO
Strongly recommended	2 NRTIs[1] **plus** lopinavir/ ritonavir or nelfinavir **or** ritonavir or nevirapine (if <3yrs) If >3yrs: 2 NRTIs[1] **plus** efavirenz	2 NRTIs[2] **plus** one PI (lopinavir/ritonavir **or** nelfinavir) 2 NRTIs **plus** 1 NNRTI (efavirenz **or** nevirapine)	If <3yrs **or** <10 kg: (ZDV or d4T) **plus** 3TC **plus** nevirapine If >3yrs **or** >10 kg: (ZDV or d4T) **plus** 3TC **plus** efavirenz
Alternative regimens	ZDV **plus** 3TC **plus** abacavir If >4yrs: 2 NRTIs **plus** amprenavir	2 NRTIs[2] **plus** abacavir	
Insufficient data to recommend	Dual or boosted PIs, with the exception of lopinavir/ ritonavir NRTI **plus** NNRTI **plus** PI **Tenofovir-containing regimens** Enfuvirtide (T-20)-containing regimens Emtricitabine (FTC)-containing regimens Atazanavir-containing regimens Fosamprenavir-containing regimens Tipranavir-containing regimens		

[1] DHHS strongly recommended NRTI combinations: ZDV + 3TC; d4T + 3TC; ZDV + ddI
  DHHS alternative NRTI combinations: ZDV + ABC; d4T + ABC; ddI + 3TC
[2] PENTA acceptable NRTI combinations: ZDV + ddI; ZDV + 3TC; ZDV + ABC; 3TC + ABC; ddI + 3TC
AVOID: monotherapy, d4T + ZDV, use of ddC. **Delay d4T + ddI unless if used with tenofovir.** d4T + ddI is effective **but** associated with a higher rate of side effects including lactic acidosis & lipoatrophy.

3. **Monitoring of children on antiretroviral therapy**
   Children on antiretroviral therapy should be followed at regular intervals, usually every 3mos.
   Clinical parameters:
   - Weight & height growth
   - Nutritional status
   - Developmental milestones & neurological symptoms
   - Adherence & side effects
   Laboratory monitoring should include: CBC with differential, CD4 % & count. If available, viral load, liver enzymes, creatinine, glucose, electrolytes, & total cholesterol should be obtained.

4. **Therapeutic drug monitoring**
   Age-related changes in drug metabolism & wide interpatient variability of drug levels along with generally low success rates suggest that therapeutic drug monitoring might be very useful for PIs & NNRTIs. In some European countries, therapeutic drug monitoring has become routine. However, there are no widely accepted consensus guidelines, limited data on target drug concentrations, & adherence & timing may influence the results. Information on laboratories & on laboratory participation in quality assurance programs is available at www.hivpharmacology.com.

5. **When to change antiretroviral therapy**
   Deciding on when to change therapy can be a complex process that takes into account the remaining options, the level of adherence, the social situation & the clinical status. The goal of initial therapy is to suppress viral load to the lowest level possible, usually below the limit of quantification, & to allow the immune system to reconstitute. Ongoing viral replication permits the selection of resistant mutants, & will lead to increasing drug resistance. When initial therapy "fails," good treatment options are usually available. With subsequent treatment regimens, the number of remaining options becomes progressively limited.
   Many children & adults with multiply drug-resistant virus will develop breakthrough viremia but still have stable or rising CD4 counts. Often the viral load remains significantly below the pretreatment baseline. In this situation, many experts weigh the option of continuing the current therapy as long as clinical & immune status are stable against the option of creating a new regimen that might exhaust remaining regimens. Clinical trial data are not available to address this decision. The decision will depend on remaining options, clinical status, family preference, & family situation.
   Considerations on when to change are divided into virologic, immunologic, & clinical. These are not absolute. Clinical changes, however, are the clearest & most non-controversial indications for change of therapy:

Virologic considerations	• Less than a minimally acceptable virologic response after 8–12wks of therapy (defined as a <10-fold (1.0 log₁₀) decrease from baseline HIV RNA levels
	• HIV RNA not suppressed to undetectable levels after 4–6mos of antiretroviral therapy
	• Repeated detection of HIV RNA in children who initially had undetectable levels in response to antiretroviral therapy. Consider observation if rebound is to low level (<5000 copies)
	• A reproducible ↑ in HIV RNA copy number among children who have had a substantial HIV RNA response but still have low levels of detectable HIV RNA. Such an ↑ would warrant change in therapy if, after achieving a virologic nadir, a >3-fold (>0.5 log₁₀) ↑

TABLE 8D (3)

	in copy number for children aged >2yrs & >5-fold (>0.7 log₁₀) ↑ is observed for children aged <2yrs
Immunologic considerations	• Change in immunologic classification. For children with CD4 of <15% (i.e., those in immune category 3), a persistent ↓ of 5 percentiles or more in CD4 % (e.g., from 15% to 10%) • A rapid & substantial ↓ in absolute CD4 count (e.g., >30% ↓ in <6mos) • Return of CD4 % to pre-therapy baseline, in absence of concurrent infection* • >50 fall from peak level of CD4 % on therapy, in absence of concurrent infection*
Clinical considerations	• Progressive neurodevelopmental deterioration* • Growth failure defined as persistent decline in weight-growth velocity despite adequate nutritional support & without other explanation* • Disease progression defined as changing from one clinical category to another (e.g., from clinical category A to clinical category B) • New opportunistic infection or malignancy* • Recurrence of prior opportunistic infections that had been well controlled*
Toxicity	• It may be desirable to control some side effects (e.g., diarrhea) rather than changing therapy. If a single drug can be associated with the toxicity, it is acceptable to change the offending agent

* Criteria marked with asterisk are from WHO guidelines (& may overlap with DHHS recommendations). These may be particularly helpful in the resource-limited setting.

6. **What to use as alternate therapy**
   There are limited data on sequencing antiviral therapy in HIV-infected children. Several general principles are useful:
   a. When treatment failure occurs, always assess adherence to the treatment
   b. Try to address adherence problems before changing regimens
   c. If adherence has been good, assume viral resistance has developed, but it may not have developed to all agents. Viral resistance testing, if available, should be considered. If possible, obtain viral resistance testing while on failing regimen. Without testing, all 3 drugs should be changed if possible.
   d. Take into account potential cross-resistance
   e. Avoid dose reduction for toxicity unless levels can be measured
   f. Treatment failure may occur due to inadequate absorption or drug levels
   g. **Never add a single drug to a regimen that is clearly failing**

First-Line Regimen	Suggested Options
ZDV + 3TC	ABC + ddI ABC + tenofovir Some would consider ZDV + (3TC or emtricitabine) + tenofovir
d4T + 3TC	ABC + ddI ABC + tenofovir Some would consider ZDV + 3TC + tenofovir
NNRTI	Protease inhibitor: • Lopinavir/ritonavir • Nelfinavir **Consider:** • **Amprenavir + ritonavir (fosamprenavir if >40kg)** • Atazanavir with or without ritonavir • Saquinavir/ritonavir
Nelfinavir	NNRTI or boosted PI • Lopinavir/ritonavir • Amprenavir + ritonavir (fosamprenavir if >40 kg) • Atazanavir + ritonavir • Saquinavir/ritonavir
Ritonavir	NNRTI or boosted PI • Lopinavir/ritonavir • **Amprenavir + ritonavir (fosamprenavir if >40 kg)** • Atazanavir + ritonavir • Saquinavir/ritonavir
Lopinavir/ritonavir	NNRTI Consider tipranavir

Enfuvirtide (T-20) can be used in children as part of a salvage regimen, but works best with 1 or 2 additional active drugs.

C. Supportive Treatment & Prophylaxis
1. Intravenous gamma globulin (IVIG)
   a. Not routinely used. Recommended for infants & children with evidence of humoral immune defects (hypogammaglobulinemia or significant recurrent infections despite antimicrobial therapy. IVIG 400mg/kg q28 days is recommended.
   b. Thrombocytopenia (<20,000/mm³) on antiretroviral therapy: IVIG 0.5–1gm/kg/dose x3–5 days *(See Table 22 for Winrho®)*
2. Immunization: *See Table 19*
3. Pneumocystis carinii: *See above, Section A*
4. Mycobacterium avium complex: prophylaxis recommended *[MMWR 46(RR-12), 1997]*. Begin if CD4 <50 for children ≥6yrs; for children 2–6yrs, begin if CD4 <75; for 1–2yrs if CD4 <500; <1yr CD4 <750. Clarithromycin 7.5mg/kg po q12h or azithromycin 20mg/kg po once weekly is preferred. Rifabutin now used as 3ʳᵈ-line, 5mg/kg po once daily (only for children ≥6yrs). Dose of rifabutin should not exceed 300mg/day.
5. Psychosocial support *(see Am Acad Pediatrics, Red Book, 1994)*: School attendance, child/foster care, adolescent education

TABLE 9E: CLINICAL SYNDROMES, OPPORTUNISTIC INFECTIONS, IN INFANTS & CHILDREN, WHICH DIFFER FROM ADULTS*

In HIV-infected infants & children, disease progression is manifest by decrements in growth & delayed neurodevelopment as well as opportunistic infections as occur in adults (*J Ped 128:58, 1996*)

CLINICAL SYNDROME	INFANT/CHILD	ADULT	CLINICAL FEATURES (in children)/COMMENTS
Central Nervous System			
Encephalopathy			General: HIV encephalopathy is a syndrome that includes motor & cognitive dysfunction seen in pts with advanced HIV. Administration of zidovudine has been shown to be beneficial in treating children with HIV encephalopathy. ZDV can effectively reverse & improve neurologic symptoms. Similar or greater results observed with HAART (*JID 174:1200, 1996*)
Static course	Common	0	25% children show cognitive & motor deficits. Most have head circumference in 10-25th percentile. Problems with verbal expression, attention deficits, hyperactivity. Mild ↑ reflexes in legs to spastic diplegia, IQ stable.
Plateau course	Uncommon	0	Infant's or child's gain of cognitive or motor skills plateaus. Motor deficits are common. IQ usually only 50-79.
Subacute progressive course	Uncommon	AIDS dementia common	Gradual progressive decline in motor, language, adaptive function. Early, child is alert, wide-eyed, with a paucity of facial movements. Endstage: mute, dull-eyed, quadriparetic. CSF: mild pleocytosis, ↑ protein, may be + for HIV antibody & virus. CT: atrophy, progressive calcification in basal ganglia (most common in infants & young children).
Focal brain diseases: seizures, focal neurologic deficits			
Infections			
Toxoplasmosis	V. rare	Common	Toxo is uncommon in infants & children since it is most often due to reactivation.
Progressive multifocal leuko-encephalopathy (JC virus)	V. rare	Common	PML is uncommon in infants & children since it is most often due to reactivation.
Endocrine			
Failure to thrive & growth retardation	Common	Wasting syndrome common	33/36 HIV+ children showed failure to thrive, not purely related to diarrhea & malnutrition. Known causes of growth failure are growth hormone deficiency, hypothyroidism, & glucocorticoid excess. 1/3 of HIV+ children have abnormal thyroid function (↑ thyrotropin, ↑ TBG) which correlates with disease progression (*J Ped 128:70, 1996*)
Eye			
Cytomegalovirus retinitis	Uncommon	Common	CMV chorioretinitis in 1.6% children vs 10-20% in adults (*Arch Ophthl 107:978, 1989*). In children it usually occurs with generalized CMV infection, viremia & multiple organ involvement. When present, ocular lesions are same as in adults, *Table 11, p98*.
Retinal depigmentation, on ZDV	~5%	0	Asymptomatic peripheral retinal depigmentation (dosages ≥300 mg/M²/day)
HIV-associated "cotton wool" spots	Rare	Common	Seen only in children >8–10yrs, while seen in 60-70% of adults.
Gastrointestinal Tract			
Mouth			
Kaposi's sarcoma	V. rare	Common	21 cases have been reported. Clinical spectrum similar to adults.
Esophagus	Uncommon	Common	When pain/difficulty occur, children more likely to refuse to eat. CMV—odynophagia. Candida—dysphagia.
Dysphagia, odynophagia			
Diarrhea	Common	Common	Most common agents: rotavirus 24% (more common in inpatient setting), salmonella (19%), campylobacter (8%) (more common in outpatients). Presence of blood &/or WBC in stool has high positive predictive value for salmonella or campylobacter (*PIDJ 15:876, 1996*).
Heart			
Cardiomyopathy	Common	Common	Abnormal ECG changes (ventricular hypertrophy & non-specific ST-T changes) in 55-93% HIV+ children.
	Common	Uncommon	Left ventricular dysfunction 29-74% (most important cardiac change). 20% transient of chronic congestive failure. Unexpected cardiorespiratory arrests in 8/81 (*JAMA 269:2869, 1993*). Pericardial effusions & tamponade have been noted frequently in children (*PIDJ 15:819, 1996*).

TABLE 8E (2)

CLINICAL SYNDROME	INFANT/CHILD	ADULT	CLINICAL FEATURES (in children)/COMMENTS
Hematologic			
Hypergammaglobulinemia	Common	Uncommon	By age 6mos, almost all HIV+ children have ↑ gamma-globulins.
Protein S (coagulation inhibitor)	Common	Common	19/26 children had ↓ levels, but risk of thrombosis low *(Ped IDJ 15:106, 1996)*. Adults, ↑ protein S in 27–73%, thrombotic complications in 12%.
Hepatobiliary	Rare	Common	Very few reports relating to children. Etiologies such as AIDS cholangiopathy, peliosis hepatis (bacillary angiomatosis) not reported. 2 cases of fatal hepatic necrosis associated with adenovirus reported *(Rev Inf Dis 12:303, 1990)*.
Lung			
Tuberculosis	Uncommon	Common	Virtually all are primary infections. Clinical: fever, cough. X-ray: often focal infiltrates with hilar adenopathy, cavitation uncommon.
Lymphocytic interstitial pneumonitis (LIP)	Common	V. rare	LIP occurs in 40% of children with perinatally acquired HIV & EBV antigens have been demonstrated in lung tissue. Usually diagnosed in children > 1yr as compared with PCP which is most common in first year. LIP has better prognosis than PCP. Median survival is ~5x shorter in children diagnosed with PCP than in children with LIP *(Lancet 348:866, 1996)*. Clinical: slowly progressive tachypnea, cough, wheezing, hypoxemia. Rales are infrequent. Clubbing of digits is characteristic. Generalized lymphadenopathy, hepatosplenomegaly & parotid swelling. X-ray: diffuse reticulonodular infiltrates associated with hilar lymphadenopathy. Bacterial superinfection is common. Diagnosis by lung biopsy. Rx: steroids may be of some benefit.
Cryptococcosis	Uncommon		Disseminated infection or localized process of the lungs. Intermittent fever is most common presenting manifestation. All pts have low CD4, history of previous OIs, & onset of cryptococcosis most commonly in 2nd decade of life *(PIDJ 15:796, 1996)*.
Congestive heart failure	Common	Uncommon	See Heart, above.
Leiomyosarcoma	Rare (but ↑)	V. rare	EBV demonstrated by PCR in tumors *(NEJM 332:12, 1995)*.
Renal			
Nephropathy	Common	Rare	Nephropathy observed in 29% children with perinatal AIDS *(Kidney 31:1167, 1987)*. In children may present with nephrotic syndrome with a course of 12–18mos *(NEJM 321:625, 1989)*. Steroid rx may be of value.
"Sepsis"	Common	Uncommon	25% of symptomatic HIV+ children will have bacteremic episodes, most due to bacteremic pneumonia or bacteremia without a focus *(Pediatric AIDS, Eds: P.A. Pizzo, C.M. Wilfert, Ch. 13, pg 199, 1991)*.
Fungemia (a nosocomially-acquired infection)	Common	Uncommon	Risk factors: central venous catheter (>90 days), prior antibiotic therapy (>3 different antibiotics, parenteral ↑ risk), parenteral hyperalimentation, hemodialysis, prolonged neutropenia, colonization by Candida species *(CID 23:515, 1996)*.
Skin			
Impetigo	Common	Uncommon	Due to Staph. aureus or Group A strep. Clinical: areas of erythema with "honey crusting." May be widespread & evolve into "cellulitis." Increasing incidence of MRSA skin & soft tissue infections

TABLE 8F: SELECTED DRUGS COMMONLY USED IN CHILDREN WITH HIV INFECTION

INDICATION/DRUG	DOSAGE	FORMULATIONS	COMMENTS
Antifungal Drugs			
Amphotericin B	0.5-1mg/kg/day IV (same as adult, see Table 12, pg117-124)	Same as adult	
Ampho B lipid complex	5mg/kg/day IV as for adults		
Fluconazole		Oral suspension (orange-flavored), 50mg/5ml (teaspoon)	
Oral/esophageal candidiasis	6-12mg/kg/day		
Systemic candidiasis	12mg/kg/day po		
Cryptococcal meningitis			
Treatment	12mg/kg po 1st day, then 6 (to 12) mg/kg/day po		
Suppression	6mg/kg/day po		
Itraconazole	3mg/kg po q24h (capsules) 5mg/kg po q24h (suspension)	Oral suspension 10mg/ml	Efficacy & safety not established. Bioavailability of capsules is low & variable. Administer suspension on empty stomach with 4-6oz of Coca-Cola.
Caspofungin	75mg/M² IV q24h loading dose then 50mg/M² IV q24h	Same as adult	
Anti-HIV Drugs[1]			
Nucleoside analogue reverse transcriptase inhibitors (NRTIs)			
Abacavir (Ziagen)	8mg/kg 2x/daily not to exceed 300mg Neonatal dose unknown	Solution 20mg/ml 300mg tablets Fixed combination 600mg with 300mg lamivudine (Epzicom) Fixed combination 300mg with 300mg zidovudine & 150mg lamivudine (Trizivir)	Hypersensitivity reaction in ~5%, may be difficult to recognize. Rechallenge may be fatal.
Didanosine (ddI, Videx)	90mg/M² q12h not to exceed 200mg per dose. Body weight 40-60kg: Videx EC 250mg once daily Body weight >60kg: Videx EC 400mg once daily Videx EC 240mg/M² appropriate in small PK study (Antivir Ther 7:267, 2002) Neonatal dose (<90days): 50mg/M² q12h	Pediatric powder (when reconstituted with antacid): 10mg/ml Delayed-release capsules (enteric-coated beadlets): Videx EC 125, 200, 250, 400mg Generic delayed-release capsules 200, 250, 400mg Chewable buffered tablets: 25, 50, 100, 150, 200mg Buffered powder for oral solution: 100, 167, 250mg	Dose on empty stomach. Reduce didanosine dose if combined with tenofovir. Do not administer with ribavirin
Emtricitabine (Emtriva)	6mg/kg 1x/day up to 33kg Neonatal use not recommended Adolescent/adult dose 200mg 1x/day	Solution 10 mg/mL Tablet 200 mg Fixed combination 200 mg with 300 mg tenofovir (Truvada)	24-wk data on emtricitabine & efavirenz once daily showed good response in children (11ᵗʰ CROI, 2004, Abst 936). Efavirenz AUC slightly ↓ than target. Emtricitabine, stavudine, & lopinavir/ritonavir was well tolerated & very effective in 82 children (Intl AIDS Conf, 2004, Abst Tu PeB 4431).

Pediatric Equivalent (column for Itraconazole):
3mg/kg
6mg/kg
12mg/kg (not to exceed 600mg/day)

Adult Dose (column for Itraconazole):
100mg
200mg
400mg

[1] Adolescents ≥ Tanner 4 should be dosed according to adult dosing (see Table 6B)

TABLE 8F (2)

INDICATION/DRUG	DOSAGE	FORMULATIONS	COMMENTS
Anti-HIV Drugs[2] *(continued)*			
Lamivudine (3TC, Epivir)	4mg/kg 2x/day Adolescent/adult dose (weight >50kg) 150mg 2x/day or 300mg once daily Neonatal dose (<30 days): 2mg/kg 2x/day	Solution 10mg/ml Tablets 100mg, 150, 300mg **Fixed combination 150mg with 300mg ZDV (Combivir)** Fixed combination 150mg with 300mg ZDV, 300mg abacavir (Trizivir) Fixed combination 300mg with 600mg Abacavir (Epzicom)	
Stavudine (d4T, Zerit)	Body weight <30kg: 1mg/kg 2x/day 30–60kg: 30mg 2x/day, >60kg: 40mg 2x/day Neonatal dose birth to 13 days 0.01mg/kg 2x/day 0.01mg/kg q8h	Solution 1mg/ml Capsules 15, 20, 30, 40mg	Better tolerated than zidovudine but more strongly associated with lipoatrophy. Combination with ddI associated with increased risk of lactic acidosis
Zalcitabine (ddC, Hivid)	Neonatal dose unknown	Syrup 0.1mg/ml Tablets 0.375, 0.75mg	Rarely used
Zidovudine (ZDV, AZT, Retrovir)	160mg/M[2] q8h or 180–240mg/M[2] q12h Adolescent/adult dose 300mg 2x/day Neonatal dose (age <6wks) 2mg/ kg po q6h; 1.5mg/kg IV q6h. Premature infant 1.5mg/kg IV or 2mg/kg po q12h. Increase to q 8h at 2wks (>30wks EGA or at 4wks <30wks EGA)	Syrup 10mg/ml Capsules 100mg Tablets 300mg Generic syrup 10mg/ml, & tablets 300mg 10mg/ml IV Fixed combination 300mg with 150mg 3TC (Combivir) Fixed combination 300mg with 150mg 3TC, 300mg abacavir (Trizivir)	
Nucleotide reverse transcriptase inhibitor (NRTI)			
Tenofovir (Vread)	Pediatric dose currently under study, not yet approved. 8mg/kg once daily for children age 2–8 Phase III study uses 175mg/M[2] target dose. Neonatal dose unknown. Adult dose 300mg 1x/day	Tablets 300mg Tablets 75mg (investigational) tablets dissolve in water, orange or grape juice Powder formulation under development Fixed combination 300mg with 200mg emtricitabine (Truvada)	↓ bone mineral density observed in young animals. ↓ BMD was prevalent in HIV-infected children before treatment; small ↓ in BMD in 5/15 at 1yr in 1 study Pediatrics 116:e846(,2005). No change compared to controls at 1yr in another (JAIDS 40:448, 2005). Use with caution & decrease dose if any renal impairment. Decrease ddI dose if used with tenofovir
Non-nucleoside reverse transcriptase inhibitors (NNRTIs)			
Delavirdine (Rescriptor)	Pediatric dose not established Neonatal dose unknown Adolescent/adult dose 600mg 2x/day or 400mg 3x/day.	Tablets 100, 200mg	Not approved for children

[2] Adolescents ≥ Tanner 4 should be dosed according to adult dosing (see Table 6B)

TABLE 8F (3)

INDICATION/DRUG	DOSAGE	FORMULATIONS	COMMENTS
Anti-HIV Drugs[3] / Non-nucleoside reverse transcriptase inhibitors (NNRTIs) (continued)			
Efavirenz (Sustiva)	**10–15kg, 200mg; 15–20kg, 250mg; 20–25kg, 300mg; 25–32.5kg, 350mg; 32.5–40kg, 400mg; >40kg, 600mg—all 1x/day** Neonatal dose unknown/not approved for infants Adult dose 600mg 1x/day	Capsules 50, 100, 200mg Tablets 600mg Liquid preparation used in PACTG 382 (contact BMS to check on availability)	Give at night to reduce CNS side-effects. Capsules can be opened & added to food or liquid but contents have peppery taste. Lowers concentration of unboosted PIs. Pregnancy Class D. Avoid if possibility of pregnancy.
Nevirapine (Viramune)	<8yrs of age, 7mg/kg 2x/day or 200mg/M[2] >8yrs of age, 4mg/kg 2x/day or 120mg/M[2] **Note:** Initiate dosing once daily x14d; if no rash, ↑ to 2x/day Neonatal dose 5mg/kg or 120mg/M[2] 1x/day x14d, then 120mg/M[2] 2x/day x14d, then 200mg/M[2] 2x/day Adolescent/adult dose 200mg 1x/day x14d then 200mg 2x/day	Suspension 10mg/ml Tablets 200mg	Do not dose-escalate in presence of rash. If rash is associated with fever, oral lesions, conjunctivitis, blistering, or hepatitis, stop medication immediately. Severe cholestatic hepatitis & Stevens-Johnson syndrome are rare but life-threatening complications that may occur in the 1st 6wks. In adults, risk of severe toxicity increased in women with CD4 > 250 & men with CD4 > 400
Protease Inhibitors			
Amprenavir (Agenerase)	Age 4–12yrs or 13–16yrs & weight <50kg: Oral solution 22.5mg/kg 2x/day (max. daily dose 2,800mg). Capsules: 20mg/kg 2x/day (max. daily dose 2,400mg). Adolescent/adult capsule dose 1200mg 2x/day or 600mg/100 mg ritonavir 2x/day Neonatal use not recommended	Oral solution 15mg/ml (contains 550mg/mL propylene glycol & 46 IU Vit E/mL)	Liquid formulation contains propylene glycol & is contraindicated for children <4yrs of age because of high exposure. Boosting with ritonavir not studied in children but may be considered if weight >50kg.
Atazanavir (Reyataz)	Pediatric dosing under study. Preliminary data from PACTG 1020a suggest boosting with ritonavir is necessary in children. Neonatal use not recommended Adolescent/adult dose 400mg 1x/day or 300mg + 100mg ritonavir both 1x/day	Capsules 100, 150, 200mg	Preliminary data suggest wide variability in levels in children with unboosted atazanavir & ↑ clearance compared to adults. Ritonavir-boosted atazanavir may give more consistent levels. Avoid in infants due to ↑ bilirubin. Do not co-administer with proton pump inhibitors. Boost with ritonavir if co-administered with tenofovir or efavirenz.

[3] Adolescents ≥ Tanner 4 should be dosed according to adult dosing (see *Table 6B*)

TABLE 8F (4)

INDICATION/DRUG	DOSAGE	FORMULATIONS	COMMENTS
Anti-HIV Drugs*/Protease Inhibitors *(continued)*			

Fosamprenavir (Lexiva)	Pediatric dosing under study (20mg/kg 2x/day)
	Neonatal use not recommended
	Adolescent/adult dose:
	Antiretroviral naïve:
	  1400 mg 2x/day
	  700 mg + 100 mg ritonavir 2x/day
	  1400 mg + 200 mg ritonavir 2x/day
	Antiretroviral experienced: 700mg + 100mg ritonavir 2x/day
		Tablet 700mg (equivalent to 600mg amprenavir)	Administer with or without food

Indinavir (Crixivan)	500mg/M² q8h Adolescent/adult dose 800mg q8h Experimental dosing: indinavir 500mg/M² + ritonavir 100mg/M² both q12h (AIDS 14; 2209, 2000)	Capsules 200, 333, 400mg	Response associated with C$_{min}$ (AAC 44:1029, 2000). Consider measuring C$_{min}$ if available & adjusting dose.
Lopinavir/ritonavir (Kaletra)	230mg/M² lopinavir/57.5mg/M² ritonavir 2x/day with food if not taking nevirapine, efavirenz or amprenavir or weight based dosing: 7–15kg: 12mg/kg lopinavir; 15–40kg: 10mg/kg lopinavir 300mg/M² lopinavir/75mg/M² ritonavir with nevirapine, efavirenz or amprenavir or weight-based dosing: 7–15kg: 13mg/kg; 15–50kg: 11mg/kg Neonatal dose investigational 300mg/M² 2x/day Adolescent/adult dose 400mg lopinavir/100mg ritonavir 2x/day	**Pediatric solution 80mg lopinavir/20mg ritonavir per ml.** Capsules 133.3mg lopinavir/33.3mg ritonavir Tablets 200mg lopinavir/50 mg ritonavir	Dose must be when used with efavirenz or nevirapine, up to 533mg lopinavir/133mg ritonavir. New tablet formulation has decreased diarrhea. For adolescents/adults who are treatment naive, tablets can be dosed as 400mg/100mg once daily Higher doses (eg 300mg/M² or 600mg/140mg 2x/day should be considered in treatment experienced patients with PI resistance mutations
Nelfinavir (Viracept)	45–55mg/kg q12h (8th CROI, 2001, Abst. 255). Approved dose of 30mg/kg q8h may lead to inadequate levels. Neonatal dose 40mg/kg q12h was inadequate. 50–60mg/kg under investigation Adolescent/adult dose 1250mg q12h	Powder for oral suspension 50mg/level scoop Tablets 250, 625mg	Large variability in levels. Crushed or dissolved tablets more reliably absorbed. Consider measuring C$_{min}$ if available & adjusting dose. Maintaining Trough > 0.8mcg/mL associated with improved response in one study. Take with meal to ↑ absorption.
Ritonavir (Norvir)	350–400mg/M² 2x/day Neonatal dose under study Adolescent/adult dose 600mg 2x/day	Solution 80mg/ml Capsules 100mg	Dose should be escalated over 1–7 days to ↓ side effects. Use lower dose as pharmacokinetic enhancer. Solution is unpleasant tasting.

⁴ Adolescents ≥ Tanner 4 should be dosed according to adult dosing *(see Table 6B)*

TABLE 8F (5)

INDICATION/DRUG	DOSAGE	FORMULATIONS	COMMENTS
Anti-HIV Drugs[5]/Protease Inhibitors *(continued)*			
Saquinavir (Invirase) Note: Soft-gel capsules no longer available.	Under study: 50mg/kg (softgel) or 33mg/kg q8h with ritonavir Adolescent/adult dose softgel capsules: 1200mg 3x/day or 1600mg 2x/day Hard or softgel: 1000mg + 100mg ritonavir 2x/day	Hard-gel capsules 200 mg Film-coated tablets 500 mg	Saquinavir levels difficult to maintain in target range when used alone, but better with nelfinavir (PIDJ 21:712, 2002; Clin Pharm Ther 71:122, 2002). Consider measuring C_{min} if available and adjusting dose. (C_{min} >100mg/ml associated with response). Hard gel caps & tablets cause less diarrhea but should only be used with ritonavir.
Tipranavir (Aptivus)	Not approved in children. Clinical trials underway but insufficient data so far to recommend dose Adolescent/Adult dose: 500mg with 200mg ritonavir 2x/day	Capsule 250 mg	Administer with food. Active against many virus strains with extensive PI resistance, & used only in patients with extensive prior experience. Most effective when given with entuviritide. Induces metabolism of other PIs & should not be co-administered with them
Fusion Inhibitor			
Enfuvirtide (Fuzeon)	6–16yrs 2mg/kg 2x/day, maximum dose 90mg (1ml) injected subcutaneously <6yrs not approved Adolescent/adult dose 90mg (1 ml) 2x/day injected subcutaneously	Injection: lyophilized powder for injection 108mg of enfuvirtide, when reconstituted with 1.1ml sterile water to deliver 90mg/ml	Most effective when started with 1–2 new drugs to which virus is sensitive. Must be reconstituted & used within 24hrs. Inject in upper arm, abdomen, anterior thigh—rotate site. Common injection site reactions include tender itchy nodules.
Antimycobacterial Drugs			
M. tuberculosis			
Ethambutol	15–25mg/kg/day po	No pediatric formulation	Not approved in children <13 yrs but can be given. Monitor for closely for visual change
Isoniazid	Neonates: 10mg/kg po q24h Infants/Children: 10–20mg/kg po q24h (maximum 300mg/day).	50 mg/5 ml syrup	Can give IM
Pyrazinamide	20–40mg/kg po q24h as 1 or more doses (maximum 2gm/day)	No pediatric formulation	
Rifampin	10–20mg/kg po q24h (maximum 600mg/day)	No pediatric formulation. Ad hoc solution can be made by pharmacy	Can give po or IV. Do not use with protease inhibitors. Reduced dose rifabutin can be substituted
Streptomycin	10–20mg IM q12h (max. 1gm/day)		
MAC—Mycobacterium avium-intracellulare complex			
Azithromycin	5mg/kg/day for treatment 20mg/kg once weekly, not to exceed 1200mg,	Oral suspension 100 or 200mg/5 ml	
Clarithromycin	15mg/kg/day divided q12h (not to exceed 500mg po q12h)	Granules for oral suspension (125 or 250mg/5 ml) [DO NOT refrigerate suspension]	

[5] Adolescents ≥ Tanner 4 should be dosed according to adult dosing (see Table 6B)

TABLE 8F (6)

INDICATION/DRUG	DOSAGE	FORMULATIONS	COMMENTS
Antimycobacterial Drugs/MAC—Mycobacterium avium-intracellulare complex (continued)			
Clofazimine	1–2mg/kg/day po to max. of 100mg/day	No pediatric formulation	
OR			
Rifabutin	10–20 mg/kg/day po (max 300mg/day)	No pediatric formulation	↓ dose with protease inhibitors, inc with NNRTI's
Antiparasitic Drugs			
P. carinii			
Prophylaxis (See Table 8D—after 4wks of age)			
TMP/SMX	150mg/M² TMP component po divided q12h on 3 consecutive days (M, T, W) each week. Abbreviated schedules: Table 8D	Oral suspension (cherry or grape flavored), 40mg TMP/ 200mg SMX/5 ml (teaspoon)	Breakthrough episodes of PCP: TMP/ SMX 3%, dapsone 15% or higher, aerosol pentamidine 15%, IV pentamidine 25% (J Ped 122:163, 1993)
OR			
Dapsone	2mg/kg/day po (not to exceed 100mg)	No pediatric formulation	
OR			
Aerosolized pentamidine—only if ≥5 yrs old	300mg with Respirgard II inhaler 1x monthly		Used as young as 8 mos (PIDJ 12:958, 1991)
Treatment			
Atovaquone suspension	30–40mg/kg po q24h. Dosing interval not established	Not FDA-approved for pediatric use	Efficacy in children not established. CNS levels <1%
Pentamidine isethionate	4mg/kg/day IV or IM ×12–14days		Start with IV in all but mildest cases
OR			
TMP/SMX	Children >2mos 20mg TMP/100mg SMX/kg/day divided q6h po or IV in same dose q6–8h		
Antiviral Drugs—other than anti-HIV			
Cytomegalovirus			
Cidofovir	No studies in children.	IV solution only	Must follow guidelines for hydration & probenecid. Dose adjust for renal disease
Induction	5mg/kg once a week for two doses		
Maintenance	5mg/kg every 14 days		
Foscarnet		No pediatric formulation	No studies reported in children. Deposited in teeth & bone of growing animals. Dose adjust for renal disease.
Induction	180mg/kg/day divided q8h		
Maintenance	90–120mg/kg IV q24h	Adult capsule or IV solution	Has potential carcinogenicity
Ganciclovir			
Induction	5 mg/kg IV q12h		
Maintenance	5 mg/kg IV q24h		
Herpes simplex virus			
Acyclovir	250–500 mg/M² IV q8h. Infuse over 1 hr		
Varicella zoster (<2yrs old)		200mg/5ml oral suspension (banana flavored) available if appropriate	Daily urine output should be 1ml/1.3mg of acyclovir
Acyclovir	500 mg/M² IV q8h		

For additional data on drugs for pain &/or nutritional management, see www.aidsinfo.nih.gov/guidelines, Supplements to Pediatric Guidelines Nov. 2004.

TABLE 8G: PROPHYLAXIS FOR FIRST EPISODE OF OPPORTUNISTIC DISEASE IN HIV-INFECTED INFANTS & CHILDREN

PATHOGEN	INDICATION	PREVENTIVE REGIMENS*	
		FIRST CHOICE	ALTERNATIVES
Pneumocystis jiroveci	HIV-infected or HIV-indeterminate infants aged 1-12mos HIV-infected children aged 1-5yrs with CD4 count <500 or CD4 percent <15%	TMP/SMX 150/750 mg/M²/day in 2 div. doses po 3x/wk on consecutive days (A2). Acceptable alternative dosage schedules: (A2) Single dose po 3x/wk on consecutive days	Aerosolized pentamidine (children aged ≥5yrs) 300mg 1x monthly via Respirgard II nebulizer (C3); dapsone (children aged ≥1 mo.) 2mg/kg (max 100mg) po q24h (C3); Atovaquone 30mg/kg po q24h for 1-3mos old & >24mos old; 45mg/kg po q24h for 4-24mos old; IV pentamidine 4mg/kg every 2-4wks if other options are unavailable (C3)
	HIV-infected children aged 6-12yrs with CD4 <200 or CD4 percent <15%	2 div. doses po q24h; 2 div. doses po 3x/wk on alternate days	
Mycobacterium tuberculosis Isoniazid-sensitive	TST reaction ≥5mm OR prior positive TST result without treatment OR contact with case of active tuberculosis	Isoniazid 10-20mg/kg (max. 300mg) po q24h x9mos. (A1) OR 20-40mg/kg (max. 900mg) po 2x/wk x9mos. (B3)	Rifampin 10-20mg/kg (max. 600mg) po or IV q24h x12mos. (B2) (Rifampin duration of rx is 4-6mos. according to 1999 USPHS guidelines.)
Isoniazid-resistant	Same as above; high probability of exposure to isoniazid-resistant tuberculosis.	Rifampin 10-20mg/kg (max. 600mg) po or IV q24h x12mos. (B2)	Uncertain
Multidrug (isoniazid & rifampin)-resistant	Same as above; high probability of exposure to multidrug-resistant tuberculosis	Choice of drug requires consultation with public health authorities	None
Mycobacterium avium complex	For children aged ≥6yrs, CD4 <50; 2-6yrs, CD4 <75; 1-2yrs, CD4 <500; <1yr, CD4 <750	Clarithromycin 7.5mg/kg (max. 500mg) po q12h (A2) OR azithromycin 20mg/kg (max. 1200mg) po 1x/wk (A2)	Children aged ≥6yrs, rifabutin 300mg po q24h (B1); <6yrs, 5mg/kg po q24h when suspension becomes available (B1); azithromycin 5mg/kg (max. 250mg) po q24h (A2)
Varicella zoster virus	HIV-infected children who are asymptomatic & not immunosuppressed Significant exposure to varicella with no history of chickenpox, shingles, or varicella vaccine	Varicella zoster vaccine Varicella zoster immune globulin (VZIG), 1 vial (1.25 ml)/10kg (max. 5 vials) IM, administered ≤96hrs after exposure, ideally within 48hrs (A2)	None

* See Table 4A for HIV classification

TABLE 9: MANAGEMENT OF EXPOSURE TO HIV-1 & HEPATITIS B/C

OCCUPATIONAL EXPOSURE TO BLOOD, PENILE/VAGINAL SECRETIONS OR OTHER POTENTIALLY INFECTIOUS BODY FLUIDS OR TISSUES WITH RISK OF TRANSMISSION OF HEPATITIS B/C &/OR HIV-1 (E.G., NEEDLESTICK INJURY) [Adapted from *MMWR 50(RR-11):1, 2001; NEJM 348:826, 2003; & MMWR 54(RR-9), 2005* (available at www.aidsinfo.nih.gov).]

Free consultation for occupational exposures: call (PEPline) 1-888-448-4911.

General steps in management:
1. Wash clean wounds/flush mucous membranes immediately (use of caustic agents or squeezing the wound is discouraged; data lacking regarding antiseptics).
2. Assess risk by doing the following: (a) Characterize exposure; (b) Determine/evaluate source of exposure by medical history, risk behavior, & testing for hepatitis B/C & HIV; (c) Evaluate & test exposed individual for hepatitis B/C & HIV

Hepatitis B Exposure [Adapted from CDC recommendations, *MMWR 50(RR-11), 2001*]

Exposed Person	Exposure Source		
	HBs Ag+	**HBs Ag−**	**Status Unknown**
Unvaccinated	Give HBIG 0.06 mL per kg IM & initiate HB vaccine	Initiate HB vaccine	Initiate HB vaccine & if possible, check HBs Ag of source person
Vaccinated (antibody status unknown)	Do anti-HBs on exposed person: If titer ≥10 milli-International units per mL, no rx If titer <10 milli-International units per mL, give HBIG + 1 dose HB vaccine*	No rx necessary	Do anti-HBs on exposed person: If titer ≥10 milli-International units per mL, no rx If titer <10 milli-International units per mL, give 1 dose of HB vaccine (plus 1 dose HBIG if source high risk)*

For known HB vaccine series responder (titer ≥10 milli-International units per mL), no rx. For known HB vaccine series non-responder (<10 milli-International units per mL,) to 1° series HB vaccine & exposed to either HBsAg+ source or suspected high-risk source—rx with HBIG & re-initiate vaccine series or give 2 doses HBIG 1 month apart. For non-responders after a 2nd vaccine series, 2 doses HBIG 1 month apart is preferred approach to new exposure [*MMWR 40(RR-13):21, 2001*].
* Follow-up to assess/address vaccine response.

Hepatitis C Exposure

Determine antibody to hepatitis C for both exposed person &, if possible, exposure source. If source +, follow-up HCV testing advised. **No recommended prophylaxis**; immune serum globulin not effective. Monitor for early infection, as therapy may ↓ risk of progression to chronic hepatitis. See Table 12 & discussion in *Clin. Micro Rev 16:546, 2003. Case-control study suggested risk factors for occupational HCV transmission include percutaneous exposure to needle in artery or vein, deep injury, male sex of HCW, & was more likely when source VL >6 log10 copies/mL (CID 41: 1423, 2005).*

HIV: Occupational exposure management *(adapted from MMWR 54(RR-9), 2005 (available at www.aidsinfo.nih.gov))*
- The decision to initiate post-exposure prophylaxis (PEP) for HIV is a clinical judgment that should be made in concert with the exposed healthcare worker (HCW). It is based on:
  1. Likelihood of the source patient having HIV infection: ↑ with history of high-risk activity—injection drug use, sexual activity with multiple partners (either hetero- or homosexual), receipt of blood products 1978–1985, ↑ with clinical signs suggestive of advanced HIV (unexplained wasting, night sweats, thrush, seborrheic dermatitis, etc.). Remember: the vast majority of persons are **not** infected with HIV (1/200 women infected in larger U.S. cities) & likelihood of infection is low if not in above risk groups.
  2. Type of exposure (approx. 1 in 300–400 needlesticks from infected source will transmit HIV).
  3. Limited data regarding efficacy of PEP (PEP with ZDV alone reduced transmission by >80% in 1 retrospective case-controlled study—*NEJM 337:1485, 1997*).
  4. Significant adverse effects of PEP drugs & potential for drug interactions.
- Substances considered potentially infectious include: blood, tissues, semen, vaginal secretions, CSF, synovial, pleural, peritoneal, pericardial, & amniotic fluids; & other visibly bloody fluids. Fluids that are normally considered low-risk for transmission, unless they are visibly bloody, include: urine, vomitus, stool, sweat, saliva, nasal secretions, tears & sputum (*MMWR 54(RR-9), 2005*)

TABLE 9 (2)

- If source person is **known positive for HIV** or **likely to be infected** & **status of exposure warrants PEP**, antiretroviral drugs should be started **immediately** (ASAP or within hours). If source person is HIV antibody negative, drugs can be stopped **unless source is suspected of having acute HIV infection**. The HCW should be re-tested at **3–4wks, 3 & 6mos whether PEP is used or not** (the vast majority of seroconversions will occur by 3mos; delayed conversions after 6mos are exceedingly rare). Advise HCW to take precautions to avoid secondary transmission during this period of monitoring following exposure to known or suspected HIV+ source. Tests for HIV RNA should not be used for dx of HIV infection because of false-positives (esp. at low titers) & these tests are only approved for established HIV infection [a possible exception is if pt develops signs of acute HIV (mononucleosis-like) syndrome within the 1st 4–6wks of exposure when antibody tests might still be negative].
- PEP for HIV is usually given for **4wks** & monitoring of adverse effects recommended: baseline **complete blood count, renal & hepatic panel** to be **repeated at 2wks** 50–75% of HCW on PEP demonstrate mild side-effects (nausea, diarrhea, myalgias, headache, etc.) but in up to _ severe enough to discontinue PEP (Antivir Ther 3:195, 2000). Consultation with infectious disease/ HIV specialist valuable when questions regarding PEP arise. **Seek expert help in special situations, such as pregnancy, renal impairment, treatment-experienced source.** [For latest CDC recommendations, see MMWR 54(RR-9), 2005 (available at www.aidsinfo.nih.gov)]

3 Steps to HIV Post-Exposure Prophylaxis (PEP) After Occupational Exposure:

Step 1: Determine the exposure code (EC)

Is source material blood, bloody fluid, semen/vaginal fluid or other normally sterile fluid or tissue (see above)?

What type of exposure occurred?

→ Yes
→ Intact skin
No PEP*

→ Percutaneous exposure
Severity

Mucous membrane or skin integrity compromised (e.g., dermatitis, open wound)
Volume

Small: Few drops
→ EC 1

Large: Major splash &/or long duration
→ EC2

Less severe: Solid needle, scratch
→ EC2

More severe: Large-bore hollow needle, deep puncture, visible blood, needle used in blood vessel of source
→ EC3

→ No
No PEP

* Exceptions can be considered when there has been prolonged, high-volume contact

Step 2: Determine the HIV Status Code (HIV SC) for Exposure Source

What is the HIV status of the exposure source?

HIV negative
No PEP

HIV positive

Low titer exposure: asymptomatic & high CD4 count, low VL (<1500 copies per mL)
HIV SC 1

High titer exposure: advanced AIDS, primary HIV, high viral load or low CD4 count
HIV SC 2

Status unknown
HIV SC unknown

Source unknown
HIV SC unknown

TABLE 9 (3)

Step 3: Determine Post-Exposure Prophylaxis (PEP) Recommendation

EC	HIV SC	PEP
1	1	Consider basic regimen[1,a]
2	1	Recommend basic regimen[1,a,b]
2	1	Recommend basic regimen[1,b]
3	2	Recommend expanded regimen[1,c]
1,2,3	1 or 2	Recommend expanded regimen[1]
1, 2, 3	Unknown	If exposure setting suggests risks of HIV exposure, consider basic regimen[1,c]

[a] Based on estimates of ↓ risk of infection after mucous membrane exposure in occupational setting compared with needlestick.

Modification of CDC recommendations:

[b] Or, consider expanded regimen[1].

[c] In high risk circumstances, consider expanded regimen[1] on case-by-case basis.

Around the clock, urgent expert consultation available from:
National Clinicians' Post-Exposure Prophylaxis Hotline
(PEPline) at 1-888-448-4911 (1-888-HIV-4911)

[1] Regimens: (Treat for 4 weeks; monitor for drug side-effects every 2 weeks)
Basic regimen: ZDV + 3TC or FTC + **TDF; or as alternative d4T + 3TC**
Expanded regimen: Basic regimen + one of the following: lopinavir/ritonavir, or as alternative atazanavir (or atazanavir/ritonavir), fosamprenavir/ritonavir, nelfinavir indinavir/ritonavir, saquinavir/ritonavir, efavirenz; can be considered (except in pregnancy or potential for pregnancy—**Pregnancy Category D**), but CNS symptoms might be problematic; [**Do not use nevirapine**; serious adverse reactions including hepatic necrosis reported in healthcare workers (*MMWR* 49:1153, 2001).]

Other regimens can be designed. If possible, use 2 antiretroviral drugs that source pt (if known) is not currently taking or for which resistance is unlikely based on susceptibility data or treatment history. Seek expert consultation if ARV-experienced source or in pregnancy or potential for pregnancy.

NOTE: Some authorities feel that an expanded regimen should be employed whenever PEP is indicated (*NEJM* 349:1091, 2003; *Eur J Epidemiol* 19:577, 2004, & *NY State AIDS Institute, 2004, the latter with ZDV+3TC+TDF*)

http://www.hivguidelines.org/public_html/center/clinical-guidelines/pep_guidelines/pep_guidelines.htm [accessed March 2006]). Expanded regimens are likely to be advantageous with ↑ numbers of ART-experienced source pts or when there is doubt about exact number of exposures in decision algorithm. Mathematical model suggests that under some conditions, completion of full course basic regimen is better than prematurely discontinued expanded regimen (*CID* 39:395, 2004). However, while expanded PEP regimens have ↑ adverse effects, there is not necessarily ↑ discontinuation (*CID* 40:205, 2005).

POST-EXPOSURE PROPHYLAXIS FOR NON-OCCUPATIONAL EXPOSURES TO HIV *From MMWR 54(RR-2):1, 2005—DHHS recommendations*

Because the risk of transmission of HIV via sexual contact or sharing needles by injection drug users may reach or exceed that of occupational needlestick exposure, it is reasonable to consider PEP in persons who have had a non-occupational exposure to blood or other potentially infected fluids (e.g., genital/rectal secretions, breast milk) from an HIV+ source. Risk of HIV acquisition per exposure varies with the act. (for needle sharing & receptive anal intercourse, ≥0.5%; approximately 10-fold lower with insertive vaginal or anal intercourse, 0.05–0.07%). Overt or occult traumatic lesions may ↑ risk in survivors of sexual assault.

For pts at risk of HIV acquisition through non-occupational exposure to HIV+ source material having occurred ≤72 hours before evaluation. DHHS recommendation is to treat for 28 days with an antiretroviral **expanded regimen**, using preferred regimens [efavirenz (*not in pregnancy or pregnancy risk—**Pregnancy Category D**)* + (3TC or FTC)] + (ZDV or TDF)] **or** [lopinavir/ritonavir + (3TC or FTC) + ZDV] or one of several alternative regimens [*see Table 6A section B & MMWR 54(RR-2):1, 2005*].

Areas of uncertainty: (1) expanded regimens are not proven to be superior to 2-drug regimens, (2) while PEP not recommended for exposures >72hrs before evaluation, it may possibly be effective in some cases, (3) when HIV status of source patient is unknown, decision to treat & regimen selection must be individualized based on assessment of specific circumstances.

Evaluate for exposures to Hep B, Hep C (see *Occupational PEP above*), & bacterial sexually-transmitted diseases [*see Sanford Guide to Antimicrobial Therapy Table 15A, & MMWR 51(RR-6):1, 2002*] & treat as indicated.

TABLE 10: PRIMARY PROPHYLACTIC ANTIMICROBIAL AGENTS AGAINST OPPORTUNISTIC PATHOGENS IN ADOLESCENTS & ADULTS

Prevention of First Episode of Disease (for 2ⁿᵈ, see Table 12). [For 2004 USPHS/IDSA Guidelines for Prevention of OIs in HIV, see *Figure 1*.]

Lowest CD4 Count	Pathogen	Primary	Preventive Regimens Alternative	Comments
All patients regardless of CD4 level See also *Table 12, pg109* [**See AnIM 137(Suppl.5), part 2), 2002]**	**Mycobacterium tuberculosis:** TST¹ ≥5 mm or prior untreated pos. TST or contact with case of active TB	[**INH** 5mg/kg/day po, maximum 300mg po q24h x9mos.] or [**INH** 900mg po q24h + **pyridoxine** 100mg po x9mos.]	**RIF**** 600mg po q24h or **RFB**** 300mg po q24h x4 mos.²	*See Table 11, pg88. No longer called "prophylaxis", but now termed treatment of latent infection with M. tuberculosis (LTBI) (AJRCCM 161:S221, 2000). Recent study suggests 2 mos. rx with RIF + PZA as effective as 12mos. of INH in HIV+ pts (JAMA 283: 1445, 2000).* **However, there are recent reports of severe & fatal hepatitis in pts on RIF + PZA** *(MMWR 50:289, 2001). Therefore, this regimen is no longer recommended for LTBI (MMWR 52:735, 2003).*
	As above but with high probability of exposure to INH-resistant TB	**RIF**** 600mg po q24h or **RFB**** 300mg po q24h x4mos.		
	Exposure to multi-drug resistant TB	Consultation recommended		
CD4 <200/mm³ REF: *CID 40* (Suppl.3), 2005	**Pneumocystis jiroveci (formerly carinii)** (see *Table 11, pg91*) DC prophylaxis when CD4 count **>200 for >12 wks in response to HAART** *(MMWR 51(RR-8):4, 2002)*. Restart if CD4 drops <200/mm³.	**Trimethoprim/ sulfamethoxazole–DS** (160 TMP) (TMP/SMX-DS) one tab po q24h OR **-SS** one tab po q24h.	**Aerosolized pentamidine** 300mg q month via Respirgard II nebulizer (if toxo pos, see below) OR [**Dapsone** 100mg po q24h + **pyrimethamine** 50mg po qwk + **leucovorin** 25mg po qwk (also effective for toxo prophylaxis)] OR [**Dapsone** 200mg po + pyrimethamine 75mg po + leucovorin 25mg po], all 1x/week] OR [Dapsone 50mg po q12h or 100mg po q24h] OR [TMP/SMX-DS 3x/wk po] OR [Atovaquone suspension 1500mg po q24h]	*TMP/SMX superior to other rx in actual practice (incidence of failure 3,000/100 person yrs) vs dapsone or inhaled pentamidine or atovaquone (0.001/100 person yrs) & odds ratio for failure 4.5, 5.8 & 6.7, respectively vs TMP/ SMX (J AIDS & HR 19:182, 1998). Atovaquone = pentamidine but had 1 rx-limiting adverse events (JID 180:369, 1999).*
CD4 <100/mm³ REF: *CID 40* (Suppl.3), 2005	**Toxoplasma gondii** (in pts with + IgG toxo, antibody/titer). DC primary prophylaxis in toxo Ab+ pts with CD4 >200 for >12wks in response to HAART.	**TMP/SMX-DS** one po q24h.	**Dapsone** 50mg po q24h + **pyrimethamine** 50mg po q week + **leucovorin** (folinic acid) 25mg po week	*Another option: Atovaquone 750mg po q6–12h + pyrimethamine 25mg q24h + leucovorin 10mg po q24h*

TABLE 10 (2)

Lowest CD4 Count	Pathogen	Preventive Regimens Primary	Preventive Regimens Alternative	Comments
CD4 <50/mm³	**Mycobacterium avium-intracellulare**[2] *(see Table 11, pg94).* **DC prophylaxis when CD4 count >100 sustained for 3 mos. in response to HAART** [*NEJM 342:1085, 2000; AnlM 133:493, 2000; MMWR 51(RR-8):10, 2002; CID 41:549, 2005].* Restart if CD4 drops <50-100/mm³	**Clarithromycin** 500 mg po q12h or **azithromycin** 1200 mg po weekly (both assoc. with emergence of resistant respiratory flora (*HIV Clin Trials 2:453, 2001*).	Rifabutin 300 mg po q24h[†] OR (**azithromycin** 1200 mg po weekly + **rifabutin** 300 mg po q24h)	*See Table 12, pg111.* Rifabutin reduced cryptosporidium-associated diarrhea (*AIDS 14:2889, 2000*). Single daily dose of 500 mg of clarithro better than rifabutin but no direct comparison available between std. q12h dosage (*AIDS 13:1367, 1999*).
	Cytomegalovirus *(See Table 12, pg128-130)* Authors feel it is reasonable to observe pts closely, rx active CMV infection. Preemptive rx of pts with CMV viremia without evidence of organ involvement generally not recommended. **May safely dc chronic suppression when CD4 count >100-150 for ≥6mos.** [*MMWR 51(RR-8):19, 2002*]. Restart if CD4 drops ≤100-150/mm³	Chronic suppression: **Valganciclovir** 900 mg po q24h *(see Comment)*	Oral **ganciclovir** 1gm po q8h	*See Table 12, pg128, primary prophylaxis:* Prophylaxis decision should include risk group: gay males 35% vs IVDA 4.7% risk of CMV during life. If plasma PCR for CMV pos., 43% risk of disease (↓ to 26% on oral ganciclovir); if PCR neg., 14% (↓ to 1% on oral ganciclovir). Therefore, some use prophylaxis in gay males when PCR pos.
	Candida species, cryptococcus Not routinely recommended prior to 1st fungal infection [*MMWR 51(RR-8):15, 2002*]	100-200mg **fluconazole** po q24h[4] **(see Comment)**	200mg **fluconazole** po once weekly; 200mg 3x/wk **Itraconazole** 200mg po q24h was effective in Thailand (*CID 34:277, 2002*)	Study of fluconazole 200 mg 3x/wk: 18% candida, 0.4% cryptococcal meningitis (*AnIM 126: 689, 1998*). Reduced incidence of histo & crypto vs placebo (p = 0.0007) but had **no effect** on mucosal candidiasis or survival (*CID 28:1049, 1999*). Did show survival benefit in 1 small study (90 pts) in Thailand (*HIV Med 5:140, 2004*).

---

[1] TST = tuberculin skin test (Mantoux); [2] Interaction with protease inhibitors to be considered; *see Table 12, pg109;* [3] Authors think it reasonable to observe pts closely, rx strongly suspected or active MAC, then institute chronic suppression *(see Table 12, pg111);* [4] Fluconazole 200 mg po q24h ↓ crypto infection from 8% to 1% (*NEJM 332:700, 1995*). Undetermined whether 100 mg q24h effective.

** See Table 12, pg109, for options regarding concurrent use of protease inhibitors & RIF or RFB.

TABLE 11A:¹ DIAGNOSIS & DIFFERENTIAL DIAGNOSIS OF CLINICAL SYNDROMES, OPPORTUNISTIC INFECTIONS & NEOPLASMS (For Treatment, see Table 12)

CLINICAL SYNDROME, ETIOLOGY, EPIDEMIOLOGY	CLINICAL PRESENTATION, DIAGNOSTIC TESTS, COURSE			

Acute retroviral (HIV) syndrome (symptomatic primary HIV infection): (see *CID 36:1447, 2004*)

Differential diagnosis includes: EBV mononucleosis, CMV mononucleosis, toxoplasmosis, rubella, viral hepatitis, syphilis, primary HSV, drug reactions

Up to __% of new infections in U.S. may now occur in adolescents *(Pediatrics 112(6):e323, 2003)*. **This infection is often mononucleosis suspected but serologic tests for mono are negative.** Accounted for 0.66%, 0.5% & 0.16% of pts presenting with fever, rash & pharangitis respectively to outpatient settings in US *(Ann Fam Med 3:400,2005)* but diagnosis only made on 1ˢᵗ visit in 17% *(Arch Intern Med 163:2097,2003)*. Mono-like syndrome also found along with dermatitis & generalized lymphadenopathy in African children infected during breastfeeding *(AIDS 16:2303, 2002)*. 4.5% of Malawi men in STD clinic had acute HIV infection; inguinal adenopathy & genital ulcers common*(AIDS 18;517,2004)*

NOTE: During acute retroviral syndrome, **individuals have very high plasma & genital secretion viral titers & are highly infectious from sexual activity & needle sticks.** Mathematical models predict that 25–60% of all HIV infections may be transmitted during the period of acute infection *(AIDS 18:1311, 2004)*.

Depending on frequency of coitus, 7–24% of partners would be expected to become infected over 2 months of acute HIV *(JID 189:1785, 2004; J Micro Imm Inf 37:271, 2004)*.

Drug-resistant virus now commonly isolated in acute retroviral syndrome *(JAMA 288:239, 2002; J Acquir Defic Syndr 38:545,2005)* although some areas report declining rates of resistant virus *(AIDS 18:1571,2004)* & some mutations (M184V) may transmit less effectively *(JAIDS 35:17,627, 2004)* Genotyping recommended in areas of resistance to ARV.

Massive depletion of CD4 memory T cells apparently occurs within days to weeks of HIV infection *(Nat Med 11:469, 2005)*.

Central Nervous System [Excellent references: *CID 29:19, 1999; J Neurovirol 8:158, 2002; J Neurovirol 9:, for European guidelines; Dx & management of neuro complications of HIV, see Eur J Neurol 11:297, 2004*] HAART produced 95% ↓ CNS AIDS-defining events *(Neurol 54:1866, 2000)*, but other CNS conditions may be increasing (immune reconstitution leukoencephalitis, chronic "burnout" VZV encephalitis, toxoplasmosis or PML)) *(J Neuropath Exp Neurol 62:429, 2003)*. In Mexico, up to 50% of AIDS-defining diagnoses involved CNS: 1/3 toxo & 1/5 crypto meningitis, 1/10 TBc, 1/10 HIVD *(Arch Med Res 31:393, 2004)*; toxo 14.8, & CMV encephalitis 7/100 person yrs *(Eur J Neurol 11:755, 2004)*. Neuroabnormalities still preHAART in South Africa *(J Neurovirol 11 s-1;17,2005)*

Symptoms: Occur in 50-90%, others have asymptomatic seroconversion. Time from exposure to sx usually 2-6wks.

Symptoms	Frequency (%)		Symptoms	Frequency (%)
Fever	>95		Headache	33
Adenopathy	75		Hepatosplenomegaly	15
Pharyngitis	75		Neuropathy	6
Maculopapular rash	70		Oral/genital ulcers	<5
Myalgias/arthralgias	50		Esophageal ulcers	<5
N, V, or diarrhea	30–60		Palpable purpura	<5
			Conjunctivitis	<5

	Lab Abnormalities	Frequency (%)
	↑ ALT, AST	50
	↓ platelets	45
	↓ lymphs (CD4)	35
	Atypical lymphs (↑↑ CD8)	35

Up to 50% have neurological manifestations from severe headache to signs of meningitis or encephalitis. Those with acute neurologic syndromes had higher CSF viral loads (4.12 vs 5.58 log₁₀ copies/ml) than those without neurologic symptoms *(CID 30:962, 2000)*. ↑ severity of symptoms associated with ↑ viral titers *(CID 34:E14, 2002)*.

Laboratory: thrombocytopenia 45%, lymphopenia, (neutropenia reported) & may be severe, ↓ CD4, ↑ CD8, often atypical lymphs,) ↑ hepatic enzymes 21% *(Eur J Intern Med 16:120,2005)* followed by lymphocytosis (↓ CD4, ↑ CD8, often atypical lymphs,) ↑ hepatic enzymes 21% *(JID 168:1490, 1993)*, pancreatitis reported *(South Med J 97:393,2004)*

Viral burden—high-level HIV viremia (10⁴-10⁷ copies/ml plasma), high p24 antigen (89% sensitive, 100% specific; *AnM 134:25, 2001)*, standard HIV antibody tests usually neg, **false-positive viral RNA in low titers reported.** (1.9–3.0% false-positive. *South Med J 93:1004, 2000)*

Course/Prognosis: symptoms usually resolve in 1–2wks & rarely up to 10wks. The occurrence of the acute retroviral syndrome, a short incubation period to symptoms (fever, fatigue, myalgias), & duration of illness >14 days correlate with more rapid progression to AIDS *(J AIDS 32:542, 2003)*. See Table 6. Effective anti-HIV CTL activity assoc. with ↑ rate of viral clearance & lower setpoint which is assoc. with ↓ rate of progression to AIDS *(JID 189:1144, 1793, 2004)*. Early rx with HAART during acute HIV was similar to VL in never-rx pts *(P Los 1:e36, 2004)*. 12 mos. after dc of HAART in a study from France, VL 12 mos. after dc of HAART was similar to VL in never-rx pts *(P Los 1:e36, 2004; AIDS Read 15:250,2005)*

Treatment remains controversial *(AIDS 18;709,2004, AIDS Read 15:250,2005)*

See pg102 for abbreviations & footnotes

TABLE 11A (2)

CLINICAL SYNDROME, ETIOLOGY, EPIDEMIOLOGY	CLINICAL PRESENTATION, DIAGNOSTIC TESTS, COURSE

Cognitive Disorders, Diffuse Brain Dysfunction

Declining mental acuity with preservation of alertness

HIV-1 associated dementia (HAD or HIVD), also known as **AIDS dementia complex (ADC)**, multinucleated giant cell encephalitis, or HIV-1-associated cognitive/motor complex. Frequency:1/3 of adults; 1/2 children with AIDS. ↑ in older pts (*J Clin Epid 54:S35, 2001; J Neurovirol 9:205, 2003*).

Stage 0: normal
Stage 1: mild, can work
Stage 2: moderate but cannot work
Stage 3: severe, cannot work, major intellectual disability
Stage 4: vegetative **(in AIDS dementia complex, a "vegetative" patient can be aroused to a level of alertness. This is an important distinction between AIDS dementia complex & many other potential etiologies.)**

HIVD may not have declined as dramatically as other CNS OIs [4.4% of initial AIDS-defining illness before HAART, but 6.5% during HAART era (*J AIDS 31:171, 2002; AIDS 16:1925, 2002*)].

Pathogenesis: (*J Neurovirol 9:222, 2003; Rev Immunol 5:69, 2005, Virus Res 111:194,2005*)
HIV appears to produce infection of brain macrophages/microglia (but not neurons or macroglia). HIV infects brain macrophages directly via CCR5 β-chemokine receptor [pts heterozygous for the CCR5 Δ32 mutation are less likely to develop HIVD than those without Δ32-4.1% vs 14.5% (*JID 180:854, 1999*)]. ↑ frequency of apoptotic & HIV-infected astrocytes assoc. with ↑ severity of HIVD (*AIDS16:1709, 2002; J Leuk Biol 71:65, 2002*). β-chemokines (MIP-1α, MIP-1β &

RANTES) themselves are ↓ in HIVD, likely indicating ongoing macrophage activation. MIP-1 was detected in CSF in 20/23 children. 18 had abnormal neurological status (*PIDJ 23:114, 2004*). These cells (monocytes /macrophages) may be newly recruited/trafficked into the CNS late in disease accounting for the demonstrated benefit from HAART (*J. Neurovirol 6:570, 2000*). CD8 T cells found in CSF express adhesion molecules & chemokine receptors which appear to play an important role in trafficking through the blood-brain barrier & to inflammatory sites (*JID 189:200*; *2004*)

The final pathway by which the cells destroy neurons is not known, but HIV-infected brain macrophages do not respond to 2° stimulation with release of neurotoxic substances (glutamate-like neurotoxins, free radicals, arachidonic acid, L-cysteine, or so-called virotoxins (*JID 186:S193, 2002*). The toxins overstimulate N-methyl-D-aspartate (NMDA) receptors, resulting in ↑ levels of neuronal calcium ion (similar to injury in stroke, trauma) (*J AIDS 31:543, 2002*).

These pts usually present with **impaired short-term memory, ↓ concentration, clumsiness, slowness, apathy, irritability, & personality changes** (*J Neurol 249:1132, 2002; Med Clin No Amer 86:537, 2002*).

Process is slowly progressive, weeks to months (usually occurs after AIDS defining diagnosis) **& CD4 count usually <200/mm³** [median 70/mm³ before HAART era, 170/ mm³ during HAART era (*AIDS 13:1249, 1999*)].

Degree of intellectual impairment & stage of ADC correlates with CSF HIV RNA (*Semin Neuro 19:223, 1999*). Higher levels of HIV RNA in CSF predict progression of neuropsychological impairment (*ArNeurol 59:923, 2002*) & postmortem evidence of HIV encephalitis (*Neurol 59:1563, 2002*).

Neuro exam: non-focal

Early		Late
Cognition	inattention	Global dementia
	↓ concentration	
	Forgetfulness, slowing of	
	thought processing	
Motor	Slowed movements	Paraplegia
	Clumsiness	
	Ataxia	
Behavior	Apathy	Mutism
	Blunting of personality	

CSF: Normal 30–50%, WBC (monos) 5–10% [CSF abnormalities: pleocytosis, protein or immunoglobulin levels reported in 30% asymptomatic HIV+ individuals (*JID 158:193, 1988*)]

MRI scan: Early is typically normal. **Cerebral atrophy, occ. with diffuse fluff ("spilled milk"), edema of antral white matter & basal ganglia, best seen on T-2 weighted imaging.** No mass effect. Normal gadolinium rules out most cases of primary brain lymphoma & toxo but does not rule out other infections (neurosyphilis, cryptococcal meningitis, MAC encephalitis). See *AIDS 12:233, 1998.*

See pg102 for abbreviations & footnotes

TABLE 11A (3)

CLINICAL SYNDROME, ETIOLOGY, EPIDEMIOLOGY	CLINICAL PRESENTATION, DIAGNOSTIC TESTS, COURSE
Cognitive Disorders, Diffuse Brain Dysfunction/ Declining Mental Acuity *(continued)*	
The **tat gene product** has been found to be excitatory & toxic to neurons in vitro & has been detected in brain tissue of pts with HIV (*J Neurovirol 6:145, 2000*). Toxic to adults activates astrocytes to trigger neuronal cell apoptosis, likely through endonuclease G (*J Neurovirol 10:141, 2004*) but also ↑ chemokine expression; mediators of inflammation (*J Neurovirol 10:86, 2004*). The **Vpr gene product** may also directly damage neuronal cells by forming ion channels &/or apoptosis by caspase-8 activity of both natural neurons & neuro precursor cells (*J Virol 74:9717, 2000; DNA Cell Biol 23:227, 2004*). **gp120**, a coat protein, appears to enhance glutamate-induced neurotoxicity by inducing apoptosis, possibly showing CXCR4 also appears to attach to neuroprogenitor cells via the same chemokine receptor & inhibit activation & proliferation of neuroprogenitor cells in vitro & hippocampal slices. CSF from demented but not non-demented pts shows similar impaired progenitor cell proliferation assoc. with ↑ VL in CSF (*JID 190:211, 2004*). Also gp120 when injected into the lateral ventricles of rat brains activates caspase-3 on neuro cells directly leading to apoptosis (*Neurotox Res 5:609, 2004*). Both gp120 & tat can induce oxidative stress leading to disruption of the blood brain barrier in vitro (*Brain Res. 1045:57, 2005*). CSF **TNF-α levels** also ↑ with ↑ severity of HAD (*Neuro 60:1388, 2003*). Levels of TNF may also be related to apoptosis; an apoptotic effect which appears to be blocked by insulin-like growth factor 1 receptor (IGF-1R) (*Viro 305:66, 2003*). TNF related apoptosis inducing ligand (TRAIL), may also play a role (*Cell Mol Immunol. 2:113, 2005*). A unique human protein, FL21909, secreted by HIV-infected macrophages, also induces apoptosis via activation of caspases 9 & 3 (*J Immunol 170:1566, 2003*). The exact mechanism by which activated macrophages kill neuronal cells remains an interesting but unknown mystery (*J Neurochem 86:1057, 2003; Mol Immunol 42:213, 2005*). Interestingly, HIV-infected macrophages are themselves protected from apoptosis, perhaps contributing to a long-lived HIV viral reservoir (*Neuropathol Appl Neurobiol 30:478, 2004*). TNFalpha was also expressed in human brain in microglia/macrophages & neurons from 2 patients with a rapidly progressive form of ADC (*J Neurol Neurosurg Psych 76:960, 2005*). Virus isolated from brain tissue from HIVD appears to express unique neurotropic genotypic/phenotypic features (*Viro 20:279, 2001*) & develop discordant drug resistance patterns from those in plasma isolates (*J Virol 79:1772, 2005*). Interestingly, minocycline reduced the severity of SIV encephalitis in 5 monkeys (*JAMA 293:2003,2005*).	Pts receiving highly active antiretroviral therapy (HAART) have fewer cognitive abnormalities than untreated pts (*AIDS Res Hum Retroviruses 18:485, 2002*), & when impaired may show marked improvement with ↑ HAART (*AIDS 15:493, 2001*). Symptoms of acute meningoencephalitis may reflect failure of HAART with ↑ CSF HIV viral load & respond to change in HAART (*CID 37:1107, 2003*). Survival in HAD pts has dramatically improved: 11.9mos to 48.2mos (*AIDS 17: 1539, 2003*). Symptoms of subacute encephalitis may reflect HAART failure showing on HAART (*J AIDS 23:380, 2000*). Presence of HIV encephalopathy on HAART correlated with delayed viral decay in CSF but not plasma. Effect not associated with drug resistance or poor CSF drug penetration (*AIDS 17:1897, 2003*). Improvement in neuropsychological testing correlated with ↓ in CSF HIV-1 RNA after initiation of HAART (*Neuro 60:1388, 2003*). Levels of HIV-RNA in CSF may fall slowly with HAART; 9/25 still had >50 HIV-RNA copies/ml after 2 mos of indinavir-containing regimen; all were <50 at 6 mos (*AIDS 17:1167, 2003*). Progressive HIV encephalopathy responded to HAART in a cohort of 126 children (*J Pediatr 146:402,2005*) & another with 146 (*Arch Pediatr Adol Med 159:651,2005*) A particularly severe form of demyelinating leukoencephalopathy has been described in HAART pts (*AIDS 16:1019, 2002; Brain Pathol 13:195, 2003*). While the impact of HAART on AIDS-associated dementia appears from most studies to be beneficial, as HIV-infected persons live longer the eventual outcome is not yet clear (*Brain Pathol 13:104, 2003*). In 2004, worrisome reports appeared of an ↑ prevalence of "mild" HIV-associated cognitive impairment in the Hawaii (*Histopath 45:549, 2004; Nat Rev Immunol 5:69, 2005; Ar Neurol 61:1687, 2004*). Presence of Diabetes was an independent predictor of dementia in the Hawaii Ageing with HIV Cohort OR 5.43 (*JAIDS 38:31, 2005*).
Progressive multifocal leukoencephalopathy (PML) in early-stage disease [see pg61]	Dementia is rare, occurs only late.
An underdiagnosed & undertreated manifestation of HIV infection that effects quality of life & response to HAART especially in women (*J. Neurovirol 11:138,2005*) & orphans in Africa (Soc.Sci Med 61:555, 2005)	Depression among the most common neuropsychiatric disorders in HIV-infected individuals 57.3% of 726 HIV-infected persons & may slow improvement of neurocognitive function response to HAART(*HIV Med 7:112, 2006*). Non-adherence to HAART correlates with ↑ severity of depression (*Psychosomatics 45:394, 2004*) & depression itself may impact response to HAART (*Psychoson Med 67:1013, 2006*). Treating depression can improve response to HAART on both individuals & populations (*J Acquir Immune Defic Syndr. 39:537, 2005*). HAART may not reverse psychosocial problems & depression (*AIDS Reader 14:514, 2004*) & may itself cause depression (*CID 41:1648, 2005*). Psychotropic therapy can also significantly improve quality of life (*CNS Spectr 8:59, 2003*). DHEA effective vs placebo in 145 pts over 8 weeks with nonmajor depression (*Am J Psych 163:59, 2006*).
Depression	

See pg102 for abbreviations & footnotes

TABLE 11A (4)

CLINICAL SYNDROME, ETIOLOGY, EPIDEMIOLOGY	CLINICAL PRESENTATION, DIAGNOSTIC TESTS, COURSE
Central Nervous System, Cognitive Disorders *(continued)*	
Declining mental acuity with concomitant depression of alertness (without focal findings)	Depression of alertness occurs only in advanced disease.
AIDS dementia complex/ADC) *(as above, Stage 3 or 4)*	**Late stage**
Cryptococcal disease (see Meningitis, *pg62; Eye, pg99*).	Often assoc. with ↑ CSF pressure
Toxoplasmic encephalitis	Usually focal findings
Progressive multifocal leukoencephalopathy (PML) *(see pg61)*	**Pts usually alert in early stages of disease; can become depressed later**
Primary CNS lymphoma *(see pg60)*	Rare when focal findings, occurs when deep structures in brain involved
Cytomegalovirus (CMV) encephalitis (CD4 <50/mm³) Frequency not well defined. Overall CMV ~20%, clinical encephalitis occurs in 1% of CMV cases, but probably much higher: 16% of brains in 1 autopsy series had CMV encephalitis *(Scand J Inf Dis 33:755, 2001)*. Most useful dx test is detection of CMV DNA by PCR in CSF *(CNS Drugs 16:303, 2002)*. Response to rx sporadic? *(Herpes 11:95A, 2004)*. CMV itself appears to be able to cause apoptosis of neuronal, glial, & endothelial cells of the Central Nervous System *(J. Clin Viro 32:218,2005)*. Certain CMV genotypes appear to selectively cause CNS infection *(AIDS 19:273, 2005)*	Onset subacute (mean 3.5wks): delirium/confusion 90%, apathy & withdrawal 60%, focal neurologic signs 50%. Metabolic abnormalities, hyponatremia, hyperkalemia, hypo-osmolality, hypernatremia secondary to dehydration. **CSF:** usually 0 cells. **PCR for CMV DNA 87% sensitive & 85% specific** *(J Clin Microbiol 38: 3061, 2000; J Clin Virol 25:559, 2002)*. **MRI with contrast: meningeal enhancement** *(CID 20:747, 1995)*, also focal (ring-enhancing), space-occupying lesions *(CID 22:626, 1996)*.
Diffuse micronodular encephalitis	
Ventriculoencephalitis	Onset of symptoms acute (mean 2wks): lethargy, disorientation, cranial nerve palsies, nystagmus. Antecedent CMV retinitis in 1/22 pts & 7/11 on anti-CMV rx. **CSF: uniformly abnormal (↑ cells, protein, mild ↓ glucose). Dx as above: CMV DNA by PCR. MRI: ventriculomegaly** *(CID 20:747, 1995; AJM 96:415, 1994)* with **periventricular enhancement with gadolinium** *(AJM 125:577, 1996)*.
Tuberculosis. See Meningitis, *pg62.*	Always consider in 3ʳᵈ World *(esp. Africa)* in pt with altered mental status, headache, lethargy or coma. Serum VDRL & FTA/ABS + in >90%. CSF VDRL sensitivity ranges from 10–89% *(CID 18:288, 1994)*.
Neurosyphilis (general paresis, meningiovascular)	MRI: cortical atrophy, infarcts. *(Curr Infect Dis Rep 7:277, 2005)*.
Herpes simplex virus (HSV) encephalitis Frequency & role still undefined but may be ↑ in HAART era *(J Neuropath Exp Neurol 62:429, 2003)*	Clinical presentation variable: confusion, fever & headache, anxiety & depression, memory loss, aphasia *(Int J STD AIDS 15:597, 2004)*. CSF: Virus seldom cultured from CSF *(J Clin Viro 25:559, 2003)*. Definitive dx requires brain biopsy or CSF PCR test for HSV DNA (98% sensitive during 1st wk of disease, antibody neg. early but... after 10–14 days *(CID 25:82, 1995)]*.
Neuropneumocystosis	7 cases reported. Most receiving aerosolized pentamidine, most had headache & confusion without focal findings. Diagnosed at postmortem in all *(CID 25:82, 1997)*.
Causes not directly related to HIV Drugs: sedative/hypnotic, alcohol, "street drugs" Hypoxemia: Sepsis; Metabolic: hypothyroidism, vitamin B₁₂ deficiency, electrolyte imbalance	Associated clinical features may suggest etiology but may be subtle, esp. in advanced HIV.

See pg102 for abbreviations & footnotes

TABLE 11A (5)

CLINICAL SYNDROME, ETIOLOGY, EPIDEMIOLOGY	CLINICAL PRESENTATION, DIAGNOSTIC TESTS, COURSE

Central Nervous System, Cognitive Disorders (continued)

Focal brain dysfunction: seizures &/or focal neurologic findings (hemiparesis, cerebrovascular abnormalities, blindness) *[see CID 34:103, 2002]*

Abrupt onset

Cerebrovascular event *(see AIDS Reader 14:515, 2004)*

Transient ischemic attack (TIA)—12/1600 AIDS pts (0.75%), RR 9.1

Cerebrovascular accident (stroke, CVA)—11/1600 AIDS pts (0.69%), Inc risk of ischemic stroke with adjusted RR of 9.1%, intracerebral hemorrhage. RR 12.7% [found in AIDS patients in Maryland *(Stroke 35,51,2003)*.

Subacute course (days)

Toxoplasmic encephalitis (TE): [In U.S. & India *(CID 36:79, 2003)*, occurs in 3–10% of patients with AIDS (median CD4 58): 15% in Malaysia *(Singapore Med J 44:194, 2003)*, in Europe & Africa occurs in 25–50% *(NEJM 329:995, 1993; CID 39:1681, 2004)*. Frequency ↓ with use of TMP/SMX prophylaxis vs P. jiroveci (carinii).] Marked ↓ incidence with HAART *(CID 33:1747, 2001)* in developed countries but not in Thailand *(Eur J Neurol 11:755, 2004)* & not all in HAART failures! *(CID 39:1681, 2004)*.

TE is likely quite common in underdeveloped world but because of inability of CT scanning, is rarely diagnosed. Seroprevalence is generally high (Thailand 25%, Senegal 40%, Central African Republic 50%, Malaysia 51%, Gabon 70%, Ethiopia 80%) & similar rates are found in animals (fowl in Egypt 70%, goats in Uganda 30%, pigs in Ghana 40%, felids from South Africa & 10.2 when CD4 100–200/mm³ vs those with CD4 >400/mm³ *(Am J Trop Med Parasit 95:587, 2001)*. **With such high infection rates, HIV pts with unexplained headache, altered mental status, focal neurological findings & CD4 <200/mm³ (or WHO Stage 3 or 4) should be considered for antitoxo rx.** *(J Neurovirol 11 s-1;17, 2005)*

Risk of focal brain lesions ↓ with HAART *(Neurol 55:1194,2000)* but most dramatic ↓ with primary CNS lymphoma,& toxo, PML slight ↓.

Most TIAs are "benign"; cause is unknown but may be associated with hypercoagulable state *(AJM 101:257, 1996)*. Exclude meningovascular syphilis, VZV, lymphoma, cryptomeningitis *(Braz J Inf Dis 8:175, 2004)*, cerebral non-HIV infection or embolic source *(Stroke 31: 2117, 2000)*. Inquire as to cocaine use with resulting risk of vasospasm ischemic events. ↑ expectancy & metabolic side effects leading to atherosclerosis from HAART; expect ↑ incidence of strokes *(Cerebrovasc Dis 15: 37, 2003)*.

Symptoms: Headache 50–70%, altered mental status 70%, hemiparesis &/or other focal signs 60%, seizures 30%. Fever, confusion, coma also seen. Symptoms may recur with immune reconstitution from HAART even with successful rx for toxo *(CID 37:e172, 2003)*.

Lab: CD4 <100/mm³ in 80%. Toxoplasma serum IgG + in essentially all pts who develop TE (frequency 85–99%) & titer predictive of development of disease. Relative risk with >150 int units/ml serum for toxo IgG 3.6. CD4 <200 20.8, & specific prophylaxis 0.2 is protective *(CID 28:575, 1999)*. PCR in CSF &/or serum for toxo DNA promising: 11/12 samples pos. vs 0/54 controls *(J Clin Micro 40:4499, 2002)*.

Scan: MRI not always necessary if multiple lesions seen on CT.

Multiple spherical ring-enhancing lesions in basal ganglia & cortex, mass effect common. Lesions often identified even without concomitant neurologic findings.

Course: >85% will respond to specific anti-toxo treatment. In one series, 86% responded by day 7 *(NEJM 329: 95, 1993)*. **If no improvement after 7–10 days of rx—biopsy.** In 22 "non-responsive" cases, primary lymphoma in 10, treatable diagnosis in 16 *(West J Med 158:249, 1993)*. [Brain biopsy indicated earlier (in <7 days) in patients with CD4 >100 or if negative toxo antibody titer; single lesion & progression of symptoms on antitoxo rx. If improvement, biopsy not required *(Ln 340:1135, 1992)*. However, in 1 longterm follow-up study (>14mos.) of 106 pts successfully rx for TE, 43 (40%) developed dementia symptoms, diagnosed by imaging & died from dementia while only 5/106 pts rx for PCP developed dementia *(Acta Neurol Scand 100:178, 1999)*.

See pg102 for abbreviations & footnotes

TABLE 11A (6)

CLINICAL SYNDROME, COGNITIVE DISORDERS, ETIOLOGY, EPIDEMIOLOGY	CLINICAL PRESENTATION, DIAGNOSTIC TESTS, COURSE
Central Nervous System, Cognitive Disorders/Focal Brain Dysfunction/Subacute Course (days) *(continued)*	
Primary CNS lymphoma *(see Hematol Oncol Clin No Amer 17:785, 2003)* ↓ incidence from 8.0/1000 person-years pre-HAART to 2.3/1000 person-yrs post-HAART, p <0.01 *(J AIDS 21:S11, 1999).* Epstein-Barr virus DNA present in nearly all *(Eur J Haematol 64:368, 2000).*	**Symptoms:** Usually afebrile. Often alert, but with mass effect may have more global mental dysfunction (60%), seizures (15%). **Lab:** CSF: Normal 30–50%, protein 10–150mg/d/L cells (monos) 0-40/ml, cytology + in <5%. **CSF PCR pos. for EBV DNA >90%** in one study *(J Clin Oncol 18:3325, 2000)* but only 33% in another *(J Clin Microbiol 38:3061, 2000).* ↑ CSF EBV DNA levels more common in both primary CNS lymphoma & CNS non-Hodgkins lymphoma than systemic NHL *(J Neurovirol 8:432, 2002)* **Scan: White matter more often involved than gray matter. One or a few weakly enhancing irregular lesions, typically in periventricular region with mass effect.** Thick-walled lesions are more common in lymphoma than in toxo *(Radiol 179:823, 1991).* Biopsy necessary for definitive diagnosis; stereotactic biopsy effective *(J Clin Neurosci 6:217, 1999).* **Course:** Response to radiation palliative but median survival time poor (9.3wks) *(Australas Radiol 44:178, 2000).* However, with HAART survival markedly improved: 6/7 alive median follow-up 667 days vs 0/18 untreated pts *(AIDS 17:1787, 2003).* No such improvement was seen in Australia *(HIV Med 5:377, 2004).* Chemotherapy for NHL did not reduce effectiveness of HAART in ↓ VL in plasma or CSF. *(AIDS Res Hum Retrovir 19:1091, 2003).*
Tuberculous brain abscess *(Meningitis, pg62)*	Evidence of extracranial infection may be absent—most common suspected cause (69%) of HIV-associated focal brain lesions in 1 study in South Africa *(QJM 97:413, 2004).*
Cryptococcoma *(Meningitis, pg62)* May coexist & be confused with toxo encephalitis	Usually concomitant with cryptococcal meningitis. CRAG of CSF & serum positive. But with an isolated cryptococcoma, CRAG (serum & CSF) may be negative.
Varicella zoster virus (VZV) encephalitis *(Am J Med Sci 321:372, 2001)* Less common complication of dermatomal zoster with HAART *(Neurovirol 9:129, 2004)*	Often associated with dermatomal zoster (71%) *(Scand J Inf Dis 32:263, 2000).* May mimic CNS lymphoma clinically & cytologically *(Leuk Lymphoma 44:1793, 2003).* CSF: Mean WBC 127/mm³, protein, lymphs, mean protein 157. **PCR sensitive & specific.** 97% *(J Clin Micro 38:2006, 2000; J Clin Virol 25:S59, 2002).* Scan: Multifocal infection of white matter similar to PML or vasculitis *(Neuroradiol 42:526, 2000).*
Cytomegalovirus (CMV) infection Aspergillosis of the CNS—39 cases reported *(Med 79:281, 2000)* • In pts with ↓ WBC & rx with corticosteroids • • Direct extension from sinuses or orbits—also from lung	MRI: May show focal ring-enhancing space-occupying lesions *(CID 22:626, 1996)* Nonspecific neuro symptoms including headache, cranial or somatic nerve weakness or paresthesias, altered mental status & seizures. Medical rx usually unsuccessful. Scan—CT reveals contrast-enhancing lesions.
Herpes simplex virus (HSV) encephalitis Bacillary angiomatosis, intracerebral	See pg58. Asymmetric encephalitis. Very rare but treatable. Associated with other lesions (skin, liver). Scan: Contrast-enhancing mass lesion. Course: Responds to erythromycin *[ArIM 116:740, 1992].*

See pg102 for abbreviations & footnotes

TABLE 11A (7)

CLINICAL SYNDROME, ETIOLOGY, EPIDEMIOLOGY	CLINICAL PRESENTATION, DIAGNOSTIC TESTS, COURSE
Central Nervous System, Cognitive Disorders/Focal Brain Dysfunction/Subacute Course (days) *(continued)*	
Chagas' Disease (Trypanosoma cruzi) *(Am J Trop Med Hyg 73:1016, 2005)*	One case report with hemiparesis. Born in El Salvador, in U.S. 6 years before onset of illness *(AJM 92:429, 1992)*. Another presented with confusion, hemiparesis, nuchal rigidity → coma, found to have rt cerebral lesion on CT *(CID 34:118, 2002)*. Rare causes such as these emphasize the importance of brain biopsy. PCR of CSF helpful for dx & rx *(CID 34:118, 2002)*.
Nocardia brain abscess	Rare complication may coexist with pulmonary nocardia *(J Inf 41:232, 2000)*.
Chronic course (weeks) *(see CID 20:1305, 1995)*	
Progressive multifocal leukoencephalopathy (PML) Frequency 4–7% of AIDS patients. Caused by JC virus (a papovavirus), which produces productive infection of oligodendrocytes, the myelin-producing cells of the CNS. JC virus may affect expression of the myelin basic protein gene leading to disruption of myelin sheaths *(J Neurovirol 6:S92, 2000)*. co-infection & activation of HIV-6 may be associated with demyelinative lesions *(J Neurovirol 5:363, 1999)*. (CD4 usually ≤100/mm³, mean 85/mm³). Specific cytotoxic T lymphocyte response to JC virus associated with favorable outcome *(J Neurovirol 7:318, 2001; AIDS 17:1557, 2003; Brain 127:1970, 2004)*. Prolonged survival & remission reported with highly effective antiretroviral rx *(Ln 349:850, 1997; AIDS 13:1881, 1999)* but not consistently *(AIDS 14:11, 1998)* & may develop during HAART *(CID 28:1152, 1999)*. In 118 Spanish pts with PML, 1/3 died despite HAART, neurologic function improved in 2/3 of survivors, baseline CD4 <100/mm³ was associated with ↑ mortality *(CID 36:1047, 2003)*. Has not ↓ as dramatically as other CNS OIs with HAART *(Neurol 55:1194, 2000; J AIDS 37:1263, 2004)*.	**Symptoms:** Develops insidiously with a single focus (limb weakness 1/3, visual defects 1/3, altered mental status 1/3) *(J Infect 32:97, 1996)* but afebrile & arousable (preservation of alertness until late in disease course). With progression, multiple foci occur. Seizures found in 20% in one series *(AJM 99:64, 1995)*. **Lab:** CSF: Normal (pleocytosis in 20%, ↑ protein 30%). **JC IgM antibody & PCR of CSF for JCV 82% sensitive, 100% specific** *(JID 160:1138, 1994; AIDS 12:581, 1998; Am Clin Lab 20:33, 2001)*. JC viral load in CSF was not predictive of disease state or progression in 1 study *(JID 160:1690, 1999)* but was in another *(Ann Neurol 45:816, 1999)*. **MRI Scan: Multiple fluffy or diffuse hypodense non-contrast enhancing lesions in subcortical white matter, no mass effect**. High signal intensity on T-2 images in hemispheric white matter, ill-defined margins (CT/MRI—clinical dissociation, images worse than pt. symptoms). May become contrast-enhancing with immune reconstitution assoc. with HAART *(AIDS 13:1426, 1999)*. Occ. inflammation present without HAART *(J Neurovirol 9(Suppl 1):25, 2003)*. Brain biopsy is definitive diagnostic procedure (demyelination, JCV on electron microscopy) *(J Neurovirol 10:1, 2004)*, sensitivity 40–96%, but not required if MRI is characteristic & JC PCR positive. **Course:** Death usual within 6mos but spontaneous sustained remissions occur in 5–10% *(Neurol 38:1060, 1988)*. Cidofovir + HAART ↑ survival & ↓ JC viral detectability in 1 study *(AIDS 14:F117, 2000; J Neurovirol 7:375, 2001)*. **Immune reconstitution with HAART may have serious consequences:** 4/9 pts on HAART developed ↑ inflammatory changes in area of PML, lesion vs 1/19 not receiving HAART; 3 of the 4 deteriorated clinically & radiologically *(AIDS 15:1900, 2001)*. 2 other pts who worsened with HAART responded transiently to steroids (high dose) but died from progressive neurological deterioration *(CID 35:1250, 2002)*. 8 Italian pts developed PML 21–55 days after starting HAART; 4 died, all 8 had ↑ CD4 counts & ↓ VL *(J Neurovirol 9(Suppl 1):73, 2003)* while those started on HAART at time of PML dx had higher 1-year probability of survival vs those continuing HAART or not treated *(AIDS 18:333, 2004)*. **No clear consensus on management of PML currently exists** *(J Neurovirol 9(Suppl 1):1/2, 2003)*.
Seizures *(See causes of focal brain dysfunction)*	
Cerebral mass lesions (32%) Encephalitis (24%) Meningitis (16%) Other or undetermined cause (28%)	In India *(J Assn Phys India 48:573, 2000)*: Toxo (30%) Tuberculoma (13%) Cryptomeningitis (18%) PML (4%) ADC (4%)	In 2 reports: toxoplasma: majority were toxoplasma. 15 S. African AIDS pts with new onset seizures had perfusion defects of the temporal lobe by SPECT/SCAN suggesting HIV-induced brain abnormalities. No other etiology identified *(J Neurol Sci 202:29, 2002)*.

See pg12 for abbreviations & footnotes

TABLE 11A (8)

CLINICAL SYNDROME, ETIOLOGY, EPIDEMIOLOGY	CLINICAL PRESENTATION, DIAGNOSTIC TESTS, COURSE
Central Nervous System, Cognitive Disorders (continued)	
Headaches	
New headache	<1wk duration: think crypto meningitis (20% in 145 HIV+ outpatients in Uganda, Kambugu 2005), toxo encephalitis, tubercular meningitis, aseptic or pyogenic meningitis, primary CNS lymphoma.
Chronic (see Focal brain dysfunction, pg59–61)	
HIV-associated, early disease	May be a presenting symptom. Not AIDS dementia complex or HIV-associated aseptic meningitis, CSF: β pleocytosis but ↑ HIV viral load in CSF (CID 30:962, 2000; Neurol 43:1098, 1993).
Nucleoside therapy	ZDV 50–60% in controlled trial, 3% in open study; ddI 1–7%, ddC 2–12%, stavudine 95% in controlled trial, 3% in parallel track program
Meningitis (headache, fever, lethargy with or without nuchal rigidity)	**See Br Med Bull 72:99, 2005 for description of current dx & therapeutic challenges.**
Cryptococcal meningitis (CD4 usually ≤100/mm³). For discussion of pathogenesis, see JID 186:522, 2002	**Symptoms: Stiff neck in only 1/4 of pts** (Bull Soc Path Exot 97:119, 2004). In Burkina-Faso, symptoms of CM: headache 3/4, stiff neck 1/4, altered consciousness 1/3, fever 1/3, seizures 1/4.
Both fluconazole use as primary prophylaxis & esp. HAART have markedly reduced incidence in developed regions (Neurol 56:257, 2001).	Seizures more common in children (38%) than adults (11%) in Zimbabwe (PID 21:54, 2002). May proceed rapidly to coma & death (Eur J Neurol 11:468, 2005). Parkinson symptoms reported (Mov
However, it is a common AIDS-defining diagnosis in 3ʳᵈ World including Uganda, Zimbabwe, South Africa, Zambia & Brazil (Aus & NZ Med 26:783, 1996; AIDS 14:2515, 2000; Postgrad Med J 77:769, 2001) along with Tb: meningitis &	Disord 118:1354, 2003). Extraneural disease in 20–60%. Skin lesions resembling Molluscum contagiosum in 3–10%, respiratory sx preceding headache common (78%). (J AIDS 9:168, 1995).
toxoplasmic encephalitis. Crypto & TbC commonly co-exist (J Med Microbiol 45: 376, 1996). Crypto caused 45% of meningitis in HIV+ persons in Zimbabwe	**Lab: CRAG (serum) >99% positive—excellent screening test** but of no value for following response to rx (HIV Clin Trial 1:4, 2000). Cryptococcal antigenemia preceded symptoms of meningitis
(AIDS 14:1401, 2000). In Uganda, it occurred at a rate of 40.4/1000 person yrs & caused 17% of AIDS-related deaths (AIDS 18:1205, 2002). In India, 31/1000	by median of 22 days (>100 days in 11%) in 77 pts in Uganda (AIDS 16:1031, 2002). Diabetes insipidus reported (Scand J Inf Dis 34:397, 2002).
person yrs (Indian J Med Sci 56:325, 2002). Dx in 20% of AIDS pts with new onset headache in Uganda (Kambugu, 2005). More common cause of chronic	**CSF:** LP opening pressure >200 in 60%. Often non-inflammatory. Median of 4 lymphs/mm³. CSF glucose normal to low, protein normal. **Increased intracranial pressure associated with blindness & ↑ mortality. If**
meningitis than tuberculosis in Thailand in HIV + (Neuroepidemiology 26:37,2005)	**opening pressure ≥250 mmH₂O, urgently rx with CSF drainage** (10–20ml CSF). Control of ↑ CSF pressure (reduction of >10 mm or no change) assoc. with improved outcome/survival as those whose pressure ↑ >10 mm, p <0.001 (CID 30:47, 2000; CID 38:1790, 2004). Selective placement of lumbar-peritoneal shunts has also been effectively used to control persistent ↑ CSF pressure (J AIDS 4:Human Retro 17:137, 1998). Dexamethasone or mannitol of no value (CID 22[Suppl 2]: S119, 1996).
	Acetazolamide use associated with ↑ serious adverse events—do not use (CID 35:769, 2002). If intracerebral mass lesion, think co-infection with toxo (Diag Microbiol Inf Dis 29:193, 1997).
	6–6.6% associated on HAART concurrent with or soon after dx of cryptococcosis developed **immune reconstitution inflammatory syndrome (IRIS)** (↑ hydrocephalus with ↑ ICP, ↑ hypercalcemia [sarcoid reaction], ↑ cavitary pneumonia & a subclavicular & subclavicular site abscess; all had neg. fungal cultures (CID 35:e128, 2002). See Table 11B. Has also presented as relapsing meningitis with pos. antigen but neg. cultures which responded to corticosteroids (AIDS 18:1223, 2004). Sterile cryptococcomas of the brain also reported (AJM 113:155, 2002; AIDS 18:349, 2004).

TABLE 11A (9)

CLINICAL SYNDROME, ETIOLOGY, EPIDEMIOLOGY	CLINICAL PRESENTATION, DIAGNOSTIC TESTS, COURSE
Central Nervous System, Cognitive Disorders (continued)	
Bacterial meningitis (occurs at any CD4 level). HIV+ have 20–150x ↑ risk vs HIV-neg. pts (J AIDS 32:345, 2003)	**Presentation similar to non-HIV+ population**. Blood cultures usually positive. Responds well to conventional antibiotic rx. Prognosis actually better than HIV-neg. pts in 1 study (CID 27:176, 1998) but 2X higher in HIV+ children in Malawi (65% vs 36%) (Ar Dis Child 88:1112, 2003). Antibiotic-resistant S. pneumo emerging as significant problem in HIV+ pts. esp. in 3rd World: 22% resistant to pen in HIV+ in South Africa (CID 33:610, 2001).
Streptococcus pneumoniae 45% Haemophilus influenzae 12% Neisseria meningitidis 14% (no ↑ risk with HIV↑) Rare: Salmonella [10 cases reported (Am J Med Sci 323:266, 2002)] Streptococcus bovis & strongyloides GI infection (Sex Tran Infect 81:276,2005) Listeria monocytogenes	Bacteria still cause of cases of meningitis in African HIV+ pts & accounted for of cases in Ghana (AIDS 14:144, 2000; E Afr Med J 75:516, 1998). Caused 1/3 of deaths in Kenyan children (An Trop Ped 22:125, 2002). Incidence of listeriosis (meningitis & bacteremia) 65–145X more common than in general population (CID 17:224, 1993). Yield from blood cultures by 'cold shock' of cultures, i.e. refrigerate overnight before incubation. HIV+ persons should avoid soft cheeses, undercooked chicken (J AIDS 8:466, 1995).
Tuberculous meningitis (Mycobacterium tuberculosis) (NEJM 351:1719, 2004) Occurs at any CD4 level but ↑ incidence in HIV+ pts: 235x ↑ in U.S. study (AIM 156:1710, 1996). Rare in developed world but common cause of meningitis in 3rd World: Zimbabwe 12% of cases (AIDS 14:1401, 2000), South Africa 18% (J Neurosci 162:20, 1999), 24% (AJM 89:497, 1996) (47%) in Spain (Ar Neurol 53:671, 1996). A study in Vietnam compared clinical & laboratory findings in 143 pts with TB meningitis with 108 with bacterial meningitis (<1/3 vs over 1/2 had duration of illness >6 days; peripheral WBC <10,200/mm³, CSF WBC <760/mm³ & after 48hrs of antibiotic rx: failure of CSF/blood glucose to ↑ by 100%, blood & CSF neutrophils at <80%, predicted TB meningitis (Ln 360:1287, 2002).	**HIV+ at ↑ risk but clinical manifestations are similar to HIV- patients** (JID 192:2134, 2005) except intracerebral mass lesions more common (AJM 93:520, 1992). Radiculomyelitis reported (CID 30:915, 2000). Meningeal involvement documented in of autopsies from pts with disseminated TB in Kenya (J AIDS 24:23, 2000). 9-mo mortality rate significantly decreased in HIV + (JID 192:2134, 2005) CSF: Lymphocytic pleocytosis, glucose ↓. Protein ↑. Direct AFB smear of CSF only 11% sensitive. culture 33%. Several dx tests on CSF show promise: Ligase chain reaction amplification 55% sens., 100% spec. (Scand J Inf Dis 34:14, 2002); radioimmunoassay 73% sens., 88% spec. (Clin Diag Lab Immunol 9:897, 2002), gen-probe rapid molecular dx (MTD) 93.8% sens., 99% spec. (Int J Tub Lung Dis 6:913, 2002). CSF-Cytospin smears for TB antigen 73% sens., 100% spec. (Clin Diag Lab Immunol 9:344, 2002) Adenosine deaminase activity ↑ in TB vs crypto or bacterial meningitis but sig. overlap between groups (Clin Neurol Neurosurg 104:10, 2002; Eur J Clin Micro Inf Dis 23:471, 2004). May resemble cryptomeningitis but CRAG⁺ neg. & tends to occur with higher CD4 counts (AJM 63:671, 1996). Mortality rate 30/58 (52%) in Gabon (J AIDS 32:345, 2003). Multiple-drug resistant TBc isolated from 30/350 (8.6%) with TB meningitis in South Africa & assoc. with poor outcome (CID 15:851, 2004). Consider in endemic areas (see pg92)
Fungal meningitis (coccidioidal & histoplasmal) CD4 usually <100/mm³	
HIV aseptic meningitis Occurs at any CD4 level	May occur early in HIV infection or relapsing throughout course. CSF: Mild lymphocytic pleocytosis, modest protein. These findings may be present in asymptomatic patient but ↑ HIV viral load in CSF (CID 30:962, 2000).
Meningovascular syphilis: syphilitic meningitis (see Curr Neurol Neurosci Rep 4:435, 2004)	May present with focal neurologic findings due to active endarteritis: depression, seizures, behavioral disorder, confusion (Braz J Inf Dis 5:280, 2001)
May co-exist with other etiologies	Rx: CSF VDRL positive (serum VDRL negative in 5–10%), >20 cells, CSF glucose may be ↓ (≥), CSF-VDRL positive (serum) in 5 pts (CID 135/mm³ in 5 pts (CID 25:673, 1997).
Candidal meningitis	May mimic tuberculous meningitis. CD4 135/mm³ in 5 pts (CID 25:673, 1997).

See pg102 for abbreviations & footnotes

TABLE 11A (10)

CLINICAL SYNDROME, ETIOLOGY, EPIDEMIOLOGY	CLINICAL PRESENTATION, DIAGNOSTIC TESTS, COURSE
Central Nervous System (continued)	
Movement disorders	**Most common clinical features:** Tremor, Parkinsonism, hemiballism, hemichorea.
Occur in 3% of HIV+ pts & up to 50% of those with advanced AIDS.	**Less common:** dystonia, chorea, myoclonus, tics, & dyskinesias.
Usually present with other clinical features: peripheral neuropathy, seizures, myelopathy, & dementia.	Often associated with OIs, particularly toxo & crypto, & may improve with specific treatment plus HAART.
Most Common Peripheral Nerve Syndromes in HIV Disease by Stage: The following are organized according to stage of HIV infection & relative prevalence *(see table on pg66)* Peripheral neuropathies are common (6–13%) in HIV/AIDS. They most commonly affect the sensory nerves & are caused by either HIV (DSP), opportunistic infections (CMV), drugs (TNA) or are idiopathic *(AIDS 16:2105, 2003; Curr Opin Neurol 16:403, 2003)*. They present as part of several discrete syndromes & vary according to stage of disease *(J Neurovirol 8/Supp.2:33, 2002)*.	
Acute retroviral syndrome	See Acute retroviral syndrome, pg55.
Neuropathy (6–8%)	Headache/retro-orbital pain, often ↑ with eye movement (30%), photophobia. Myelopathy, peripheral neuropathy, brachial neuritis, facial palsy, cauda equina & Guillain-Barre syndrome reported *(Neurol India 51:559, 2003)*
	Course: Usually self-limited, but persistence reported.
Early (asymptomatic HIV)	
Inflammatory demyelinating polyneuropathy (IDP) (occurs <5%) (see below)	Ascending paralysis with preservation of sensory function—global limb weakness. Probably represents autoimmune phenomenon. Nerve conduction studies show demyelinating features.
Subacute (Guillain-Barre syndrome) or acute inflammatory demyelinating polyradiculoneuropathy (AIDP) *(J Neurol Sci 208:39, 2003)*	One pt with CMV-associated Guillain-Barre responded to ganciclovir + HAART *(J Chemother 13:575, 2001)*. May be associated with immune reconstitution *(CID 36:e111, 2003)*
Chronic (chronic inflammatory demyelinating polyneuropathy) (CIDP or IDP) (may also occur late)	Progressive weakness in arms & legs, paresthesias with minor sensory loss, may be asymmetrical, absent DTRs
	Demyelinating polyneuropathy, CSF ↑↑ protein, mild to moderate lymphocytic pleocytosis (10–50cells/mm³). EMG shows demyelination.
Mononeuritis, multiplex (MM) (also occurs late) (rare)	Facial weakness, foot or wrist drop
	EMG, multifocal axonal neuropathy, multifocal cranial & peripheral neuropathies, thought to be immune mediated or vasculitis.
Multiple sclerosis-like syndrome (rare)	Waxing & waning course, multifocal defect, may rarely represent immune reconstitution syndrome (RIS) *(Curr Neurol 52:39, 2004)*.
Late (symptomatic HIV), CD4 <200/mm³	
Weakness/spasticity:	
Vacuolar myelopathy (occurs in as many as 40% of patients at autopsy) & is the most common form of spinal cord disease in HIV-infected individuals; under-recognized clinically *(Serum Neurol 22:133, 2002)*. Other infectious causes of myelopathies: HTLV-1, herpesviruses (VZV, HSV2, CMV), enteroviruses, T. pallidum, TBc, various fungi, & parasites.	Progressive painless gait disturbance with ataxia & spasticity. Also rarely occurring in upper extremities. + Babinski; may involve bowel & bladder. Imaging usually normal. Use of somatosensory-evoked potentials in pts with absent ankle DTRs valuable as tool in differential dx of myelopathy from neuropathy. CSF normal or ↑ protein, 5–10cells/mm³. Abnormalities in tibial central conduction time correlated with myelopathy *(Neurol 11:1477, 2000)*.
Progressive polyradiculopathy: CMV (**lumbosacral polyradiculopathy/myelitis** (also VZV, syphilis, spinal lymphoma) (cauda equina syndrome) *[see below]*	Subacute onset. Back & radicular pain, ascending weakness, areflexia, bladder & sphincter dysfunction, variable sensory loss but may produce "saddle anesthesia." May progress rapidly to flaccid paralysis. Myelitis + radiculitis can also be caused by varicella zoster *(Scand J Infct Dis 32:263, 2000)*.

See pg102 for abbreviations & footnotes

TABLE 11A (11)

CLINICAL SYNDROME, ETIOLOGY, EPIDEMIOLOGY	CLINICAL PRESENTATION, DIAGNOSTIC TESTS, COURSE
Central Nervous System *(continued)*	
Mononeuritis multiplex due to CMV *(AIDS 16:1341, 2002)*	Multifocal sensory & motor deficits in major peripheral or cranial nerves (esp. laryngeal nerves & upper > lower extremities—acute onset over 1mo), usually painful. CD4 <50 Rx: *See Table 13, pg145-146*
Numbness/burning: Distal sensory loss with neuropathic pain (most common neuropathy) *(AIDS 16:1341, 2002)*	Hyperesthesia, **burning feet**, painful, may affect walking, distal numbness with ↓ ankle DTR, stocking/glove sensory loss.
Distal predominantly sensory symmetrical polyneuropathy (DSP) *(see table below)* (occurs in up to ⅔ of pts with late-stage HIV). Risk factors include age >40 *(Ar Neurol 61:546, 2004)* (OR 1.17), diabetes (OR 2.1), white race (OR 1.33), nadir CD4 <50 (OR 1.64) & plasma HIV-1 RNA levels *(AIDS 16:407, 2002)*. Suppression 50->199 (OR 1.40). VL >10,000 copies/ml at 1ˢᵗ measurement of HIV may improve symptoms. ETOH abuse, drugs (vincristine, INH & thalidomide, used to rx aphthous ulcers) & ritavirin *(CID 40:148, 2005)*. ↓ incidence with HAART *(CID 40:148, 2005)*. Etiology unknown but HIV gp120 shown to attach to CXCR4 receptor on Schwann cells which release RANTES which induces dorsal root ganglion neurons to produce TNF assoc. with subsequent neurotoxicity *(An Neurol 54:287, 2003)*.	Severity of symptoms (pain) correlates with plasma HIV-1 RNA levels *(AIDS 16:407, 2002)*. Suppression of HIV may improve symptoms.
Toxic neuropathy from antiretroviral drugs (TNA) *(also see Table 6C)* (ddI > d4T > 3TC) (occurs >5%) but has been reported to occur in up to 30% of pts on d4T. Frequency usually associated with dose & duration of exposure: for d4T, 13% for <24 mo. rx vs 29% for >24mos. *(Adv Ther 19:1, 2002)*. Others have found that d4T alone or in combination with ddI doubles risk. *(Antivir Chem Chemother 14: 281, 2003, AIDS 19: 1341, 2004)*. FDA warning for ritavirin + ddI ± d4T assoc. with mitochondrial toxicity *(CID 38:e79, 2004)*. It appears that disease progression & host factors (mitochondrial haplogroup & age) all predispose individuals to neurotoxic effects of antiretroviral drugs *(CID 40: 148, 2005, AIDS 19:1341, 2005)*. Etiology appears to be associated with NRTI selective inhibition of γ-DNA polymerase leading to depletion of mitochondrial DNA & degeneration of mitochondria of neurons & Schwann cells *(Lab Invest 81:1537, 2001; HIV Med 5:11, 2004; AIDS 18:137, 2004)*.	**Aching feeling of feet, burning sensation.** ↑ serum lactate levels discriminated d4T neuropathy from DSP neuropathy (90% sensitivity, 90% specificity) *(AIDS 17:1094, 2003)*. EMG: axonal neuropathy; symptoms (pain) may worsen for up to 4wks after discontinuation of rx. In 54% of pts, able to continue drugs with full or reduced dose & in most (42/50) neuropathy improved or resolved. Substantial portion of pts continue to experience debilitating pain. **Lamotrigine** (an anticonvulsant drug) ↓ pain vs placebo in 227 pts. Rash a common side effect *(Neurol 54:2115, 2002)*. Results confirmed in 92 pts receiving antiretroviral rx but no difference from placebo in 135 pts with DSP without ART. Rash similar in Lamotrigine & placebo groups *(Neurol 60:1508, 2003)*. Coenzyme Q actually ↑ pain in 25 HIV+ pts with TNA *(CID 39:1371, 2004)*. But rx with acetyl-L-carnitine (1500mg q12h po) up to 33mos. assoc. with ↓ symptoms & peripheral nerve regeneration in 21 HIV+ pts with TNA *(AIDS 18:1549, 2004)*. Capsaicin was ineffective in relieving pain (Cochrane Database Syst Rev CD003937,2005)
Weakness/myalgias:	
Myopathy: HIV, zidovudine [ZDV + ddC > ZDV + ddI *(AIDS 12:2425, 1998)*]	Weakness without sensory finding, DTRs intact with myalgias. EMG: irritative myopathy, ↑ CPK, muscle biopsy; myofibril degeneration + inflammation

See pg102 for abbreviations & footnotes

TABLE 11A (12)

DIRECT COMPARISON OF THE 4 MAJOR HIV-ASSOCIATED NEUROPATHIES WITH RX SUGGESTIONS (J Peripher Nerv Syst 6:8, 2001)

	DISTAL SYMMETRIC POLYNEUROPATHY (DSP)/TOXIC NEUROPATHY FROM ANTIRETROVIRAL DRUGS (TNA)	INFLAMMATORY DEMYELINATING POLYNEUROPATHY	PROGRESSIVE POLYRADICULOPATHY	MONONEURITIS COMPLEX
Distribution:	Stocking/glove	Extremities—ascending	Cauda equina distribution	Cranial nerve + multiple peripheral nerves
Symptoms:	Hyperesthesia, pain, paresthesia with contact, "burning feet"	Muscle weakness; few if any sensory complaints	Radiating pain in distribution of cauda equina; leg weakness. Bladder/bowel dysfunction (urinary retention)	Cranial & peripheral nerve complaints; motor & sensory
Findings:	↓ response to pain, temperature, vibration; ↓ ankle DTRs; normal strength	Facial nerve paresis; ascending weakness; generalized ↓ in DTRs	Flaccid paraparesis; mild sensory loss; absent leg DTRs, anal wink	Typical nerves involved: facial, median, lateral cutaneous femoral, ulnar, peroneal
Possible etiology(ies):	Toxic; metabolic; nutritional; drugs: nucleoside reverse transcriptase inhibitors	Idiopathic; CMV implicated; CSF—lymphocytic pleocytosis: ↑ protein	CMV—PMNs in CSF Lymphoma—monos in CSF	Can be due to CMV or idiopathic (vasculitis)
Treatment:	Symptomatic (e.g., analgesics, tricyclic antidepressants). If receiving NRTIs, dc. If not, start HAART, ↓ viral load may ↓ symptoms (see above for experimental treatments)	Similar to Guillain-Barré: corticosteroids, plasmapheresis, IVIG	For CMV—ganciclovir, valganciclovir For lymphoma—chemotherapy	Ganciclovir if CMV

CLINICAL SYNDROME, ETIOLOGY, EPIDEMIOLOGY — CLINICAL PRESENTATION, DIAGNOSTIC TESTS, COURSE

Electrolyte & Metabolic Abnormalities

Hyponatremia — About 20% of ambulatory & 50% of hospitalized patients have serum Na of < 135mmol/L. On admission due to GI loss & hypovolemia. During hospitalization 1/2 due to SIADH (2° bacterial pneumonias, CNS infection). Patients are edema-free, with hypertonic urine with low serum osmolality & high urinary sodium (AJM 94:169, 1993).

  Volume depletion 2° to diarrhea
  Syndrome of inappropriate secretion of antidiuretic hormone (SIADH) (2° to pulmonary or CNS infections)
  Adrenal insufficiency, primary
  Hyporeninemic hypoaldosteronism
  Nephrotoxic drugs: pentamidine, amphotericin B, foscarnet.
  Nephrogenic diabetes insipidus: ganciclovir

Hyperkalemia — 20–53% pts on TMP/SMX or TMP + dapsone for treatment of PCP develop hyperkalemia. TMP is a sodium channel inhibitor & functions as a K-sparing diuretic agent (NEJM 328:703, 1993).

  Trimethoprim
  Hypoaldosteronism
  Adrenal insufficiency
  Ketoconazole

Hypercalcemia — Lab: ↑ serum 1,25-dihydroxy vitamin D concentrations with ↓ levels of intact parathormone.

  Lymphoma (South Med J 92:924, 1999 & 93:894, 2000)
  Granuloma formation associated with immune reconstitution (HAART) in pts with MAC

Hypocalcemia — Neuromuscular irritability, carpal or pedal spasm. Foscarnet forms complex with ionized calcium. Ketoconazole can block formation of 1,25-dihydroxy vitamin D (NEJM 317:1360, 1992). Ampho B & aminoglycosides may lead to Mg⁺⁺ wasting with inhibition of parathyroid hormone release & action (AJM 151:1441, 1991).

  Drug-related: Foscarnet, ketoconazole, amphotericin B, aminoglycosides

Lactic acidosis/hepatic steatosis (see Table 6C).
Lipodystrophy (lipoatrophy or lipohypertrophy) (see Table 11F & Table 6Q).
Immune reconstitution (IRIS) or HIV-associated metabolic syndrome (see Table 11E & Table 6Q).

See pg102 for abbreviations & footnotes

TABLE 11A (13)

CLINICAL SYNDROME, ETIOLOGY, EPIDEMIOLOGY	CLINICAL PRESENTATION, DIAGNOSTIC TESTS, COURSE
Endocrine System: 7/13 asymptomatic randomly tested had abnormal endocrine function: pituitary-adrenal, pituitary-thyroid, & pituitary-ovarian axis. 6 had menstrual irregularities (*Gynecol Endocrin* 16:33, 2002).	
Pituitary gland Infectious involvement of anterior pituitary: CMV, P. jiroveci (carinii), Toxoplasma gondii	25% of advanced but non-AIDS HIV+ patients have ↓ pituitary reserve (*AJM Sci* 305:321, 1993). Functional pituitary insufficiency is very uncommon but reported (*AJM* 77:760, 1984). Useful diagnostic tests: Corticotropin-releasing hormone (CRH) test; testing for several hormones simultaneously: insulin + thyro-tropin-releasing hormone (TRH) + gonadorelin (GnRH); measure glucose, cortisol, GH, TSH, prolactin, LH, FSH & ACTH.
Thyroid gland Chronic illness	Lab: ↓ T_3 with reciprocal ↑ rT_3 (reverse T_3), T_4 usually normal. Useful diagnostic tests: T_3, T_4, thyroid-binding globulin, rT_3.
HIV infection	Lab: 16% of 350 HIV-infected French pts tested had hypothyroidism: 2.6% were overtly hypothyroid, 6.6% had subclinical hypothyroidism, & 6.8% had ↓ free T_4. In multivariate analysis, d4T tx & ↓ CD4 count associated ↓ T_4; hypothyroidism (*CID* 37:579, 2003). 1632 Italian children (35%) had thyroid abnormalities: 16 isolated ↓ T_4; T_4 level correlated positively with CD4% & duration of HAART (*PIDJ* 23:235, 2004). Similar findings in Thai children: 10/37 (28%) had abnormal thyroid function assoc. with advanced disease (*J Ped Endo Metab* 17:33, 2004).
Graves' disease—1 report assoc. with immune reconstitution from ↓HAART [*AIDS Read* [*AIDS Res Hum Retrovir* 20:157, 2004].	
Adrenal gland (the most commonly affected endocrine gland)	**Addison's disease: fever, hypotension, abdominal pain, hyponatremia, hyperkalemia**
Primary adrenal insufficiency, causes include: • CMV adrenalitis (found in 33–88% of AIDS pts at autopsy) • HIV infection of adrenal	Overt Addisons disease is uncommon, although blunted responses to ACTH are common. In 28 critically ill HIV+ pts, 6 (21%) had stress cortisol levels & low-dose (1mcg) corticotropin stimulation test levels of <18
• Infiltration by Kaposi's sarcoma, lymphoma or infection (MAC, crypto, histo, pneumocystis)	μg/dl & dx of adrenal insufficiency; 21/28 (75%) had adrenal insufficiency if 25mcg/dl was used as diagnostic threshold (*Crit Care Med* 30:1267, 2002). CMV antigenemia assoc. with adrenal insufficiency. Suboptimal response to ACTH stimulation & ↓ stress cortisol serum levels should receive stress doses of
• Drug-induced: ketoconazole (impairs steroid synthesis), fluconazole (1 report: 800 mg q24h x68 days, *J Microbol Immun Inf* 37:250, 2004), rifampin (induces hepatic enzymes which ↑ metabolism of steroids), megestrol (prolonged use) (*AnIM* 122:843, 1995) • Pituitary insufficiency (see above)	corticosteroids where there is infection, trauma, etc. (*Endocr J* 49:641, 2002). Useful diagnostic tests: AM, PM plasma cortisol levels (AM level <275 suggests adrenal insufficiency (normal single dose Cosyntropin stimulation test level [but a single normal response may not rule out adrenal insufficiency (*Am J Med Sci* 321:137, 2001)]; plasma ACTH levels, ↑ basal serum cortisol & ↓ dehydroepiandrosterone is actually more common than in HIV-neg. persons, but rarely assoc. with features of Cushing syndrome (*AnIM* 162:1095, 2004).
Pancreas **Pancreatitis**	
Drug-associated: pentamidine, didanosine (ddI) 2-6%, zalcitabine (ddC) <1%, stavudine (d4T) 1%, lamivudine (3TC) 1% but 15% in children.	Typical presentation (nausea, vomiting & abdominal pain). Type I diabetes mellitus may develop.
Hyperglycemia: Insulin resistance common in HAART; see *Table 6C*	Other diabetogenic drugs frequently taken by HIV+ patients: dapsone, rifampin, sulfamethoxazole in patients
Drug-induced (especially protease inhibitor 6%, megestrol acetate & corticosteroids) [*J AIDS & Human Retro* 17:46, 1998)]. See *Tables 6B & 6C*	with renal failure, octreotide, ganciclovir (*AnIM* 118:529, 1993). Protease inhibitors produced symptomatic diabetes mellitus in 6/105 pts (*ICAAC 1997, LB-8*).
Hypoglycemia Drug-induced [Pentamidine (IV), 2%]	During destruction of islets, insulin release may cause hypoglycemic coma.

See pg102 for abbreviations & footnotes

TABLE 11A (14)

CLINICAL SYNDROME, ETIOLOGY, EPIDEMIOLOGY	CLINICAL PRESENTATION, DIAGNOSTIC TESTS, COURSE
Gonads	
Testes	
Primary testicular failure (see *CID 33:857, 2001*).	↓ libido & impotence common. Gynecomastia found in 1.8% of 2275 HIV+ men; related to hypogonadism; ↓ free testosterone index vs controls (*CID 39:1514, 2004*). Efavirenz also assoc. with gynecomastia in a retrospective
Drug-associated: ketoconazole	case-controlled study in 23 pts (*AIDS Reader 14:29, 2004*). HAART itself may ↓ libido in males assoc. with ↑ estradiol serum levels (*Int J STD AIDS 15:234, 2004*).
	Lab: ↓ free testosterone levels, ↑ LH & FSH, normal GnRH response. Approx. 30% of men with HIV infection & 50% with AIDS are hypogonadal, ↑ with late stage disease (*CID 41:1794, 2005*). Testosterone replacement useful in muscle wasting (*AIDS Reader 13:51, 2003*).
	Found to ↑ muscle mass in low-wt HIV-infected men (*AIM 164:897, 2004*). Others have shown that testosterone rx for depression not different than placebo in a prospective randomized double-blind placebo-controlled trial in 123 men (*J Clin Psychopharm 24:379, 2004*).
Ovaries	
Menstrual irregularities are common, esp. with advanced HIV/AIDS (CD4 <200/mm³) & wasting.	In 69 HIV-infected women, weight loss >10% max. weight was significant predictor of low free testosterone serum level, thus ↓ androgen level common in women with wasting (*CID 36:499, 2003*). Testosterone replacement (patches 2x/wk) ↑ testosterone levels but had little physiological effect in a randomized double-blind study in 52 women (*JCEM, Dec. 21, 2004*).
Eye: Ocular manifestations occur in up to 75% of HIV infected pts (*Ocul Immunol Inflam 8:263, 2000, SADJ 60:386, 2005*). **Acute loss of vision**—diff. dx: CMV papillitis, VZV—rapidly progressive retinal necrosis (*AIDS 16:1045, 2002*), syphilis, cryptococcal meningitis, TBc; toxo (*Ophth 111:716, 2004*), endophthalmitis (bacterial or fungal) (*CID 26:34, 1998*). Up to 10–20% of HIV-infected worldwide will lose vision in 1 or both eyes from CMV (*Bull WHO 79:181, 2001*). 1/2 of 162 African children with HIV infection had ophthalmic involvement; most common finding was perivasculitis of peripheral retinal vessels (38%) (*Ocul Immunol Inflam 8:263, 2000*). 10% of 1250 HIV+ Ugandan adults screened with Schnellen test had visual impairment (*Othl, personal communication; IDI, Mulago Hospital*). Introduction of HAART has significantly reduced significance of ocular disease but has introduced immune-recovery uveitis associated with CMV (*Ocul Immunol Inflam 13:219,2005*). Rev.: *Curr Opin Ophthal 13:397, 2002*.	
Anterior Segment Infections	
Chronic follicular conjunctivitis due to Molluscum contagiosum	Lesions larger, more numerous, more rapid in onset than in immunocompetent individuals. Solitary lesions of molluscum contagiosum may persist after HAART (*Br J Ophthal 87:1427, 2003*) but may regress with pronounced injection (IRIS) (*Graefes Ar Clin Exp Ophth 242:951, 2004*).
Corneal microsporidiosis (Encephalitozoon hellum) (*J Infect 27:229, 1993*).	Photophobia, dry eyes, foreign body sensation, blurred vision. Punctate keratopathy. Pets, esp. birds, suspected source. Nasal sinus epithelium occasionally involved. Dx: epithelial scrapings (*Am J Ophth 115:285, 1993*).
Fungal keratitis, candida sp., nocardia (*Jpn J Ophth 48:272, 2004*).	Often no history of trauma, sporotrichosis & bilateral ulcers. Dx based on corneal scrapings & culture.
Herpes simplex virus keratitis	Predilection for peripheral rather than central involvement. Lesions take longer to heal & recurrences common. Dx: Fluorescein ± epithelial "dendrites" (*Ophthalmologica 214:337, 2000*).
Varicella-zoster virus keratitis.	Most pts have H. zoster lesions in trigeminal nerve (1st div) distribution, 2/3 have keratitis, usually punctate.
Eyelids	
Herpes zoster ophthalmitis, Kaposi's sarcoma, Molluscum contagiosum	Solitary lesions of molluscum contagiosum may persist after HAART (*Br J Ophthal 87:1427, 2003*) or may regress with pronounced injection (IRIS) (*Graefes Ar Clin Exp Ophth 242:951, 2004*).
Posterior Segment Infections	
At least 12 infectious agents identified as causes of retinal or choroidal disease in HIV+ patients (*ID Clin NA 6:909, 1992*). Considerations include more common or major entities. Bacterial retinitis: Mycobacterium avium-intracellulare, Rhodococcus equi reported.	Prompt ophthalmologic consultation indicated; etiologic diagnosis usually dependent on clinical characteristics rather than laboratory findings.

See pg10 for abbreviations & footnotes

TABLE 11A (15)

CLINICAL SYNDROME, ETIOLOGY, EPIDEMIOLOGY	CLINICAL PRESENTATION, DIAGNOSTIC TESTS, COURSE
Eye/Posterior Segment Infections *(continued)*	
Candidal endophthalmitis Prevalence in HIV+ pts unclear. It is rare with only mucocutaneous candidiasis, but may be associated with candidemia with IV lines & neutropenia. Choroid tubercles (choroidal granulomas) Choroidal pneumocytosis	Well-demarcated yellow to white lesions that protrude into vitreous, not associated with hemorrhage & usually unilateral. Found in 2.8% of pts with disseminated tuberculosis & AIDS in Malawi *(Br J Ophth 86:1076, 2002).* **All choroidal lesions have had P. jiroveci (carinii) pneumonia & prophylaxis with aerosolized pentamidine. Creamy to orange choroidal lesions, usually bilateral without vitreous inflammation. Visual acuity usually not affected.**
Cryptococcosis: choroiditis, endophthalmitis In one series 9/27 (33%) pts with crypto meningitis had neuro-ophthal. signs *(Ophth 96:1092, 1989).*	Course: Response to systemic rx, usually good. Rapid visual loss with optic nerve involvement. May be due to ↑ intracranial pressure, a medical emergency; rx with CSF drainage. Multifocal white lesions with optic nerve edema usually without vitreous inflammation seen. Dx usually based on systemic &/or meningeal crypto. With rx, progressive optic atrophy may occur.
Cytomegalovirus (CMV) retinopathy: Rx: See *Table 12, pg128* Occurs in 20-30% of AIDS patients. Found in 32/191 (17%) pts with AIDS in Malawi *(Br J Ophthal 86:1076, 2002).*	**Peripheral retinitis, CD4 count is <50/mm³.** Course: Usually begins with unilateral "floaters" to ↓ visual acuity to blindness. **Ophthal. exam: Findings are usually initially in the periphery, moving centrally until macula &/or optic disc involved. Lesions are large creamy to white areas with granular borders & perivascular exudates & hemorrhages ("cottage cheese & ketchup" appearance) with little overlying vitreous reaction. If redness of the outer eye, photophobia & irregular-shaped pupil develops, suspect infection other than CMV retinopathy.**
Marked reduction with HAART *(J AIDS 22:228, 1999; HIV Med 2:255, 2001),* but less so with advanced disease *(MMM 135:17, 2001).* **HAART markedly improves survival & success of anti-CMV rx.** *(J AIDS & HR 19:13, 1998; AIDS 12:613, 1998)* but vision loss from immune recovery uveitis (epiretinal membrane, cystoid macular edema or cataract) reported in up to 63% *(Retina 25:633, 2005)* (see *Table 11B*)	Dx: Based on clinical features. CMV DNA+ in serum; ↓ with effective anti-CMV rx *(CID 15:1756, 2001).* ↑ CMV-specific CD4 &/or CD8 cells predict prevention of recurrence after HAART *(AIDS Res Hum Retrovir 17:1749, 2001; JID 184:256, 2001),* while failure to ↑ CMV-specific CD4 response assoc. with multiple relapses *(JID 183:1285,2001).*
	Mortality from CMV correlates with CMV DNA in plasma *(JCI 101:Y97, 1998).* CMV genome not found in aqueous humor by PCR in immune recovery uveitis *(Ophthalmologica 218:43, 2004).* **Rapid ↓ in visual acuity.** Swelling of optic nerve head, atrophy within 4wks. Consider pulsed systemic steroids + ganciclovir or foscarnet *(Am J Ophth 108:691, 1989).*
Primary CMV papillitis	Dx & rx: See *CMV peripheral retinitis*, above, & *Table 12, pg128.*
	May also be associated with cutaneous zoster.
Herpes zoster/simplex virus (VZV) retinitis (mean CD4 24) 5/10 pts presenting to eye clinic in Nigeria with HZ ophthalmicus were HIV+ *(West Afr J Med 22:186, 2003).*	1) **Acute retinal necrosis (ARN) syndrome:** rapidly progressive necrosis of peripheral retina (often 360 °) with occlusive vasculopathy, marked vitreous & anterior chamber inflammation, optic neuritis & scleritis. Complete visual loss in involved eye in 1/3 pts both eyes involved *(Am J Ophth 112:119, 1991; Am J Ophth 110:341, 1990; CID 26:34, 1998).* May be associated with retrobulbar optic neuritis *(Am J Neuroradiol 25:1722, 2004).* 2) Ill-defined areas of peripheral retinal whitening without granular borders, minimal vitreous reaction, no pain or foveal lesions (confused with CMV).
HIV-associated "cotton wool" spots (CWS) CWS occurs in about 50% of patients with non-infectious microvascular retinopathy. Nonspecific findings & seen in many other conditions *(Med 82:187, 2003).*	Usually asymptomatic but occur more in late-stage disease. Ophthal. exam: Small fluffy white lesions with indistinct margins without exudates or hemorrhages. Lesions do not progress & usually regress spontaneously, do not require treatment. CWS may indicate ↑ risk for onset of CMV retinitis.
Iritis secondary to cidofovir *(CID 25:337, 1997).*	Common with intravitreal injection but recurrent episodes with IV also reported.

See pg102 for abbreviations & footnotes

TABLE 11A (16)

CLINICAL SYNDROME, ETIOLOGY, EPIDEMIOLOGY	CLINICAL PRESENTATION, DIAGNOSTIC TESTS, COURSE
Eye/Posterior Segment Infections (continued)	
PEG interferon alfa-2b—ribavirin ocular changes	8/23 (35%) receiving PEG IFN-Rib for Hep C rx developed visual/ocular abnormalities, including cotton wool spots, cataracts, ↓ color vision (AIDS 18:1965, 2004).
Retinal depigmentation	5% of children's Cx developed retinal depigmentation. Asymptomatic.
Retinal deposits of clofazimine	Clofazimine deposits in pigmented tissues. May result in brownish refractile crystals in retina.
Ribabutin-associated uveitis	Becoming ↑ common in AIDS pts with use of protease inhibitors (↑ rifabutin serum levels) in Western world but rare (1/191) in Africa (Br J Ophthal 86:1076, 2002) (see Table 16, Drug/Drug Interactions). Also in non-HIV infected (Eye 14:344, 2000).
Reported in 1–2% pts on 600 mg/day (NEJM 330:438, 1994). Also rarely on 300 mg/day (AJVM 121:510, 1994).	
Syphilis: iridocyclitis, vitreitis, optic neuritis, chorioretinitis, or combinations of these. (Eye June 3, 2005)	**In HIV+, syphilitic ocular disease is more common, more severe & often bilateral. Necrotizing retinitis with mucocutaneous lesions may be confused with CMV. Cream-colored posterior plaques may be seen with mucocutaneous lesions in 2° syphilis. Rule out neurosyphilis.**
Uveitis in HIV: Think syphilis (Int J STD AIDS 12:754, 2001)	Lab: Positive VDRL & FTA/ABS on serum.
Focal anterior scleritis with retinitis caused by syphilis uncovered with Immune reconstitution (Clin Exp Ophthalmol 32:526, 2004).	Course: Rx failures reported.
Toxoplasmic chorioretinitis	Pre-existing chorioretinal scars usually absent. Hemorrhages are absent or minimal. Vitreitis & iridocyclitis (red, painful eye) are common. May occur without intracranial lesions.
Ocular involvement uncommon in AIDS. Lesions may be single or multifocal, usually discrete, perivascular in location. Found in 15/132 pts with new onset vision impairment in Uganda (J. Ortiz, personal communication).	Lab: PCR for toxo DNA in vitreous fluid may be of value (Ophthal 111:716, 2004). Course: Response to rx usually good; prolonged suppression required. Oral steroids not used.
Fever of Unknown Origin (FUO)	
Prolonged fever is common in AIDS pts. The etiology varies with geography (AIDS 16:909, 2002); frequency ↑ with ↓ CD4 counts & ↓ with HAART (Eur J Clin Micro Inf Dis 21:137, 2002).	In 704 HIV+ pts with fever at SFGH: **18% blood cultures + in hospitalized pts.** Predictors of + culture: pneumonia, UTI, abscess, central line or neutropenia. Without 1 predictor, only 1.5% were +. **Sensitivity of AFB is related to CD4 count:** <100 19% +, 101–200 7% +, >200 0% + 17% of febrile pts in Malawi had pos. AFB blood cultures (Micr J Tuberc Lung Dis 6:1067, 2002).
Etiology of FUO in AIDS:	Chest x-ray of value when respiratory sx present 85–95% sensitive but specificity only 16–30%.
In U.S. **MAC (31%),** Pneumocystis jiroveci (carinii) pneumonia (13%), bacterial pneumonia (9%), sinusitis (6%), Rhinol 39:136, 2001), lymphoma (7%), catheter infection (1–10%), drug allergy (2–5%), disseminated histoplasmosis (7%).	**Urine culture** of value when dysuria.
Bartonella (8.5% of FUO pts, sirusitis (6% & B. henselae or B. quintana & 68/382 (18% AIDS pts in San Francisco had Bartonella infection dx by IFA or PCR (CID 37:559, 2003), & CMV (11%), unexplained in 15–30%. Immune reactivation (RIS) & drug fever have ↑ (15% with HAART (Int Med 21:335, 2004).	In pts with abn LFTs, **liver bx** revealed cause of fever in 13/24 pts (CID 20:606, 1995). **Diagnostic value of bone marrow aspirate & biopsy appears to vary from study to study, geographical location, & likely availability of other dx tests. Bone marrow** bx pos. in 52/123 FUO pts in Spain but could have probably been dx through other means (AnM 157:1577, 1997). In Brazil, specific dx in 33/99 with AFB in 12, histo 5, & lymphoma 6 (Pathol Res Pract 200:591, 2004). In 72 pts with AIDS & FUO in U.S., BM exam of low diagnostic yield even with abnormal hematological parameters (J AIDS 7:1699, 2004). In endemic areas, histoplasmosis: 32% had pos. bone marrow stain for histoplasmosis vs 8% with LDH <600 (South Med J 93:692, 2000). In pts with high prolonged fever &, ↑ bilirubin, bone marrow aspiration, biopsy & culture more sensitive & rapid for dx mycobacteria & histo than blood cultures (Am J Hematol 67:100, 2001).
In **Spain, TBc identified in 42%,** leishmaniasis in 14% (less common with HAART: CID 37:373, 2003) & MAC in 14% (CID 30:872, 1996).	
In **Thailand, TBc 63%,** crypto, Penicillium marneffei (Sante 13:149, 2003).	When fever assoc. with hepatosplenomegaly & pancytopenia: think leishmania in endemic areas; bone marrow smear pos. for amastigotes (Hum Pathol 31:75, 2000). Think lymphoma with prolonged fever, cytopenias & hemophagocytic syndrome (AIDS Pt Care STDs 17:495, 2003).
In **Africa, TBc most common by far:** crypto, malaria, others include histoplasmosis, salmonella bacteremia, bacterial pneumonia (S. pneumo common isolate from blood cultures), Rhodococcus sp. (J Infect 41:227, 2002; think TBc & Burkitt's lymphoma (Int J Cancer 92:687, 2001)	
In **India, TBc 63%,** crypto 10%, PCP 7%, others include bacterial pneumonia, amebic liver abscess, histoplasmosis, & cerebral toxo (Natl Med J India 16:193, 2003; BMC Inf Dis 22:52, 2004)	**High resolution sonography** revealed multiple microabscesses in 32 pts with FUO in Spain: 14 TBc, 7 leishmania, 5 MAC, 2 salmonella, 2 lymphoma, 1 histoplasmosis (Eur J Clin Microbiol Inf Dis 18:374, 1999). When fever remains unexplained, think MAC, lymphoma, Bartonella, PCP or fungus.

See pg102 for abbreviations & footnotes

TABLE 11A (17)

CLINICAL SYNDROME, ETIOLOGY, EPIDEMIOLOGY	CLINICAL PRESENTATION, DIAGNOSTIC TESTS, COURSE

Fever of Unknown Origin *(continued)*

In areas of high prevalence, malaria should be ruled out, but HIV+ pts with fever are frequently +ve for malaria delaying dx of above. Co-infection with both common; frequency in HIV+ patients malaria fever 1 wk; >wk CD4 count (*D 1929;84, 2005), *Ln 362:1008, 2003*). Malaria assoc. with ↑ VL (*Lancet 365:233, 2005*).

M. avium is the most common cause of FUO in the U.S. when CD4 count <50. It appears to be rare in East Central Africa (*JID 162:208, 1990; J AIDS 8:195, 1995*) but point prevalence 10% in South Africa (*CID 33:2069, 2002*). Infection due to Mycobacterium avium-intracellulare complex [M. avium 52%, M. intracellulare 21%, M. xenopi 7%, M. fortuitum 2% (*CID 20:73, 1995*)] M. genavense, an unrelated organism which clinically behaves like MAC].

M avium usually presents as disseminated infection with symptoms of **fever, weight loss, night sweats, diarrhea, anemia & neutropenia**, but may be asymptomatic even with positive blood cultures. Highest concentration of organisms (6.7 log₁₀/gm) in mesenteric nodes (*JID 173:942, 1996*). Lab: Colonization of respiratory secretions & GI tract is common & may precede disseminated disease. When symptomatic, blood cultures are usually positive for MAC (BACTEC system is very sensitive). Dual infection with M. tbc recognized. Prevalence of MAC but not MTB has declined in HAART era in Brazil (*Braz J Infect Dis 9:469,2005*) but isolated from 6% of deaths from AIDS in France (*Scand J Infect Dis 37:482:2005*)

Gastrointestinal Tract

Mouth (*Int Dis Clin No Amer 13:879, 1999, Bull World Health Organ 83;700, 2005, Top HIV Med 13:143, 2006*)
Oral manifestations very common in HIV-infected persons worldwide (*Oral Dis 8:90, 2002*). 90% of 101 HIV+ Cambodians had oral lesions: oral candidiasis 52%, hairy leukoplakia 36%, necrotizing ulcerative gingivitis 28% (*J Oral Pathol Med 31:1, 2002*). In Kenya, all of oral candidosis, 13% KS (*East Afr Med 78:398, 2001*). In Mexico, 47% of 1000 HIV-infected individuals had oral lesions; erythematous & pseudomembranous candida (38%), hairy leukoplakia (22.6%), most common (*Med Oral 8:39, 2003*). Similar to findings in 500 pts in Nigeria (*Int J STD AIDS 14:395, 2003*), 87 & 237 pts in Thailand (*Med Micro Immunol 192:157, 2003; Oral Dis 10:138, 2004*), 161 pts in Brazil (*Int Dent J 54:131, 2004*), & 1000 pts in India (*An Acad Med Singapore 33/4 Suppl):37, 2004]. Oral manifestations ↓ with HAART (*Oral Dis 10:145, 2004*).

Oral lesions without soreness (or mild soreness)

Acute retroviral syndrome (see Acute HIV, pg20)

Oral ulcerations (apthous) in 12/30 pts (40%), enanthemas (40%), 5 pts had both (*CID 17:59, 1993*).
Oral candidiasis (12%) (*JID 168:1490, 1993*).
Lab: Thrombocytopenia 74%; HIV antibody test initially + in 7/30 (23%).

Candidiasis

Response to HAART with ↓ oropharyngeal candidiasis (31% at baseline to 1% after 48wks HAART) (*AIDS 14:979, 2000*). The presence of Oral Candidiasis predicted immune failure in patients on HAART (AIDS patient Care STDS 19;70, 2005).

Cigarette smoking a risk factor for OC; OR 2.5 in 631 adults (Community Dental Oral Epidemiol 33:35, 2005).

   Pseudomembranous form (thrush) (most common form)
   (58% had CD4 <200)

Small 1-2mm to large white plaques on any mucosal surface. Can be wiped off, leaving erythematous to bleeding base.
Lab: Dx established by KOH prep of scraping & culture.
Oral candidiasis was predictor for TB in Thailand (*J Oral Pathol Med 31:163, 2002*).

   Erythematous form (58% had CD4 <200)

Smooth red patches on soft or hard palate, dorsal tongue &/or buccal mucosa.
Lab: Dx established as above.

   Angular cheilitis (60% had CD4 <200)

Erythematous cracks & fissures at corner of mouth.
Lab: Dx established as above.

   Hyperkeratotic form (candidal leukoplakia)

White lesions on tongue, palate &/or buccal mucosa that cannot be wiped off. Clinically resembles hairy leukoplakia (see below).
Lab: KOH prep of lesion will show fungi.

See pg102 for abbreviations & footnotes

TABLE 11A (18)

CLINICAL SYNDROME, ETIOLOGY, EPIDEMIOLOGY	CLINICAL PRESENTATION, DIAGNOSTIC TESTS, COURSE
Gastrointestinal Tract/Mouth/Oral lesions without soreness (or mild soreness) *(continued)*	
Kaposi's sarcoma (100% had CD4 <200) Oral shedding of HHV-8 (KS-assoc. herpesvirus) found in 22% of 196 HIV+ MSM (*J AIDS* 35:233, 2004), & 32% of 174 HIV+ CSWs in Kenya (*JID* 190:484, 2004) without KS. ↑ HHV-8 VL also found in oral secretions in HIV-pos. & -neg. pts with KS (*AIDS Res Hum Retrovir* 20:704, 2004).	Red to purple macules, papules or nodules, occasionally the same color as adjoining tissue, on tongue, palate or buccal mucosa. Usually asymptomatic but may become painful with ulceration & inflammation (*Oral AIDS 8 (Suppl.2):88, 2002*). Sublingual lesion in HIV+ children in Zimbabwe may be Ranula; biopsy! (*Oral Dis* 10:229, 2004). Lab: biopsy necessary for dx since bacillary angiomatosis also reported (*J Oral Pathol Med* 29:91, 2000).
Hairy leukoplakia (HLP) (66% had CD4 <200) Epstein-Barr virus can be detected by immunochemistry, in situ hybridization or EBV-DNA by PCR in nearly 100% of lesions (*J Oral Pathol Med* 29:-118, 2000; *Am J Clin Pathol* 114:395, 2000). EBV produces both replicative & non-productive infection in tongue epithelial cells from pts with hairy leukoplakia (HLP) (*JID* 190:387, 2004), transcription of specific EBV genes appear to be assoc. with expression of HLP (*JID* 190:396, 2004), & active infection assoc. with ↓ oral epithelial Langerhans cell count, thereby evading local mucosal immune response (*JID* 189-1656, 2004).	Lesions usually asymptomatic. White thickening of oral mucosa &/or lateral tongue margins with vertical folds or corrugations. Lesions range from few mm to covering entire dorsal surface of tongue. ↑ frequency in smokers (*J AIDS* 21:236, 1999). Lab: Biopsy: epithelial hyperplasia with thickened parakeratin layer with hair-like projections & vacuolated prickle cells. Rx: Usually not treated, but can be rx with high-dose acyclovir (*see Table 13, pg146, & Table 12, pg132*). Lesions respond but recur. 10/10 pts responded to one application of topical podophyllin resin within 4-5days; remissions of 2-28wks (*J AIDS* 4:543, 1991).
Warts [human papillomavirus (HPV)] Oral warts may ↑ in size & frequency in response to HAART (*Oral Dis* 8 (Suppl.2):91, 2002). *(AIDS Pt Care STD 18:443, 2004; Am J Med Sci 328:57, 2004).*	Usually asymptomatic. Present as single or multiple papilliform warts with multiple white spike-like projections, or as pink cauliflower-like projections, or as flat lesions resembling focal epithelial hyperplasia. Lab: Biopsy: Types 7, 13 & 32, but usually not 6, 11, 16 & 18 which are associated with anogenital warts. Rx with topical cidofovir gel 1% successful in 1 recalcitrant case (*Cutis* 73:191, 2004).
Secondary syphilis (often multiple) (*Med Oral* 9:33, 2004) Lymphoma	Dx by VDRL &/or biopsy of lesion Lab: Biopsy. May be EBV+ (*Oral Oncol* 38:96, 2002).
Carcinoma, squamous cell	Squamous cell carcinoma of tongue reported in HIV disease. Lab: Biopsy.
Cytomegalovirus (CMV) oral ulcers	A rare manifestation of CMV (*AnIM* 119:924, 1993). Usually with disseminated infection. Lab: Biopsy & immunohistochemistry.
Histoplasmosis, Geotrichosis, Cryptococcosis, Penicillium marneffei. Oral histo was a clue to presence of HIV infection in Brazil (*Oral Surg, Oral Med* 93:654, 2002) & found in 3% of 733 HIV+ pts in Argentina (*J Oral Pathol Med* 33:445, 2004). In endemic areas, think oral leishmaniasis (*Oral Dis* 8:59, 2002).	Rare in occurrence. Lesions painless, clean ulcerations on palate, gingiva & oropharynx. Lab: Biopsy; organism identified on culture & stains.
Sore mouth without discrete lesions	
HIV-associated gingivitis & periodontitis. Common with advanced HIV. Pts at all stages of HIV infection have ↑↑ numbers of PMNs & mast cells throughout the gingiva & ↑↑ cells with ↑ expression of HIV receptors/co-receptors/ α defensins perhaps ↑ susceptibility of HIV infection via oral route (*J Dent Res* 83:371, 2004). Was associated with ↑ aggregations of spirochetes (87%), yeast (65.6%), & "herpes-like viruses" (56%) in 1 study (*J Periodontal Res* 38:147, 2003).	Marked halitosis, spontaneous bleeding & deep-seated gingival pain are usual. Gingiva show fiery red margins with necrosis & ulceration of interdental papillae. May rapidly progress to loss to gingival soft tissue & destruction of supporting bone leading to loss of teeth & necrotizing stomatitis. Is similar to noma (gangrenous stomatitis). Dx based on clinical features. Cultures not helpful. Entamoeba gingivalis has been isolated. ? Significance (*CID* 27:471, 1998). Rx: Start with curettage/debridement, followed by topical povidone-iodine (Betadine) irrigation, then chlorhexidine gluconate (Peridex) mouthwash + oral antibiotics effective against anaerobes (metro-nidazole, clindamycin. AM/CL).

See pg10 for abbreviations & footnotes

TABLE 11A (19)

CLINICAL SYNDROME, ETIOLOGY, EPIDEMIOLOGY	CLINICAL PRESENTATION, DIAGNOSTIC TESTS, COURSE
Gastrointestinal Tract/Mouth *(continued)*	
Oral lesions, painful	
Recurrent aphthous ulcers (RAU)	Recurrent crops of superficial painful ulcers (1mm to 1cm) on non-keratinized oral or oropharyngeal
More common in HIV disease, last longer & produce more painful symptoms than in immunocompetent persons (*Am J Clin Dermatol 4:669, 2003*)	mucosa. Bx: shows only non-specific inflammation Rx: Topical steroids in 50%. Orabase may ↓ pain & swelling. Thalidomide (200mg po q24h x14d), 13/14 pts responded (*CID 20:250, 1995*). In ACTG 251, 14/23 healed with thalidomide rx vs 1/22 on placebo but had significant side-effects (*CID 28:892, 1999*).
Herpes simplex virus (HSV)—See rx, pg134	Recurrent crops of small painful vesicles that ulcerate, usually on palate or gingiva. Usually heal but
HSV-1 most common cause, rarely HSV-2; both can be shed in oral secretions (*Sex Trans Inf 80:272, 2004*)	tend to recur. Herpetic geometric glossitis [extremely tender longitudinal fissures occur, heal with acyclovir IV (*NEJM 329:1859, 1993*)].
	Lab: Smears from lesions reveal multinucleate giant cells, + for HSV on immunofluorescent staining.
Drug-associated lesions	Painful mouth lesions occur in 10-15% of patients on zalcitabine (ddC).
Xerostomia (dry mouth)	Clinical: Dry mouth occurs in 2% of patients on didanosine (ddl).
Sjögren's-like syndrome—may be drug-associated	See Salivary gland enlargement, below. Rx: Saliva substitutes (Orex®, Xero-Lube®, Moi-Stir®, Salivart®) (electrolytes in carboxymethylcellulose base), & nasal spray, may help.
Salivary gland enlargement	Presents as painless (80%) bilateral parotid swelling due to infiltration with CD8 + T lymphocytes.
Benign parotid lymphoepithelial lesions (diffuse infiltrative CD8 lymphocytosis syndrome or DILS)	Submandibular glands not involved. 80% have generalized lymphadenopathy, bilateral cervical. Resembles Sjögren's syndrome with sicca symptoms (dry mouth & eyes). Associated findings may
CD4 counts 200–500/mm³	include lymphocytic interstitial pneumonia (60%), aseptic meningitis. Most black pts were HLA-DR5. In
↑ prevalence in Africans with HIV infection reported (*Arch Path Lab Med 124:1773, 2000*)	contrast to Sjögren's, none had sm anti La/SS-A or anti La/SS-B antibodies, rheumatoid factor usually negative. Dx based on fine needle aspiration. More common in children. All initially responded to radiation but 11/12 relapsed after 5 months.
Other possibilities: CMV (17%), PCP, adenovirus, lymphoma, Kaposi's sarcoma, tuberculosis; 10 cases reported (*J Oral Pathol Med 34: 407, 2005*), MAC, sarcoid.	Uni- or bilateral parotid swelling (*CID 22:369, 1996*). KS present as painless mass in parotid or submandibular region (*Cancer 88:15, 2000*).
Esophagus¹: Esophageal motility disorders common (16/18, 88%) with or without symptoms of dysphagia or odynophagia (*Dig Dis Sci 48:962, 2003*)	
Dysphagia (difficulty swallowing with a sensation of food sticking)	
Candidiasis	X-ray. Barium swallow: typically evidence of plaques & ulceration ('moth-eaten' appearance). Find-
Frequency 50–70%, decline in HAART era (*Am J Gastro100:1455, 2005*)	ings supportive but not diagnostic.
In HIV + pt with new onset dysphagia/odynophagia, especially if oral thrush present, fluconazole 100 mg po q24h x2 weeks in non-responders.—See below (*Dig Dis Sci 45: 1301, 2000; AJM 154:2705, 1994*). Annual incidence of fluconazole-refractory mucosal candidiasis 4.2% (*CID 30:749, 2000*) (See Table 12, pg12). The most common cause of dysphagia in HIV+ patients (45-79% of pts)	Endoscopy: Large yellow-white plaques usually seen throughout the esophagus. Biopsy/brushing: Will show tissue-invasive pseudomycelia. Secondary prophylaxis: Recurrence rates (20–80%) in 45–90days. Fluconazole: dosage not defined; 100 mg po biweekly, 10% recurrence over median of 9mos (*32nd ICAAC Abst 1116:297, 1992*). 150mg po weekly, 42% recurrence over 6mos (*Med J Aust 158:312, 1993*).
Drug-associated	Dysphagia occurs in 2-3% of patients on zalcitabine (ddC).

See pg102 for abbreviations & footnotes

TABLE 11A (20)

CLINICAL SYNDROME, ETIOLOGY, EPIDEMIOLOGY	CLINICAL PRESENTATION, DIAGNOSTIC TESTS, COURSE
Gastrointestinal Tract/Esophagus *(continued)*	
Odynophagia (pain on swallowing) or esophagospasm (retrosternal episodic pain without swallowing)	
Cytomegalovirus (CMV) esophagitis Frequency 5–15% Common 9–13% HIV+ pts.	Symptoms are odynophagia, usually without dysphagia, weight loss. Endoscopy: Large solitary (>10cm² in surface area), shallow, superficial ulcers especially in distal esophagus. (AJM 98:169, 1995). Histology necessary to establish diagnosis. If no inclusions, was aphthous ulcer. Present in 24/74 pts who had failed antifungal rx for odynophagia (AM 101:599, 1996). Rx: Therapeutic trial with ganciclovir in symptomatic pts may be warranted. 27/35 pts responded, relapse rate high, 5/6 non-GCV responders responded to foscarnet (AJM 98:169, 1995). Stricture may occur after healing. Pts present with odynophagia. Differential diagnosis: CMV, HSV, drug-induced ulcers. Found in 25/74 pts who failed antifungal rx for odynophagia (AJM 101:599, 1996).
Idiopathic (aphthous) esophageal ulceration (IEU) Frequency 10–30% In one series, __ pts of esophageal ulcers due to IEU.	Endoscopy: Large discrete ulcers. Rx: Prednisone 40mg po q24h; taper by 10mg/wk, total course 4wks. 11/12 pts responded clinically (AJM 93:131, 1992). Thalidomide (200mg po q24h x14d), 5/5 pts healed or improved, 1 relapsed (CID 20:250, 1995). In a randomized double-blind controlled trial of 200mg/day x4wks, 8/11 had complete healing vs 3/13 placebo (p <0.03). Side effects: 4 somnolence, 2 rash, 2 peripheral neuropathy (JID 180:61, 1999).
Herpes simplex virus (HSV) esophagitis Frequency 5–10%	Clinical: Acute onset, intense pain, widespread involvement. May be associated with oral herpes (AIDS Clin Care 7:2, 1995). Median CD4 15/mm³ (CID 22:926, 1996). Endoscopy: Shallow erosive ulcers (like reflux esophagitis) Rx: Acyclovir
Esophageal ulcers associated with acute HIV infection	Clinical: Acute retroviral syndrome (fever, myalgia, maculopapular rash) (pg56) + odynophagia or dysphagia. Lesions heal spontaneously. Pts are not predisposed to recurrent esophageal ulceration. Endoscopy: One or more discrete ulcers. On biopsy: retroviral virions. Rx: Viscous lidocaine may ↓ symptoms.
Lymphoma, Kaposi's sarcoma, squamous cell carcinoma, histoplasmosis	Clinical: Occur occasionally in esophagus in HIV (South Med J 97:383, 2004).
Stomach: nausea, vomiting, early satiety, hematemesis, melena;	
Gastritis 2° to Helicobacter pylori Dig Dis 49:1836, 2004	Gastritis more severe in 102 HIV+ pts with H. pylori than 107 HIV-neg. (p <0.0001). CD4 counts higher in H. pylori pts with HIV than those without H. pylori (p <0.0001). Usually asymptomatic, occasional hematemesis.
Kaposi's sarcoma (KS) Occurs in 40% of patients with cutaneous or nodal KS.	Endoscopy: Submucosal reddish nodules with intact overlying mucosa. Biopsy necessary to confirm dx but many lesions (3/4) cannot be biopsied because of submucosal location & limited depth of endoscopic biopsies. Assoc. with phlegmonous gastritis from Gp A strep in 1 case (A Pathol Lab Med 128:801, 2004). May produce obstructed gastric outlet syndrome or hemorrhage (hematemesis, melena). In HIV lymphomas often multifocal with disease throughout abdomen.
Lymphoma J Clin Oncol 22:4227, 2004	**X-ray: Larger masses often show 'target lesions' with central umbilicated ulcerations.** Endoscopy: Mass lesions, biopsy.
Cytomegalovirus (CMV) gastritis Drug-induced abdominal pain	Endoscopy: See CMV esophagitis above, lesions are similar. Consider antiretroviral drugs as the cause: zidovudine (500mg/day, dyspepsia 6%), didanosine (250mg q12h, abdominal pain 7%), zalcitabine (0.75mg q8h, abdominal pain 3%), foscarnet (60mg/kg IV q8h, abdominal pain 16%); drugs for opportunistic infection: TMP/SMX, ketoconazole, fluconazole, pentamidine, other drugs, especially NSAIDs.

See pg102 for abbreviations & footnotes

TABLE 11A (21)

CLINICAL SYNDROME, ETIOLOGY, EPIDEMIOLOGY	CLINICAL PRESENTATION, DIAGNOSTIC TESTS, COURSE
Gastrointestinal Tract/Stomach (continued)	
Leishmaniasis (stomach, duodenum)	Dysphagia, odynophagia, epigastric & abdominal pain, diarrhea, GI bleeding reported in AIDS pts with CD4 <100/mm³ in endemic areas (CID 19:49, 1994).
– Gastric ulcers caused by Strongyloides stercoralis reported in HIV+ pts (Dig Liver Dis 36:760, 2004).	
– Gastric ulcers/nodules caused by bacillary angiomatosis producing bacteremias reported (Int J Surg Path 11:241, 2003).	
Abdominal pain, acute onset (J Emerg Med 23:111, 2002)	APACHE II criteria best predicted outcome in severe cases—accuracy 75% (Glasgow 69%, Ranson 48%); similar to pancreatitis in non-HIV infected populations (Am J Gastro 98:1278, 2003).
Pancreatitis. (See pg97)	
• Drug-associated most common (46%), e.g., didanosine, pentamidine; lamivudine (3TC) in children	
• Infection common (90%) in 109 postmortem on AIDS pts in Brazil: mycobacterium 22%, toxoplasmosis 13%, CMV 9%, Pneumocystis jiroveci (carinii) 9%, & HIV p24 antigen in macrophages 2%—all had normal serum amylase premortem (AIDS 14:1879, 2000).	
Bowel perforation/peritonitis	AIDS pts with perforation usually febrile, with rigid abdomen, rebound tenderness. Perforations most common in large bowel. Also lymphoma, typhlitis, KS, tuberculosis, salmonellosis (Emerg Med Clin NA 7:575, 1989).
Most common cause is CMV in advanced HIV infection	Immune reconstitution from HAART assoc with perforation of ileocecal TB (Dis Col Rect 15:977, 2002).
Small bowel disease: cramping paraumbilical abdominal pain, weight loss, large volume diarrhea	
Diarrhea	toxin. If above negative, consider endoscopy of colon & small bowel for treatable causes such as CMV, MAC, KS, lymphoma (Rev Gastroenterol Disord 2:176, 2002). The frequency of chronic diarrhea is ↓ in pts receiving HAART (Am J Gastro 94:3553, 1999); however, these antiretroviral drugs themselves have become a common cause of diarrhea (CID 28:701, 1999; Epidemiol 128:73, 2002; CID 39:717, 2004) & reduce the quality of life (Qual Life Res 13:243, 2004). In Brazil, diarrhea
Diarrhea occurs in 30–96.6% (after 3yrs) of U.S. & Euro. HIV+ pts & approx. 90% in developing countries (AIM 151:1567, 1991). Have diarrhea ... with ↓ CD4 (J AIDS 20:154, 1999). AIDS-defining diarrhea persists for >5 days, evaluation should include microscopic exam of stool (wet mount for Isospora & E. histolytica, modified acid-fast stain for cryptosporidia & cyclospora, modified trichrome for microsporidia, cultures for routine pathogens & C. difficile	
	& wasting were associated with ↓ serum levels of d4T & ZDV. Most common causes of diarrhea were cryptosporidium & Isospora belli (Braz J Inf Dis 7:16, 2003). Glutamine & alanyl-glutamine & ↑ ARV drug levels (CID 38:1764, 2004). But saquinavir (hardgel) absorption (AUC serum level) actually ↑ in pts with diarrhea &/or wasting (AAC 48:538, 2004).

Acute infectious diarrhea¹ (for specific treatment, see Table 12) [Major site of infection may be small bowel or colon) (Gastro Clin N.A. 26:259, 1997] Mean annual incidence of bacterial diarrhea, 7.2 cases per 1000 person-yrs in 9 major US cities from 1992-2002 (CID 41:1621, 2005)

Agent	Prevalence/CD4 Stage	Clinical Features	Diagnostic Clues/Comments
Campylobacter jejuni, C. coli, C. upsaliensis (Emerg Inf Dis 8:237, 2002)	4–15% (isolated from 7/43 pts with diarrhea, CID 24:1107, 1997) & was most common bacterial pathogen (20%) isolated from HIV+ pts in South African study (J Health Popul Nutr 20: 230, 2002). Any CD4	Watery or bloody diarrhea, fever, ± fecal WBC	Stool culture, most labs cannot detect C. cinaedi, C. fennelli, ↓ sensitivity using membrane filter technique on non-selective blood agar.
Clostridium difficile	4.1 cases per 1000 person-years **Most common cause of bacterial diarrhea among persons infected with HIV** (CID 41:1621, 2005) Any CD4	Watery diarrhea, fecal WBC, fever, leucocytosis, cramps, hypoalbuminemia, disease spectrum: nuisance diarrhea, colitis, megacolon. Endoscopy usually shows pseudo-membranous colitis but may be normal. C difficile toxin usually positive. CT scan shows colitis with thickened mucosa. May present with leukemoid reaction (South Med J 97:388, 2004).	Antibiotic exposure: most common—cephalosporins, clindamycin, ampicillin; rare—TMP/SMX, ZDV, albendazole, rifampin

See pg102 for abbreviations & footnotes

TABLE 11A (22)

Agent	Prevalence/CD4 Stage	Clinical Features	Diagnostic Clues/Comments
Enteric viruses: Rota, adeno, corona, astro, picobirna, & calicivirus *(Molecular Med Today 6:483, 2000)*	4-15% Any CD4	Acute diarrhea but 1/3 become chronic. Adenovirus isolated in 16% of pts with diarrhea & associated with ↑ mortality in 1 study *(J Med Virol 58:280, 1999)*	Stool electron microscopy: detection of viral particles has limited value because viruses produce a self-limiting infection & are untreatable *(J AIDS & HR 13:33, 1996)*
Enteroadherent E. coli Enteroaggregative E. coli & entero-invasive E. coli also found more commonly in HIV pts with diarrhea than those without in Senegal *(p = 0.00001) (JID 189: 75,2004)*	10-20%. Common cause of diarrhea in Central African Republic & in19% of pts in Senegal *(J Clin Micro 40:3086, 2002; Int J Inf Dis 5:192, 2001).* Any CD4, mean 26	Watery diarrhea, weight loss, ↓ D-xylose absorption, acute but may be chronic, usually in right colon, most pts on TMP/SMX prophylaxis	Adherence to Hep-2 cells (research labs only). Cytotoxic phenotypes assoc. with diarrhea in AIDS pts *(Trans R Soc Med Hyg 97:523, 2003).*
Idiopathic	25-40%. Variable CD4. Non-infectious causes, rule out drugs, diet, inflammatory bowel disease, anxiety, food poisoning		Negative studies include culture, ova & parasites, C. difficile toxin assay. Lacto-bacillus no better than placebo in controlling diarrhea in placebo-controlled crossover study *(HIV Clin Trials 5:183, 2004).*
Salmonella S. enteritidis S. typhimurium	5-15% 100x when compared to general population, any CD4 count, more common with lower CD4	Watery diarrhea, fever, ± fecal WBC	Blood culture, stool culture (sensitivity approx. 90%)
Shigella	2% Any CD4	Watery or bloody diarrhea, fever, fecal WBC	Stool culture

Certain parasites may also cause acute diarrhea including Isospora belli & Entamoeba histolytica/dispar *(Int J STD AIDS 14:487, 2003) (see below & next page)*

Chronic infectious diarrhea 10% of pts with CD4 <200/μl—unchanged with HAART but with change in etiology. ↓ OI (53 to 13%) & ↑ non-infectious causes (30 to 70%) *(Am J Gastro 95:3142, 2004).* A 2-wk course of albendazole given to 153 HIV+ pts with chronic diarrhea in Zambia resulted in 60% complete or partial response & cleared parasites in 46% of those pos. (cryptosporidium 7%, isospora 37%, & microsporidium 16%) *(Aliment Pharm Ther 16:592, 2002).* TMP/SMX ↓ mortality & diarrhea episodes in 509 HIV+ individuals in Uganda *(Lancet 364:1428, 2004).*

Cryptosporidia See *NEJM 346:1723, 2002 & CID 36: 903, 2003).* Appear to be spread sexually between men who have sex with men *(Sex Trans Inf 79:412, 2003).* Most frequent cause of diarrhea in HIV+ pts in Peru *(JID 191:4, 2004).*	13-20% *(E Afr Med J 80:398, 2003)* CD4 <150	Entoritis, watery diarrhea, noninflammatory diarrhea (fecal WBC neg.), afebrile, malabsorption, wasting, large stool volume with abdominal pain, remitting symptoms for months, years	Water-borne, low infectious dose, in healthy adults only 132 oocysts *(NEJM 332:855, 1995).* AFB smear of stool to show **oocyst 4-6 μm**. In pts with CD4 >180/mm³, C. parvum cleared spontaneously in 7-28days; with CD4 <180, 87% persisted. Rx with HAART was associated with clearance of or-ganism from stools except when oocyst-positive *(5th Conf Retrovir & OIs 1998, Abst 480).* Nitazoxanide effective in Zambian children who were HIV-neg. **but not in HIV+** *(Ln 360:1375, 2002).* Rx: See Table 12
Cyclospora cayetanensis	US <1%, Haiti 11% CD4 <100	Enteritis, watery diarrhea, up to 18x q24h for 10mos. *(World J Gastro 10:1844, 2004).*	AFB smear: **oocyte 8-10 μm**, resem-bles cryptosporidia *(CID 23:429, 1996; NEJM 328:1308, 1993; AnIM 121: 654, 1994)*

See pg102 for abbreviations & footnotes

TABLE 11A (23)

Gastrointestinal Tract/Chronic Infectious Diarrhea *(continued)*			
Agent	**Prevalence/CD4 Stage**	**Clinical Features**	**Diagnostic Clues/Comments**
Cytomegalovirus (CMV)	13-20%, CD4 <100	Fever, fecal WBC, ± blood, enteritis, colitis, perforation with toxic megacolon, solitary rectal ulcer, small bowel mass. Most common cause of GI bleeding (AIDS Pt Care 13:343, 1999). Bleeding may be massive & assoc. with focal ischemia (AIDS Pt Care STD 18:497, 2004).	Sigmoidoscopy with rectal biopsy (best initial invasive test), 10-30% of CMV colitis will affect only right side, further steps include colonoscopy with small bowel biopsy, CT segmental lesions or pancolitis. Failure of ganciclovir rx may be due to drug resistance mutations (J Gastro 138:643, 2003). Rx: See Table 12
Entamoeba histolytica	1-3%. Infection in HIV+ women in Tanzania assoc. with ↓ birth weight in neonate (Curr Int Dis Rep 4:124, 2002). Any CD4 count	Colitis, bloody stool, cramps, pos. fecal WBC, most are asymptomatic carriers (AIDS 13:2431, 1999). Course may be protracted (J Clin Gastro 33:64, 2001)	Travel history (Latin America, SE Asia). Stool ova & parasites. Was overdiagnosed by microscopy when compared to DNA amplification: 91/232 pos. with only 21/91 confirmed (Trans R Soc Trop Med Hyg 97:309, 2003).
Giardia	1-5%. ↑ isolation from HIV-neg. pts in Bahia, Brazil *(Braz J Inf Dis 5:339, 2001).* Any CD4 count	Enteritis, watery diarrhea, flatulence, bloating, malabsorption	History of drinking mountain stream water. Stool ova & parasites.
Idiopathic	More common with lower CD4 (<200)	Watery diarrhea, malabsorption, no fecal WBC	Biopsy shows villous atrophy, crypt hyperplasia, no identifiable cause despite endoscopy with biopsy & electron microscopy for microsporidia
Isospora belli	U.S. 1.5%, developing countries 10 - 12%. Caused diarrhea in 17% of 94 Indian HIV+ pts (Natl Med J India 15:72, 2002), 14/107 in Malawi (E Afr Med J 80:398, 2003). CD4 <100	Enteritis, watery diarrhea, wasting, noninflammatory diarrhea (no fecal WBC), no fever	Food/water-borne infection spores 1-2 μm. AFB stool smear: oocytes 20-30 μm
Microsporidia Septata intestinalis Enterocytozoon bieneusi hellum	20% CD4 <50 HIV pts more susceptible to clinical disease (JID 180:2003, 1999). Isolated from HIV+ Thai children & 17.4% of Ugandan children (SE Asian J Trop Med Pub Health 33:241, 2002; Ann J Trop Med Hyg 67:299, 2002).	Enteritis, watery diarrhea, noninflammatory diarrhea (fecal WBC neg.). Fever is uncommon, remitting disease over years, malabsorption, wasting common. Pts improve with response to HAART. May disseminate detected in urine & may respond to albendazole (8/12 bu 2) (HIV Med 1:155, 2000). Rx with furinagilin 60mg po q24h x2wks cleared stool in 6/6 vs 0/6 placebo, ↑ absorption of D-xylose & ↓ diarrhea, 3/6 had side-effects (NEJM 346:1963, 2002)	Food/water-borne infection spores 1-2 μm, fluorescence with calcofluor (excellent screening test), confirmation with Giemsa stain. Special trichrome stain also diagnostic. Complications: disseminated disease, biliary disease.
Mycobacterium avium (cause & effect for diarrhea not always clear)	10% CD4 <50	Enteritis, watery diarrhea, no fecal WBC, common fever & wasting, diffuse abdominal pain in late stage	Stool culture unreliable, colonization may occur without diarrhea. Diagnosis: positive blood cultures, biopsy may show changes like Whipple's disease, hepatosplenomegaly, adenopathy, thickened small bowel
Small bowel bacterial overgrowth		Watery diarrhea, malabsorption, wasting, often associated with hypochloridia.	Hydrogen breath test, culture of small bowel aspirate

See pg102 for abbreviations & footnotes

TABLE 11A (2)

CLINICAL SYNDROME, ETIOLOGY, EPIDEMIOLOGY	CLINICAL PRESENTATION, DIAGNOSTIC TESTS, COURSE
Gastrointestinal Tract (*continued*)	
Diarrhea due to alternative mechanisms (↑ to 70% with HAART)	Considerations. HIV disease per se, autonomic denervation, Crohn's disease, pancreatic insufficiency (*HIV Med 1:33, 2005*), overgrowth of normal microbial bowel flora, & antiretroviral drugs (may now be most common cause). Rx of latter: d/c or some success reported with oat bran, psyllium, loperamide, $CaCO_3$, Sp303, & pancrelipase (*CID 30:908, 2000*).
Typhlitis (acute cecitis, inflammation of cecum)	Clinically resembles acute appendicitis, but involves the cecum, which is ulcerated, edematous, necrotic. Associated with *Clostridium septicum* & *Pseudomonas aeruginosa* (*AnIM 116:998, 1992*). Can be a manifestation of C. difficile. Consider especially in severely neutropenic patients.
Colorectal disease: left lower quadrant &/or suprapubic cramping, rectal urgency (tenesmus), frequent small volume stools, occasional proctalgia & dyschezia (painful defecation)	
Drug-associated diarrhea (*CID 28:701, 1999*)	See adverse effects. *Tables 6B & 13*. **Diarrhea is a common complication of rx with antimicrobial agents (including antiretroviral agents).** May be a direct effect of drug on GI motility (macrolides), overgrowth of GI flora (clinda), C. difficile.
Infectious agents (as above)	Adenovirus has been found on biopsy & easily overlooked, may be assoc. with symptoms (*Arch Path Lab Med 125:1042, 2001*).
Idiopathic (aphthous) proctitis	Endoscopy—large, discrete ulcers. Biopsy to exclude other causes. Thalidomide (200mg po q24h x21d), improvement in 2/2 pts (*CID 20:250, 1995*). See *Table 12, pg136*.
Cytomegalovirus (CMV)	Endoscopy—focal ischemic colitis with submucosal hemorrhages & discrete shallow ulcers in distal colonic mucosa. Ganciclovir is effective in most patients. Rx: See *Table 12*
Herpes simplex virus (HSV) Types 1 & 2	Painful recurrent small to persistent progressive large necrotizing ulcers in perirectal area. Emergence of acyclovir-resistant strains on rx is common. Lab: Smears from lesions reveal multinucleate giant cells, + for HSV on immunofluorescent staining.
Mycobacterium tuberculosis	Tuberculosis in ileocecal area & colon may be seen in HIV patients without evidence of pulmonary TBc on chest x-ray. 14% of diarrhea caused by TBc in India (*CID 23:482, 1996*). Immune reconstitution from HAART assoc. with perforation of ileocecal TB (*Dis Col Rect 15:977, 2002*).
Other considerations: idiopathic inflammatory bowel disease (ulcerative colitis)	Kaposi's sarcoma may be confined to the rectum & present as hemorrhagic rectocolitis (*Clin Imaging 28:33, 2004*).
Kaposi's sarcoma, lymphoma, epidermoid carcinoma & other neoplasms	Lab: Numerous PMNs on smear of exudate. Specific diagnosis depends on laboratory studies.
Proctitis	Empiric rx for GC & chlamydia recommended but should also consider herpes & lues (*CID 38:300, 2004*).
Neisseria gonorrhoeae	
Herpes simplex virus	
Syphilis, primary or secondary	
Lymphogranuloma venereum (LGV)	
Chlamydia trachomatis (non-LGV immunotypes)	
Human papillomaviruses	
Cytomegalovirus	
Enteric pathogens, e.g., Shigella, Entamoeba histolytica, Campylobacter	

See pg102 for abbreviations & footnotes

TABLE 11A (25)

CLINICAL SYNDROME, ETIOLOGY, EPIDEMIOLOGY	CLINICAL PRESENTATION, DIAGNOSTIC TESTS, COURSE
Genital Tract: acute sexually transmitted diseases associated with ↑ HIV viral load (*JID 182:459, 2000*)	
Anogenital warts (Condylomata acuminatum) (*see CID 35:439, 2002*)	Soft, moist, pink or red swellings that grow rapidly. Usually several in same area & look like cauliflower.
Genital warts [human papillomavirus (HPV) types 6, 11, 16 & 18]. The most common STD in the U.S. in 1998; present in 30/481 HIV+ women in New York City (*Ln 359:108, 2002*). Anal warts assoc. with HPV with abn cytology; surprisingly common in sexually active U.S. adolescents (*AIDS 17:311, 2003*).	Identified clinically. Exclude condyloma lata of secondary syphilis. If atypical or persistent, biopsy to exclude carcinoma. Women with cervical warts should not be treated until result of Pap smear available. Correlation between Pap smear & colposcopy good in 189 HIV+ women (*CID 42:662, 2006*)
Secondary syphilis, condyloma lata	Rx: **Podophyllin or podofilox** (*See Table 12, pg135*).
Carcinoma	May be missed on Pap smear, colposcopy better (*Ob Gyn 78:84, 1991*). Cervical cancer: HIV-infected
Cervical dysplasia (*See NEJM 348:518, 2003*)	& are more likely to have advanced disease (*J AIDS & HR 18:241, 1998*) (*see Table 8A*) & is the most common cause of sexually-transmitted disease-related deaths in women. The prevalence of
Cervical intraepithelial neoplasia (CIN) associated with human papillomavirus (type 16, 18, or 31 in 80-90%).	cervical intra-epithelial lesions in HIV-infected persons is reduced with HAART (*AIDS 12:459, 1998*)
In one study 14/35 HIV+ had intraepithelial lesions vs 3/32 HIV− women (*J AIDS 3:896, 1990*).	**Intravaginal 5-fluorouracil (5-FU) cream** (2%) applied biweekly for 6mos in HIV+ pts with CIN after standard surgery for high-grade lesions reduced recurrence rate 28% vs 47% in placebo, # with recurrence of advanced disease 8% vs 31% (p = 0.01) & time to recurrence of CIN (p = 0.04). Toxicity was minimal (*Ob Gyn 94:954, 1999*).
Chancroid (Haemophilus ducreyi) Culture from edge of lesion or bubo on medium supplemented with patient's own serum	Genital ulcers are exquisitely tender. Usually associated with suppuration of inguinal nodes. Upon exposure to HIV+ contact, HIV seroconversion occurred in 2.9% of men with genital ulcers vs 1.0% in those without ulcers (*ArIM 119:1181, 1993*). Rx failure with either ciprofloxacin (single dose) or erythromycin (x1wk) was 3x greater in HIV+ pts but equal for Rx groups (*JID 180:1886, 1999*).
See **Primary syphilis**	Rx: See *Table 12, pg106*.
Genital herpes simplex (HSV) [usually type 2, but may be type 1 (~5% but especially in developing countries) (*Sex Trans Infect 75:377, 1999*)]. Associated with ↑ HIV transmission from men → women (*AIDS 16:451, 2002*). Transmission of HSV-2 can be significantly ↓ between discordant couples by treating the infected partner with once-daily suppressive rx with valacyclovir (*NEJM 350:11, 2004*).	Small painful vesicles, usually in clusters. Ulcerate & may coalesce into large lesions. Inguinal nodes usually slightly enlarged & tender. Usually heal in 10-20 days without scarring. In AIDS pt, recurrent genital lesions may require continuous antiviral rx to prevent spreading, disabling & atypical lesions. In a prospective study of 72 women with HSV-2 pos. in 29% of pos., there was no apparent genital lesion, cultures were more common HSV2 pos. in 29% of pos., there was no apparent genital lesion, cultures were more common in advanced HIV infection. Acyclovir resistance is common: 12/226 (5.3%) in survey of 14 U.S. cities.
See **Primary syphilis below**	Rx: See *Table 12, pg134*. HIV can be consistently isolated from active ulcers (*JAMA 280:61, 1998*).
Genital ulcers, general Etiology varies according to geographical area (*Sex Trans Dis 26:55, 1999*), % from a series of 158 patients from Jamaica (*CID 28:1086, 1999*) & 143 pts from Mississippi (*JID 178:1060, 1998*): Herpes simplex 52-31%, Hemophilus ducreyi 23-39%, Treponema pallidum 10-19%, lymphogranuloma venereum 6%, mixed infection 8%, idiopathic "aphthous-like" Prevalence of H simplex as cause of GUD increased from 23% in 1993 to 58% in 2002 in Botswana (*CID 41:1304, 2005*).	Various multiplex polymerase chain reaction (M-PCR) tests now available for HSV, H. ducreyi & T. pallidum. See individual organisms for dx tests, etc. Presence of GUD at time of primary infection with HIV-1 appears to be associated with ↑ rate of rise of HIV viral load (*JID 189:303, 2004*).
Gonorrhea (urethritis, cervicitis) Rectal gonorrhea (↑ in gay men in San Francisco): Rates in 1997—40/100,000, up from 20/100,000 in 1993 & similar to pre-1980. ↑ rate follows ↓ in condom use.	Spontaneous purulent discharge. Lab: Urethral smear usually shows >95% PMNs. 50% of patients with gonorrhea have concomitant C. trachomatis. Urethritis assoc. with ↓ HIV shedding (*AIDS 15:105, 2001*). Urethritis assoc. with ↑ seminal HIV RNA but was ↓ on HAART (*AIDS 16:219, 2002*)
	Rx: See *Table 12, pg113*

See pg102 for abbreviations & footnotes

TABLE 11A (26)

CLINICAL SYNDROME, ETIOLOGY, EPIDEMIOLOGY	CLINICAL PRESENTATION, DIAGNOSTIC TESTS, COURSE
Genital Tract (continued)	
Granuloma inguinale (Calymmatobacterium granulomatis) See *primary syphilis*. Rare in the U.S.	Initially a painless red nodule which slowly increases in size & ulcerates. No associated lymphadenopathy. Lab: Giemsa stain of scraping. Donovan bodies, intracytoplasmic bacilli in macrophages. *Rx: See Table 12, pg106*
Idiopathic genital ulcers: "Aphthous-like" *(J AIDS & Human Retro 13:343, 1996)*	Painful, shallow ulcers with negative workup including bx for syphilis & herpes simplex. 37% had coexistent oral ulcers & 19% of genital ulcers progressed to fistula formation. Rx: Most responded to topical, intralesional or systemic steroids.
Lymphogranuloma venereum (LGV)—caused by Chlamydia trachomatis "Viral syndromes", influenza (predominance of constitutional symptoms) Ulcerative proctitis. Maybe on ↑ with recent outbreak in The Netherlands *(CID 39:996, 2004).*	Small, transient non-indurated vesicular lesion which heals quickly & may be unrecognized. 1st symptom usually unilateral tender enlargement of inguinal nodes (avoid biopsy—may fistulate) which progresses to inflammation of overlying skin, multiple sinuses. Constitutional symptoms: fever, malaise, headache, joint pains are common. If rectum involved, bloody purulent rectal discharge (see *MMWR 53:986, 2004)*. HIV + proctoscopic findings & WBCs in anorectal smear were predictive of LGV in MSM (CID 42:186, 2006). *Rx: Table 12, pg106*
Non-gonococcal urethritis, cervicitis Non-gonococcal urethritis: C. trachomatis (50%), other known causes (10–15%); Ureaplasma urealyticum. In women: Herpes simplex virus, trichomoniasis, candidiasis. Hormonal contraception ↑ risk of C. trachomatis in HIV+ women in Kenya *(AIDS 18:2179, 2004).* Pediculosis pubis (Phthirus pubis) (crabs)	Urethral discharge usually not spontaneous (no "drip"), thin, watery in character. Milk urethra or exam 1st morning void before voiding or exam urethral smear usually shows >80% PMNs + epithelial cells. Pos. fluorescent antibody (FA) test vs. C. trachomatis. Rapid EIA tests have sensitivity of only 52–74% (do not warrant widescale use) *(JAMA 273:9, 1995).* New NA-amplified test on urine, 90–95% sensitive, 98–99% specific *(J Clin Microbiol 36:391 & 3220, 1998).* 6–10% of ureaplasma are resistant to tetracycline (doxycycline). Itching in anogenital region. Scrotal dermatitis (excoriation) usually present. Ova (nits) attach to the skin at the base of the hairs. Minute brown spots on undergarments (louse excreta) may be seen.
Reiter's syndrome (See *Musculoskeletal System, pg95*) Salpingitis-pelvic inflammatory disease (PID), salpingitis, tuboovarian abscess Pelvic inflammatory disease: gonococcus, chlamydia, anaerobes (Bacteroides fragilis & other species). Enterobacteriaceae, streptococci (especially Group B).	PID is more serious in HIV+ women (7–17% require hospitalization). Indications for hospitalization: compliance as an outpatient unlikely, pregnant, peritonitis, suspected pelvic (tuboovarian) abscess, diagnosis uncertain. Need for laparoscopy to clarify diagnosis, failure to respond on outpatient rx in 72hr. Isolation of Trichomonas vaginalis from lower genital tract ↑ risk of PID (p = 0.002) *(CID 34:519, 2002).*
Scabies (Sarcoptes scabei) ("Norwegian scabies") *(See Skin, pg99)* **Syphilis**. *(MMWR 53:575, 2004)* Syphilis cases ↑ 6-fold in the U.K. *(Sex Trans Inf 80:159, 2004)* & around the world. Tracts with HCV & HIV in IVDU populations world wide (Addiction 101:252, 2006)	
[Syphilis in the HIV + pt has been described with fulminant presentations, irregular serologic findings, rapid progression, irregular serologic findings *(Dermatol 198:362, 1999)*, & failure of standard penicillin therapy. Yet others have reported that HIV has not altered clinical syphilis *(AnM 118:350, 1993).* Uveitis, retinitis more likely in HIV. The serological response is less predictable to penicillin rx & while clinical relapses appear to be rare, serologically defined rx failures were higher in HIV+ pts for primary: 17% vs 6% for HIV-neg, at 3 mos. & 14% vs 8% at 12 mos.; & secondary syphilis 36% vs 15% at 3 mos. vs 8% at 12 mos. of 563 pts. Current recommendations for rx syphilis appear to be adequate *(NEJM 337:307, 1998).* Asymptomatic syphilis most common presentation of new HIV + cases in UK (Sex Transm Infect 81:217, 2005)	
Primary syphilis (chancre): other etiologies that cause ulcerative lesions—herpes, chancroid, scabies, granuloma inguinale, trauma. Uncommon: tuberculous ulceration, Behget's, CMV. Drug reaction: foscarnet. Idiopathic (aphthous) genital ulcers reported in women: 1/2 had similar lesions in mouth *(J AIDS & HR 13:343, 1996).*	Syphilitic chancre not exclusively tender. Dual infections, syphilis & herpes, not uncommon. All genital ulcers should be considered syphilitic until proven otherwise. Lab: RPR does not become + until 3–6wks after initial infection. An early negative test does not exclude syphilis. If negative, repeat at 6wks. The FTA/ABS becomes + at 3–4wks. *Rx: Table 12, pg116.* Acute infection ↑ VL & ↓ CD4 counts *(AIDS 18:2075, 2004).*

See pg102 for abbreviations & footnotes

TABLE 11A (27)

CLINICAL SYNDROME, ETIOLOGY, EPIDEMIOLOGY	CLINICAL PRESENTATION, DIAGNOSTIC TESTS, COURSE
Genital Tract/Syphilis *(continued)*	
Secondary syphilis: Can mimic most skin diseases. Common misdiagnoses include: drug-induced eruption, rubella, infectious mononucleosis, fungal infection, acute HIV. Condyloma lata confused with warts. Alopecia areata, scalp lesions resembling ringworm. (*Cutis* 76;361, 2005)	Usually associated with generalized lymphadenopathy. Patient often febrile. May show findings of hepatitis &/or nephritis. Ulceronodular syph with vesicular lesions (Lues Maligna) reported (*CID* 20:387, 1995). 10 cases of multiple excavating pulmonary nodules in HIV infected individuals reported (*CID* 42;e11, 2006). Lab: Positive darkfield. The RPR & FTA/ABS virtually always positive. In pts with suggestive clinical findings & non-reactive RPR or VDRL, dilute serum to exclude possible prozone phenomenon (*ArIM* 153:2496, 1993). Biological false-positive VDRL 4–6% in HIV+ vs 0.2–0.8% in HIV–, but in some (5%), BFP proved to be true pos. active syphilis (*JID* 176:1397, 1997). Treatment requires close follow up. monitoring & adequate compliance (Expert Opin Pharmacother 6:2271, 2005).
Latent [early, <1yr duration; late, >1yr duration); indeterminate; neurosyphilis	The dx of neurosyphilis in HIV+ individuals is problematic. All HIV+ pts with or without neurologic symptoms, or individuals with serum FTA/ABS antibody titer ≥1:32, or individuals who will not be rx with penicillin should have an LP. *See Table 12, pg716. (MMWR 42:(RR-14) 39, 1993).* In 5x neurosyphilis, CSF VDRL is usually pos.; however, false-negative tests have been reported, so neg. VDRL on CSF does not rule out neurosyphilis. May revert to pos. after penicillin rx. Pts with reactive serum RPR & FTA/ABS (or VDRL & MHA-TP) & CSF pleocytosis or ↑ protein are considered to have presumptive neurosyphilis. But in HIV+ individuals with no evidence of syphilis, 30% have CSF pleocytosis or ↑ protein (*CID* 18:288, 1994; *Indian J Med Res* 122:249, 2005). Therefore, if rx based on pleocytosis or ↑ protein alone, many pts without syphilis will be treated (*for rx issues, see Table 12, pg116*). 33% of pts with HIV & neurosyphilis present with early neurosyphilis syndrome (*JID* 177:931, 1998).
Vaginitis	
Candidiasis	Candida vaginitis, recurrent &/or refractory, initial symptom of HIV infection in about 1/4 of women (*AJM* 89:142, 1990). Pruritus, thick cheesy discharge, pH 4.5, hyphae on KOH prep.
Trichomoniasis	Copious foamy discharge, pH 5–7. T. vaginalis on isotonic saline prep.
Bacterial vaginosis, caused by complex vaginal bacterial flora (*NEJM* 353:18, 2005)	Malodorous discharge; pH 5–6. wet prep shows cells covered with organisms 'clue' cells. Fishy odor when secretions rx with KOH.
Heart Incidence of cardiovascular disease specifically related to HIV is low (pericarditis & pulmonary hypertension most common) (*Review in ArIM 160:602, 2000*) but ↑ during HAART era (*Am.J Cardiovasc Drugs 4:315, 2004*).	Usually asymptomatic (↑ cardiac silhouette on CXR), may have chest pain, rub.
Pericarditis/Pericardial effusion Effusion found in 20–40% of 181 HIV-infected pts, 15% moderate to severe; ↑ risk in pts with advanced HIV, heart failure, TB, KS, other pulmonary infections (*Chest 115:418, 1999*). Etiology: Infection—viral (CMV, HSV), fungal (crypto, histo), HIV, **TB [37%, by far most common cause in Africa** (*Cardiovasc J S Afr 14:231, 2003*)], & various bacteria (S. aureus, pneumococci, nocardia, listeria, rhodococcus). Less common: chlamydia, HIV, myco-bacteria), tumor, Kaposi's sarcoma, lymphoma & leishmaniasis (*Scand J Inf Dis 34:151, 2002*) (*for TB rx, see Heart 84:183, 2000*) In 185 pts reported with tamponade, etiology: **Mycobacterium in 78%**, bacteria in 11% (S. aureus, streptococci, pseudomonas, listeria, klebsiella, & rhodococcus), lymphoma in 8%, KS in 7%. Less common pathogens were crypto, nocardia, aspergillus, CMV, HSV. In 26%, no cause found (*Angio 54:469, 2003*). *See pg102 for abbreviations & footnotes*	For tamponade, most common symptom may be dyspnea followed by fever, cough, chest pain & cardiac arrest (*Angio 54:469, 2003*). Pericardial effusion is sign of poor prognosis (6 mos. mortality 34–64%) (*Circ 92:2229, 1995*). Echocardiogram: Pericardial effusion in 30–38%. Value of corticosteroids for the pericarditis in HIV pts promising but not proven (*QJM 96:593, 2003*).

TABLE 11A (28)

CLINICAL SYNDROME, ETIOLOGY, EPIDEMIOLOGY	CLINICAL PRESENTATION, DIAGNOSTIC TESTS, COURSE
Heart (continued)	
Primary pulmonary hypertension Estimated incidence 0.5–2% (CID 39:1549, 2004) Etiology: Seems to be related to chronic HIV infection in most cases (83%) but not to CD4 count or to of pulmonary infections (Mayo Clin Proc 73:37, 1998). HIV itself was not found in endothelial cells by PCR but 2 HIV proteins, GP 120 which stimulates endothelin-1 & TNFα production & fat in combination with TNF, activate endothelial cells to release EGF & other growth factors. These cascades may explain the pulmonary vascular pathology (Chest 118:1136, 2000). HSV-8 was found in 10/18 lung specimens in non-HIV infected pts with sporadic primary hypertension (NEJM 349:1113, 2003).	Dyspnea, right sided heart failure. Lung biopsy. Most common finding is plexiform arthropathy of pulmonary vasculature. Impact of HAART controversial: some demonstrated improvement with ↓ incidence & improved hemodynamics (CID 38:1178, 2004) while others did not (CID 39:1549, 2004). Rx with bosentan, an endothelin receptor antagonist, improved hemodynamics & exercise tolerance in 16/16 pts after 16 wks (AJRCCM 170:1212, 2004). Inhalation of a prostacyclin analog, iloprost, also improved hemodynamics (Eur Resp J 23:321, 2004).
Myocarditis/Cardiomyopathy **Infectious:** Toxoplasmosis, CMV, EBV, Chagas. 1 case of fulminant myocarditis during HIV seroconversion reported (Ital Heart J 5:228, 2004).	Prevalence depends on definition. Autopsy: focal myocarditis 15–50% (Curr Prob Cardiol 15:575, 1990). Echo: 0–40% develop evidence of LV dysfunction. Clinical cardiomyopathy in 1–3% AIDS pts. Rule out alcohol, cocaine. Reactivation of Chagas with cardiomyopathy reported (Am J Cardiol 94:1102, 2004).
Idiopathic (15.9 cases/1000 HIV-infected patients) (Prog Cardiovasc Dis 43:151, 2000) Etiology: HIV nucleic acid sequences detected in 58/76 pts (NEJM 339:1093, 1998). HIV itself appears to cause heart muscle disease. gp120 HIV envelope protein) found in cardiac macrophages, endothelial cells & cardiomyocytes with evidence for apoptosis of cardiomyocytes found (Cardiovasc Toxicol 4:97, 2004). HIV viral protein R (Vpr) also implicated (Lab Invest, Dec, 2004).	**Biventricular dilatation with pathologic features of myocarditis.** Average ejection fraction 33% (J Am Coll Cardiol 13:1030, 1989). Viral sequences of adenovirus & CMV were found in 11 pts with myocarditis (histologically) at autopsy in children (J Am Coll Cardiol 34:857, 1999). No causal relationship to malnutrition, immunologic mechanisms. Rx is after load reduction & diuretics.
Coronary & carotid artery disease associated with HAART (See Table 6C)	
Endocarditis (See Table 6C) Non-bacterial, thrombotic (marantic): (see Sanford Guide to Antimicrobial Therapy).	Sterile thrombi common, may be on any valve & embolize systemically. Opportunistic pathogens not a common cause of endocarditis in HIV+ patients (although there are case reports). Response of HIV+ patient to rx is similar to non-HIV+ patient.
Infective Consider in injection drug users, reported in 4–10%. More common with advanced HIV: odds ratio = 2 for CD4 200–500; OR = 3.6 for CD4 <200/mm³ & ↑ frequency of infections; OR = 3.15 for < daily use; OR = 6.07 for ≥ daily use in non-IVDU pts; more common in advanced HIV, etiology similar to non-HIV population (QJM 96:217, 2003; AIDS Rev 6:97, 2004).	Clinical features similar in HIV+ & -neg (Am J Med Sci 328: 145, 2004). Pts tolerated valve replacement well when indicated (Clin Micro Inf 9:45 & 1073, 2003; Cardiol Clin 21:167, 2003).
Malignancy (See Table 18) Kaposi's sarcoma Lymphoma	Lesions are clinically silent but may produce irritability with arrhythmias. Cardiac involvement with Kaposi's sarcoma of lymphoma usually occurs only with widespread disease.
Hematologic Abnormalities⁹ Hematopoietic abnormalities including anemia, cytopenias & cytopenias are very common in HIV-infected individuals & likely involve HIV-initiated altered stem cell differentiation (Curr HIV Res 2:275, 2004)	

See pg102 for abbreviations & footnotes

TABLE 11A (29)

Anemia (see *CID 38:1454, 2004 for treatment guidelines*). Occurs in up to 85% of AIDS patients; severity of anemia is an independent predictor of ↓ survival (*CID 34:260, 2002; CID 37(Suppl.4):S293, 2003*). However, HAART is effective rx of HIV-associated anemia; rise of >1g/dl of hemoglobin in 1 year rx (*J AIDS 29:54, 2002; Am J Hematol 70:318, 2002; J AIDS 37:1245, 2004*). If anemia persists after HAART initiated, once weekly epoetin alfa 40,000 units/wk was effective (↑ in Hb 2.5-2.9g/dl over 8wks) & assoc. with improved quality of life measurements (*J AIDS 34:368, 2003; Postgrad Med 79:367, 2003; AJM 116(Suppl 7A):27S, 2004; CID 37:1221, 2004; AIDS Res Hum Retrovir 20:1037, 2004*).

CLINICAL SYNDROME, ETIOLOGY, EPIDEMIOLOGY	CLINICAL PRESENTATION, DIAGNOSTIC TESTS, COURSE
Hematologic Abnormalities (continued)	
Anemia of chronic disease (impaired erythropoiesis) due to HIV, OI, malignancy. Degree of anemia correlates with concentrations of cytokines (TNFα, MIP-1α, & IL-1β) & cytokine receptors in bone marrow aspirates (*J Invest Med 47:471, 1999*). Autoantibodies to erythropoietin have also been detected & correlate with anemia. Iron deficiency anemia secondary to GI bleeding (Kaposi's sarcoma, lymphoma, carcinoma)	• Normochromic, normocytic. • ↓ reticulocyte counts • ↓ erythropoietin levels (inappropriately low for degree of anemia) • ↑ serum iron, ↓ total iron-binding capacity (TIBC), normal to ↑ serum ferritin — bone marrow iron stores — • Microcytic, hypochromic. • ↓ serum iron, ↑ TIBC, ↓ serum ferritin • ↓ bone marrow iron stores
Infiltration of the bone marrow (especially Mycobacterium avium-intracellulare)	Anemia often profound (hematocrit 15-20%), WBC & platelets might be ↓. Visceral leishmaniasis reported (*CID 39:1088, 2004*). Occur in 20%. Most likely due to altered serum transport. Anemia usually not due to or compounded by B_{12} deficiency.
Decreased B_{12} levels	Direct Coombs test commonly positive. Hemolysis is rare.
Antibody-mediated hemolysis	
Pure red cell aplasia due to parvovirus B-19. Found in 16% of autopsies in 1 series. Can also cause neutropenia (*Abst 172, 3rd CRV, 1996*) & papular-pruritic skin lesions (*J Am Acad Derm 43:916, 2000*). May also cause persistent infection in HIV-infected children without anemia (*AJM 189:847, 2004*).	Bone marrow shows maturation arrest at pronormoblast stage. Rx with IV immune globulin has resulted in remission in most patients, enabling administration of full ZDV dosage (*J Hamedov, Guide of AIDS, 6th Edition, pg269*). HAART may reverse chronic infection (*Am J Hematol 60:164, 1999*).
Drug-induced anemia • G6PD deficient: hemolysis; common: dapsone, primaquine; uncommon: INH, sulfonamides, TMP/SMX (common in pts of African & Mediterranean origin) • Zidovudine & stavudine (*CID 29:459, 1999*) produce megaloblastic anemia • Myelosuppression: ganciclovir, valganciclovir, foscarnet, flucytosine, sulfonamides, trimethoprim, trimetrexate, pyrimethamine, pentamidine, amphotericin (*J Microbiol Immun Int 31:233, 1998*) • Indinavir (hemolytic anemia (*Postgrad Med J 75:313, 1999; AIDS Reader 14:555, 2004*).	**Zidovudine**: May respond to epoetin alfa if endogenous serum erythropoietin levels <500 mU/ml. Patients with erythropoietin levels >500mU/ml do not respond (*Table 22*). Use of EPO for HIV anemia in general may be effective in ↑ Hct & associated with ↑ survival while transfusions are not (*CID 29:44, 1999*). Foscarnet: anemia in 1/3 pts but <1% required discontinuation. Severe anemia 2° to ZDV & valproic acid drug interaction reported (*AIDS 16:851, 2002*).
	Nevirapine: Single dose to mother to prevent maternal-child transmission of HIV at birth, assoc. with ↓ Hgb, Hct, WBC & platelets at 6wks of age vs untreated neonates (*AIDS 18:e38, 2004*).
Malaria is a common cause of anemia in endemic areas with or without HIV infection (*Central Af J Med 46:5, 2000*).	Particularly severe in HIV+ pregnant _ (*Am J Trop Med Hyg 71:41, 2004*)
Granulocytopenia (occurs in up to 50% of AIDS patients) (*AIDS 13:52, 1999*). • Ineffective granulopoiesis • Antineutrophil antibodies • Antineutrophilic antibodies • Drugs: • Zidovudine >>cdC & ddI. • Ganciclovir & valganciclovir. • Flucytosine. • Foscarnet. • Sulfonamides. • Dihydrofolate reductase inhibitors: trimethoprim, pyri-methamine, trimethoprim. • Pentamidine. • Antineoplastic therapy. • Interferon alfa	May respond to granulocyte-macrophage colony-stimulating factor (GM-CSF) or granulocyte-colony stimulating factor (G-CSF). Suggest determining degree of granulocytopenia & using alternative agents rather than G-CSF or GM-CSF. These growth factors may be of particular value in antineoplastic chemotherapy regimens during nadir of neutropenia (*CID 30:256, 2000*). Use may be associated with Sweet's syndrome & activation of HIV (see Table 22). Infection most likely when profound neutropenia (<100 neutrophils/mm3) associated with chemotherapy or lymphoma (*Abst 194, 3rd CRV, 1996; J Hemato Ther Stem Cell Res 8:S1 8, 1999*). Acute HIV-assoc. hemophagocytic syndrome reported with ↓ WBC, ↓ Hct, ↑ ALT & AST & hepatosplenomegaly (*AIDS 17:1792, 2004*).

See pg102 for abbreviations & footnotes

TABLE 11A (30)

CLINICAL SYNDROME, ETIOLOGY, EPIDEMIOLOGY	CLINICAL PRESENTATION, DIAGNOSTIC TESTS, COURSE
Hematologic Abnormalities (continued)	
Thrombocytopenia (occurs in 11%) (*Br J Haematol 105:1086,1999 for diff dx*)	Usually occurs in early HIV infection & platelet counts increase as HIV infection progresses. Studies
Early stage HIV-associated thrombocytopenia (ITP) (*CID 21:415, 1995*)	show ↓ platelet production & ↓ platelet survival (*Ln 343:479, 1994*).
Antineoplastic therapy Lopinavir/ritonavir & indinavir	Rx: • Treatment may not be necessary; incidence of significant bleeding is low, spontaneous
Drugs: (*Int J Int Dis 8:315, 2004*)	remissions in 10–20%.
• Interferon alfa	• In a Swiss study, ZDV therapy increased platelet counts by 50,000 to 100,000/mm³.
• Beta-lactam antibiotics	Studies show spontaneous response in 10% (may take 3wks) but ↑ in platelet counts.
• Most other drugs above that cause neutropenia	• IV immune globulin (400 mg/kg q24h x5-d) will usually lead to transient ↑ in platelet counts,
• May improve with HAART (*NEJM 341:1239, 1999; AIDS 13:1913,*	but is expensive. IV anti-D (anti-Rh) antibody: response in 75% (may take 3wks) but
1999)	sustained in <10%. Not effective in Rh-negative or pts with splenectomies (*Transfusion*
	34:759, 1994). See Table 22.
HIV quasi species with distinct phenotype appear to be associated with thrombocy-	• Splenectomy. Rarely indicated; 2/3 of patients will respond if other therapies fail.
topenia (*J Virol 73:3497, 1999*). In addition, megakaryocytes & platelets both	
express the HIV coreceptor CXCR4 CD4 & (*Br J Haematol 104:220, 1999*).	
Thrombotic thrombocytopenia (TTP). hemolytic uremic syndrome (HUS)	Fever, neurologic abnormalities, renal abnormalities, microangiopathic hemolysis (schistocytes on
TTP & HUS described in 150 HIV+ individuals since 1986; cause unknown (*Infection*	peripheral smear), & thrombocytopenia [was found in 7% of 350 consecutive AIDS pts admitted to
27:12, 1999), reported with valacyclovir rx (*AnIM 160:1705, 2000; Ann Hematol, Sept.*	Johns Hopkins Hospital 1996-97. 24% had schistocytes (*Am J Hematol 60:116, 1999*)]
23, 2003) & abacavir (*J Intensive Care Med 18:156, 2003*)	Rx: Primary—plasma exchange. Splenectomy, steroids, dextran for salvage rx. Rx for CMV effective in 1
	pt with ↓ PCR for CMV (*Scand J Int Dis 36:234, 2004*).
Thrombotic events (*see CID 39:1214, 2004*): May be 10x ↑ with HIV	30/650 HIV-infected persons had 43 venous or arterial thromboses (lower extremity deep vein
	thrombosis & PE in 2/3). Med. age was 43. 77% smoked cigarettes, 57% dyslipidemia, 43% had
	malignancies (KS). Most common lab findings were: (1) phospholipid antibodies, (2) thrombophilia,
	(3) ↓ levels of protein C, S, & antithrombin III, (4) ↑ levels Factor VIII, (5) ↑ levels homocysteine. **Most**
	had CDC C3 but with ↓ CD4 (median 290/mm³).
Eosinophilia [HIV infection itself may induce proliferation of eosinophils (*UID 174:615,*	(*S Card J Int Dis 30:530, 1998*). No correlation between eosinophil count & CD4
1996; Immunology & Allergy Clin N.A. 17:207, 1997).	or viral load (*AIDS 34:1264, 2004*).
Allergic diseases, drug reactions: Zalcitabine (3–5% pts), ganciclovir (≤1% pts),	TMP/SMX (also eosinophilic meningitis (*S Card J Int Dis 30:530, 1998*). IL-2; other drugs such as
dapsone. Zidovudine (2 pts reported with fever, eosinophilia (8%, 19%) & cutaneous leukocytoclastic vasculitis (8%-24wks of ZDV (*AnIM 152:850, 1992*). Intractable pruritus &
eosinophilia reported in 6 pts assoc. with TMP-SMX, IgA, IL-4, IL-5 & ↓ interferon production by mitogen-stimulated PBMCs—all had high viral load, etiology unknown (*Allergy 54:266, 1999*).
Extensive workup of pts with eosinophilia & cutaneous disease not warranted since diagnostic yield vanishing low (*AJM 102:449, 1997*).	
Parasitic infections: Strongyloides. Isospora belli (in contrast to cryptosporidia & giardia which are not associated with ↓ eos).	
Ecto-parasitic infections: Norwegian scabies;	
Neoplasms: Hodgkin's disease	
Pulmonary lymphoid hyperplasia, seen in children;	
Fungal infections: coccidiodomycosis	
Coagulation abnormalities: prolonged partial thromboplastin time (PTT), lupus	An incidental finding in HIV+ patients, not associated with either excessive bleeding or thrombosis in
anticoagulant/antiphospholipid antibodies (present in 20-66% HIV+, *Blood Rev 7:121,*	this population. Invasive procedures have been performed without bleeding complications. However,
1993)	it may also have systemic lupus erythematosus (25 cases of SLE + HIV reported. Semin Rheum
	30:418, 2001). Antiphospholipid syndrome noted for 3,789 pts with antiphospholipid syndrome from Spain &
	Latin America (*QJM 38:1009, 2004*); clinical features: avascular bone necrosis 59%, cutaneous
	necrosis 16%, peripheral thrombosis 16%, stroke 12%, PE 9%, ↓ platelets 6%.

See pg102 for abbreviations & footnotes

TABLE 11A (31)

CLINICAL SYNDROME, ETIOLOGY, EPIDEMIOLOGY	CLINICAL PRESENTATION, DIAGNOSTIC TESTS, COURSE
Hepatobiliary Disease (↑ transaminase levels in 2–3.8% asymptomatic HIV+ pts)	
Acalculous cholecystitis: Prevalence ↑ in AIDS patients. Pseudocholelithiasis Infectious Idiopathic (55%)	Right upper quadrant pain, fever in 2/3 but jaundice uncommon (18%). R/O "pseudocholelithiasis" [2] to ceftriaxone, symptomatic in 9% pts with "sludge" in gallbladder by ultrasound. More likely in pts on ≥2 gm/day, or total parenteral nutrition, or younger patients on ≥28 days rx. Lab: Increase in alkaline phosphatase >other LFT abnormalities. Biopsy: In some cases, histologic sections have shown CMV, cryptosporidium, Isospora belli *(AnIM 121:663, 1994)* & Cyclospora cayetanensis *(CID 21:1092, 1995).* Rx: Appropriate surgical intervention when indicated
AIDS cholangiopathy (sclerosing cholangitis, intra- & extrahepatic) (obstructive biliary tract disease). Cause is uncertain; the following have been associated: Cryptosporidium Cytomegalovirus Microsporidia Kaposi's sarcoma Mycobacterium avium-intracellulare (MAC). Lymphoma	Clinical: Fever, pain, right upper quadrant pain. Median survival of 20 pts was 7mos *(Gut 34:116, 1993).* Lab: Alkaline phosphatase ↑ 2–20x normal; alk p'tase >1000 assoc. with poor prognosis *(Am J Gastro 98:2176, 2003)* Ultrasound or ERCP: Prominent or dilated intrahepatic &/or extrahepatic bile ducts down to periampullary area with marked thickening of ductal walls. Papillary stenosis in _ patients, sphincterotomy may relieve symptoms in these patients *(AJM 99:600, 1995).* Cryptosporidia or CMV in 9/15 patients (60%) *(NEJM 328:95, 1993).* Another series (20 pts): cryptosporidia 13, CMV 6. Enterocytozoon bieneusi found in 8/8 patients in whom cryptosporidia or CMV not found *(NEJM 328:95, 1993).*
Hepatic parenchymal disease, *see Viral hepatitis, below* Liver failure causes 5% of in-hospital deaths *(J AIDS 24:211, 2000).* Endstage liver disease is now one of the leading non-AIDS related deaths in HIV+ pts *(CID 15:1030, 2003)* & liver-related conditions the most common cause of serious & life-threatening events (Grade 4) *(J AIDS 34:379, 2003).* Causes of infiltrative disease identified in about 40% of patients. Infections: Cytomegalovirus 1–14%, MAC 11–17%, chronic active hepatitis 12%, C. neoformans 2%, H. capsulatum 1%, M. tuberculosis 1–3%, C. albicans 0.6%, Penicillium marneffei *(see Comments)* Neoplasms: Kaposi's sarcoma 0.4–9%, non-Hodgkin's lymphoma 1–2.5%	Hepatocellular abnormalities usually reflect systemic infection or malignancy. Histologic findings rarely of diagnostic value *(CID 23:1302, 1996).* Hepatic histology abnormal in 90% of pts with AIDS: steatosis 42%, portal inflammation 35%, congestion 22%, poorly formed granulomata 14% *(Hepatology 7:927, 1987; AJM 52:404, 1992; J AIDS 11:170, 1996).* Fever, weight loss, hepatosplenomegaly in pt with travel to Southeast Asia: consider Penicillium marneffei *(CID 23:125, 1996).* Amebic liver abscess reported in 3 HIV+ pts with protracted course in Taiwan *(J Clin Gastro 33:64, 2001).*
Hepatomegaly with severe steatosis, lactic acidosis in patients on antiretroviral therapy Occurs predominantly in women, majority overweight, at least 4 mos of antiretroviral rx (all NRTIs). *See Table 6C (lactic acidosis)*	**Clinical:** Tachypnea, abdominal pain, hepatomegaly. **Lab:** Hepatic transaminases 3–10x normal, ↑ triglycerides; mortality >50%. Incidence <0.4% *(AIDS Clin Care 6:17, 1994).* Biopsy: severe macrovesicular steatosis; ↓ arterial ammonia, lactic acidosis; ↑ PTT.

See pg102 for abbreviations & footnotes

TABLE 11A (32)

CLINICAL SYNDROME, ETIOLOGY, EPIDEMIOLOGY	CLINICAL PRESENTATION, DIAGNOSTIC TESTS, COURSE
Hepatobiliary Disease (continued)	
Peliosis hepatis (bacillary angiomatosis) (see *J. Koehler in MEDICAL MANAGEMENT OF AIDS, 6th Edition, 1999)*	**Clinical:** Fever, abdominal pain, weight loss, hepato- & splenomegaly. About 1/2 pts will have skin lesions: painful, erythematous plaques or nodules. 1/2 have lymphadenopathy. 2/3 pts give history of cat bite or scratch *(JAMA 269:770, 1993).* Lab: Alkaline phosphatase ↑ *(hepatocellular tests).* Etiologic agent: Bartonella henselae (usual), B. quintana (uncommon). Can be isolated from blood, 5-15days incubation of lysis-centrifugation cultures on blood agar under CO₂ *(J Clin Micro 30:275, 1992).* Rx: Can be rx with erythromycin, clarithromycin, azithromycin. Doxycycline may also be effective *(NEJM 323: 1581, 1990).* Patients respond clinically (↓ fever, ↓ symptoms) in 3–4days, but require up to 2mos for LFTs to become normal. Lifelong suppression with macrolide or doxy may be necessary *(see Table 12).* X-ray: May be associated with bone lesions (punched-out appearance). CT/MRI findings: characteristic intrahepatic vascular lakes. Rx: Table 12, pg106.
Drug-associated hepatic dysfunction *[see J AIDS 34(Suppl 1):S34, 2003; CID 38(Suppl 2):S43, 2004]* (Avoid acetaminophen) Multiple drugs used in HIV patients are associated with abnormalities in LFTs; among these are: TMP/SMX (1/2 pts), acyclovir, nevirapine, didanosine (ddI), ZDV, ddC, all Pls, esp. high-dose ritonavir *(Semin Liver Dis 23:183, 2003)*, hydroxyurea, ganciclovir, foscarnet, ketoconazole, fluconazole, INH, rifampin *(see Table 12).* Most require dose reduction or discontinuation if abnormalities exceed about 5x normal values.	**Clinical:** NRTIs more likely (7.9%) to cause hepatic enzyme (ALT) elevations (>200 int'l units/l) than dual PIs (4%, p < 0.01). In 26 pts switched to nevirapine from PI-containing regimen, serum GTP within 3 mos. & hepatic necrosis & death has been reported with nevirapine. **Nevirapine hepatotoxicity may be severe, esp. in pts with ↑ CD4 counts.** ↑ ALT also noted at 6wks in neonates who received nevirapine at birth *(AIDS 16:851, 2002).* **Co-infection with Hep B & C, ↑ baseline ALT elevation & previous hx of parenchymal liver disease ↑ likelihood of drug toxicity** *(CID 30:S77, 2000)*, esp. ritonavir *(J AIDS 29:41, 2002).*
Viral hepatitis *(See Int Dis Clin North Am 14:741, 2000)* **Hepatitis A** (HAV) Hep A in HIV-infected persons is clinically indistinguishable from Hep A in uninfected persons, however is assoc. with prolonged HV viremia (med. days 53 vs 22 in non-HIV infected). ↑ HAV serum titers (p < 0.001). ↓ ALT (1955 vs 2918 int'l units/L) & ↑ alk phosphatase (413 vs 216 int'l units/L) *(CID 34:380, 2002).*	Clinical: HAART is more likely (7.9%) to cause hepatic enzyme (ALT) elevations (>200 int'l units/l). HAV has ↑ in frequency in homosexual men in U.S., Canada, Australia *(MMWR 45:155, 1992).* Outbreaks also reported in IDUs *(Am J Pub Health 79:463, 1989).* Hepatitis A vaccine, inactivated, licensed in U.S. in 1995. FDA-approved indications include: **persons engaged in high-risk sexual activity,** IDUs.
Hepatitis B (HBV) Risk factors for HIV & hepatitis B are the same (80–90% HIV+ pts are + for HBV markers *(AnIM 117:837, 1992).* Rate of acute Hep B infection was 12.2/1000 person yrs in 16,248 pts followed 1998–2001 in U.S.; ↑ risk in black subjects (RR 1.4); alcoholism (RR 1.7), IVDU (RR 1.6) & AIDS-defining condition (RR 1.5); & ↓ risk with HAART with or without lamivudine (RR 0.6) *(JID 188:571, 2003).*	Co-infection with Hep A may ↑ HIV RNA in plasma & ↓ CD4 counts. Risk of becoming Hep B chronic carrier (20%), HIV+ pts respond less well to Hep B vaccine & about lose antibody after 4 years *(NEJM 316:630, 1987; CID 18:339, 1994).* In Hep Bs antigen positive patients, progression of HIV appears to be markedly accelerated *(J AIDS & HR 19:198, 1998).* Rx with lamivudine (3TC) as part of antiretroviral rx also showed inhibition of HBV RNA (86% at 2mos., 47% 2yrs). however, 3TC resistance (550 mutation) emerged at rate of 20%/yr *(Hepatol 30:1302, 1999) (see pg130).* Withdrawal of 3TC may result in flare of hepatitis *(CID 28:1032, 1999)* & 7/12 who seroconverted experienced relapse after cessation of treatment *(CID 38:490, 2004).* Acute bouts of clinical hepatitis may occur in pts with chronic active hepatitis B in response to HAART immune reconstitution *(Eur J Gastroenterol Hepatol 15:95, 2003).* HBV infection ↑ rate of hepatic toxicity of HAART (esp. ritonavir): OR 27.81 (p < 0.0001 at 24 mos. of rx) *(J AIDS 29:41, 2002).* Rx: Table 12, pg130.

TABLE 11A (33)

CLINICAL SYNDROME, ETIOLOGY, EPIDEMIOLOGY	CLINICAL PRESENTATION, DIAGNOSTIC TESTS, COURSE
Hepatobiliary Disease/Viral Hepatitis (continued)	
Hepatitis C (HCV) (See CID 30:577, 2000 & Ln 360:584, 2002). The USPHS/IDSA Guidelines recommend that all HIV-infected individuals be screened for HCV infection & those pos. be treated if indicated (MMWR 51:1, 2002). HCV co-infection becoming much more frequent: Italy 90% HIV+ IDUs, Denmark 4% in HIV+ homosexual men, 1/3 of HIV+ in USA (CID 23:1117, 1996; Infect 31:232, 2003; CID 36:1313, 2003; JID 189:292, 2004). HCV-infected pts more likely to be HIV-infected: 30.5% of 446 HCV-infected in Madrid, Spain (ICAAC 2002, Abst. H746). ↑ HCV assoc. with sharing needles & drug-preparation equipment & exchanging sex for drugs 186:1558, 2002). Co-infection with HCV & HIV ↑ risk of perinatal transmission of HIV to infant. Rx: Table 12, pg131–135.	**In HIV-HCV co-infected pts, the course of Hep C is accelerated, the hepatotoxicity ffrom HAART is increased, & HCV-related liver disease is becoming a common cause of death** (JID 192; 992, 2006). Co-infection produces a higher degree of HCV viremia &↑ rate of HCV antibody loss. 19/100 HIV+ pts who were HCV Ab-neg. had + HCV RNA + , HIV-neg. controls were HCV Ab-neg. (Hepatol 30: 1054, 1999) but did ↑ progression to new AIDS diagnosis & death & blunted CD4 response to HAART in Swiss HIV cohort study (Ln 356: 1800, 2000). 125 Canadian HIV-coinfected HIV+ pts experienced no clearcut benefit from HAART compared to 1076 HIV+ pts without HCV infection (J AIDS 33:365, 2003). HIV appears to accelerate course of Hep C-induced liver fibrosis (Hepatol 30:1054, 1999). Histological improvement in liver pathology to interferon rx similar to HIV-neg. (40% vs 36%); however, sustained response rate was lower in HIV+ (6% vs 30%) (AIDS 16:441, 2002). HAART for HIV associated with ↑ in HCV RNA but without change in hepatic transaminases in 2 series (JID 180:2027, 1999; AIDS 16:1915, 2002). **HCV infection ↑ rate of hepatic toxicity of HAART** (esp. ritonavir): OR 12.14 (p=0.0001) (J AIDS 29:41, 2002). The main hematological side-effects of HAART (↓ WBC, with interferon) & ↓ Hgb (with ribavirin) may be more severe in HIV+ pts, esp. when also receiving HAART (Ln 360:584, 2002). **Endstage liver disease from Hep C is becoming a common cause of death in the HAART era** (33% > 1998 vs 2–10% from 1988–1998 in 383 Spanish hemophiliac pts (Haemophilia 9:605, 2003; AIDS 17:1803, 2003). HAART reduces progression of liver fibrosis attributed to HIV infection (CID 42:262, 2006). Prolonged antigenemia, ↑ liver injury (CID 18:339, 1994).
Hepatitis D (delta agent)	
Antibodies to delta agent in 25% of HIV+, HBV– individuals	HEV antibodies by EIA found in 33/162 (20%) homosexual men (Italy), 60/198 (30%) (Spain) (Ln 344:1433, 1994; ibid, 345:127, 1995). Despite some technical non-specificity, an ↑ prevalence of HEV in endemic areas is suggested. In the U.S., where HEV prevalence is <1% this may not be true.
Hepatitis E (HEV)	
	Clinical: No significant consistent correlation between active infection with Hep G as determined by HGV RNA in serum & either hepatocellular necrosis (↑ ALT), fulminant hepatitis or hepatocellular carcinoma has been found (Blood 94:1460, 1999; Am J Neph 19:317, 1999). The virus appears to infect lymphocytes & not hepatocytes (J Gastro 34:680, 1999). Serum HGV RNA reduced by interferon alfa but not ZDV (JID 180:1334, 1999). Infection (past or current) with HGV associated with ↑ CD4 counts & **better AIDS-free survival rates** in one study of 131 hemophilia pts (NEJM 345:707 & 715, 2001; AnM 139:26, 2003; CID 38:405, 2004).
Hepatitis G (see Semin Liver Dis 23:137, 2003). Appears to be transmitted by parenteral or sexual route (CID 34:1033, 2002). ↑ IVDUs (75%), following blood transfusions & in hemophiliacs (38%), hemodialysis pts (17%), homosexuals (55%) (J Med Virol 58:373, 1999).	There are isolated reports of hepatitis associated with other viruses: EBV (PIDJ 7:383, 1988), HSV (JID 157:597, 1988), VZV (J Inf 25:107, 1992), adenovirus (RID 12:303, 1990).
Hepatitis, viral, other	
Influenza-like Symptoms: Acute & self-limited illness (lasting <10 days) consisting of fever, myalgias, malaise with either sore throat + cervical adenopathy, rhinitis, or conjunctivitis	Viruses were detected in 15 (50%) & Mycoplasma pneumoniae in 9 (30%) of 30 HIV+ pts during such episodes but in only 12 (40%) was isolation in close temporal relationship. These include CMV in 6, M. pneumoniae in 3, herpes simplex virus in 3, & enterovirus in 1. Pts with ↑ CD4 counts were more likely to have "flu-like" symptoms than those with advanced disease (↓ CD4 counts). No cases of influenza were identified even though an epidemic of influenza A was present in the geographical area of study (AIDS 12:751, 1998).
Lipomatosis/Lipodystrophy (See Tables 6C & 11B)	

See pg102 for abbreviations & footnotes

TABLE 11A (34)

CLINICAL SYNDROME, ETIOLOGY, EPIDEMIOLOGY	CLINICAL PRESENTATION, DIAGNOSTIC TESTS, COURSE
Lung Most common causes are Pneumocystis jiroveci (carinii) pneumonia, bacterial pneumonia, tuberculosis (Ln 348:307, 1996) (See Sanford Guide to Antimicrobial Therapy for non-HIV pulmonary infections). Viral pneumonia dx increasingly common in older adults but not unique in HIV infected patients (CID 42:518, 2006) see Curr Opin Infect Dis 18:165, 2005, review of HIV pneumonia	
Bronchitis, bronchiectasis, bronchiolitis obliterans (BOOP) In addition to mycoplasma & respiratory viruses, H. influenzae, S. pneumo, & P. aeruginosa were cultured from sputum in 1 study; relationship to etiology not proven (AnM 154:2087, 1994).	Mean: CD4 600/μl. In pts with chronic productive cough or recurrent pneumonia in same site, consider bronchiectasis. Dx based on CXR, most evident on CXR in 84% (Quart J Med 85:875, 1992; J Comp Asst Tomo 17:260, 1993). Whether prevalence is ↑ has not been defined but suspected (AnIM 154:2086, 1994). Acute bronchitis most common dx on HIV clinic pts in Kenya (Int J STD AIDS 15:120, 2004). BOOP rare in HIV+ but described (J Int 49:159, 2004).
Emphysema-like bullous disease	On high-resolution CT scan, 42% HIV pts had bullous lesions (Radiol 173:23, 1989). Pulmonary function tests: ↑ residual volume, ↑ functional residual capacity, ↓ diffusing capacity but no airflow obstruction (AnIM 116:124, 1992). 40 pts with HIV infection & emphysema were found to have ↑ disease in upper lobes with ↑ concentrations of glutathione, suggesting a response to excessive oxidant stress vs non-HIV infected individuals (Chest 126:1439, 2004).
Pneumonia (infiltrate on CXR) (Good review of lab evaluation of Ols of lung, AnIM 124:585, 1996; Clinics in Chest Dis 4:713, 1996)	
Any CD4 level	Clinical presentation varies with stage of HIV infection.
Community-acquired bacterial: Attributable mortality 9.3%; shock, CD4 <100, pleural effusion, cavity & multiple lobe involvement ↑ mortality (AJRCCM 162:2063, 2000)	Clinical presentation: cavity, cavity & multiple lobe involvement ↑ mortality (AJRCCM 162:2063, 2000)
Mycobacterium tuberculosis (common) **ANY PT SUSPECTED OF TB SHOULD BE ISOLATED** (private room, negative pressure, health care workers (HCW) & visitors entering should wear high efficiency disposable masks). [See Table 23]. In the Western world the number of new cases of HIV-associated TBc & MDR TBc has declined (1998–2001), likely due to the implementation of rigorous infection control measures & Directly Observed Therapy (DOT). (CID 29:1138, 1999; AnIM 130:971, 1999).	• **Upper lobe disease most common.** Extrapulmonary disease uncommon. PPD (5 TU) is + (≥5 mm induration) in 80%. • **Later HIV infection** (CD4 <400/mm³). Either reactivation or progressive primary disease (30–50%). Clinical: fever, cough (may be absent), shortness of breath, weight loss, night sweats. 1/2 to 2/3 involve extrapulmonary sites, especially lymph nodes & bone marrow (granulomas in 50% of bone marrow biopsies). A papulopustular rash reported (CID 27:205, 1998). Mycobacterial blood cultures + in 1/4 to 1/2 of patients. (BACTEC system is sensitive & rapid). Caution: patients reported with blood + for both M. tbc & MAC. Cultures of urine, sputum, CSF, liver, GI mucosa & ascites may also be +. Mass lesions of brain (tuberculoma) may mimic CNS toxoplasmosis. PPD (5 TU) positive (≥5mm induration in <23% with clinical AIDS). Malnutrition ↑ severity of pulmonary TB in Malawi (Int J Tuberc Lung Dis 8:211, 2004).
In the 3rd World TBc & HIV are closely linked: 50% of pts who have TBc in parts of sub-Saharan Africa are also infected with HIV (Int J Tuberc Lung Dis 5:225, 2001) & likewise TBc was found in 50% of autopsies done in AIDS pts (J AIDS 20:23, 2000). Point prevalence of active TBc in 100 hospitalized pts with HIV in South Africa was 54% (CID 33:2068, 2002) & the leading cause of death in Botswana (Int J Tuberc Lung Dis 6:55, 2002); 48% had TBc in Malaysia (Jpn J Int Dis 56:187, 2003); 26% in New Delhi, India (Int J STD AIDS 14:411, 2003); 47% in Guatemala (Int J STD AIDS 14:810, 2003) & 14% in Cambodia (Int J Tuberc Lung Dis 6:55, 2002). The proportion of new cases of TB attributed to HIV was 72% in men in northern Thailand (J AIDS 31:80, 2002). Incidence of TB & mortality similar with HIV-1 & HIV-2 (AIDS 18:1933, 2004).	**X-ray: Mediastinal-hilar adenopathy most common with progression to diffuse, somewhat coarse interstitial densities or localized infiltrates,** especially in mid or lower lung fields. Pleural effusion in 10–20%. Disseminated (reticulonodular) infiltrates, not classic 'miliary' since 'millets' are granulomata, usually not seen (when CD4 low) the most common with CD4 <200/mm3. Hilar/peritracheal adenopathy uncommon with PCP or bacterial pneumonia, common in TB. Cavity formation ↑ with multidrug-resistant disease (J Comput Asst Tomo 28:366, 2004). In 1 study in Ethiopia, 10% of sputum-pos. cases had normal chest x-ray (Infection 32:333, 2004). Smears + for acid-fast bacilli in 40–50% of pts with pulmonary TB, BAL + in 50–60%, culture + in 80–90%. The "string test" used to retrieve enteropathogens (giardia or salmonella) was used to obtain swallowed sputum; 14 pts pos. by string test vs 8 from induced sputum (p 0.03) (Lancet 365:150, 2005).

See pg102 for abbreviations & footnotes

TABLE 11A (35)

CLINICAL SYNDROME, ETIOLOGY, EPIDEMIOLOGY	CLINICAL PRESENTATION, DIAGNOSTIC TESTS, COURSE
Lung/Pneumonia/Mycobacterium tuberculosis (common) (continued)	

Lung/Pneumonia/Mycobacterium tuberculosis (common) (continued)

Tuberculosis often occurs before pt has AIDS-defining illness, but HAART sig. ↓ risk (AIDS 14:1985, 2000). Most cases due to reactivation but primary tuberculosis being recognized with increasing frequency: 10% of HIV+ individuals are tuberculin (+). **Rate of development of TB in the 1st year in PPD+ patients is reduced to 0.51% following INH prophylaxis for 12mos** (AIDS 13:2069, 1999). Average CD4 count at TB dx = 375/mm³. TBc has been shown to accelerate the course of HIV (AIDS 14:1219, 2000). ↑ HIV viral load (JID 190:1627, 2004) & induces expression of CXCR4 on alveolar macrophages while suppressing CCR5 by ↑ CC chemokine expression, thus encouraging switch from macrophage-trophic to lymphocytotrophic HIV phenotype which is assoc. with acceleration of disease progression (J Immunol 172:6251, 2004).

Other etiologies of community-acquired pneumonia (AIDS 16:85, 2002)

• Bacterial etiologies:
  Streptococcus pneumoniae (common, 35–70%; 25% in Cameroon & 31% in Uganda (CID 36:652, 2003))
  Haemophilus influenzae (common, 3–40%)
  Staphylococcus aureus (7%) (uncommon except with IDU, right-sided endocarditis)
  Moraxella catarrhalis (<1%) (J Chemo Ther 12:406, 2000)
  Pseudomonas aeruginosa (3–10%) most common pathogen in one series (30%) (Chest 117:1017, 2000) but has ↓ in era of HAART (Postgrad Med J 79:691, 2003)
  E. coli (6–7%)
  Serratia marcescens (<1%) (Eur J Clin Microbiol Inf Dis 19:428, 2000)
  Other Gram-negative (7–9%)
  Prevalence not defined:
  Mycoplasma pneumoniae, Chlamydia pneumoniae, Legionella sp. (rare) (J Inf 45:199, 2002; AIDS Reader 14:267, 2004). See below

• Multiple etiologies not uncommon due to 1/3 of cases); early bronchoscopy encouraged (The AIDS Reader, July/Aug 1997, p. 112)

• Bacterial pneumonia ↑ in HIV (5.5 cases/100 person years vs 0.9/100 OR 0.22 person years), mortality 4x ↑; TMP/SMX prophylaxis ↓ pneumonia by 67% (NEJM 333:845, 1995; JID 181:158, 2000).

• Cigarette smoking ↑ risk of bacterial pneumonia (RR 1.57), oral candidiasis (RR 1.37) & AIDS dementia complex (RR 1.80) (J AIDS & Human Retro 13:374, 1996).

• HIV RNA copies: ↑ from a median of 60,000 copies/ml plasma to 245,000 copies/ml in 13 pts with bacterial pneumonia. Titers dropped to baseline after recovery (J AIDS & HR 13:23, 1996).

Rx with HAART resulted in immune reconstitution inflammatory syndrome (IRIS) characterized by worsening of chest x-ray after 1–5wks in 45% of 31 pts receiving antituberculous rx; 23% were severe. 4/7 of the latter converted PPD to + (Am J Roentgenol 174:43, 2000). Severe respiratory failure reported. Rx determined primarily by drug interactions with ARV. Corticosteroids provide rapid clinical improvement but HIV concern with IRIS (see below). Some authorities recommend starting ART in pts with very advanced disease (CD4 <100/mm³) & delaying HAART until continuation phase (>2mos.) for those who are clinically stable (CD4 <100/mm³) (AIDS 16:75, 2004). However, AIDS events more common during 1st 2mos of anti-TB rx in those with CD4 <100, suggesting early rx with HAART could be beneficial (CID 190:1670, 2004). IRIS assoc. with ↑ CD4, ↑ ratio of CD4 to CD8 1 month after HAART & with dissemination of TB (CID 39:1709, 2004).
Rx: Table 12, pg107–109.

Pneumococcal pneumonia is common in HIV+ patients (CID 38:1623, 2004). (86% S. pneumo serotypes isolated included in pneumococcal vaccine, Table 20.) In several studies pneumococcal immunization reduced risk of pneumonia by 50–70% even when vaccine given to pts with <100 CD4 cells (AIDS 13:1971, 1999; ArlM 160:2633, 2000; Vaccine 22:2006, 2004). Annual incidence of invasive disease due to S. pneumo is 1100 per 100,000 men with AIDS, age 25–44yrs (JAMA 265:3275, 1991). In African-Americans & CD4 <200. In Uganda, surprisingly ↑ of all-cause pneumonia in vaccine group, but a survival advantage in vaccine group (AIDS 18:1210, 2004). Others have also found insignificant protective effect of pneumococcal vaccine in HIV+ persons in Spain (J Med Virol 72:517, 2004; Lancet 363:1, 2004). Prevalence of multidrug-resistant Strep. pneumoniae among HIV+ individuals is increased (24 vs 6.4%) & more likely to be invasive (40x ↑) vs non-HIV. In resource-restricted areas; in 217 pts in Malawi, mortality of those with meningitis was 65%, pneumococcemic pneumonia 26%, & pneumococcemia without localizing signs 26% (AIDS 16:1409, 2002).
Clinical: Typical presentation with fever, chills, productive cough, pleuritic chest pain & dyspnea can be seen at all stages of HIV infection. **Most (up to 95%) of HIV+ patients with pneumococcal pneumonia will have positive blood cultures** (Chest 117:1017, 2000). Leucocytosis may not occur, but look for left shift bands. Although value of sputum cultures controversial, they were of value in establishing dx in 1 study in Africa (Eur J Clin Micro Inf Dis 21:362, 2002).
X-ray: Usually consolidation (homogeneous densities) with either segmental or lobar distribution (41/50 had lobar). Also similar in HIV+ & HIV-neg. in Kenya study (AIDS 16:2095, 2002; COPD 10:183, 2004).
Course: Response to appropriate antibiotics is usually prompt (48–96hrs to become febrile, radiographic resolution is much slower, as it is in non-HIV+ patients). If patient fails to respond as above, consider concomitant PCP or TBc. CD4 ↓ during acute S. pneumo infection (Clin Microbiol Int 10:587, 2004).
Rx: Table 12, pg108.

Haemophilus influenzae pneumonia/bacteremia: occurs with ↑ frequency. Incidence of invasive disease is 80/100,000. In one series, most pts (57%) had bilateral pneumonia, in another only 30% had pneumonia. 1/3 to 1/2 isolates are type b. 15/15 reported were ß-lactamase negative. Response to appropriate antibiotics is prompt. Mortality is 11.5% (CID 30:461, 2000).

See pg102 for abbreviations & footnotes

TABLE 11A (36)

Lung/Pneumonia *(continued)*

CLINICAL SYNDROME, ETIOLOGY, EPIDEMIOLOGY	CLINICAL PRESENTATION, DIAGNOSTIC TESTS, COURSE
	Pseudomonas aeruginosa: Pneumonia 8.7%/year. Clinical: median CD4 9/µl. 1/2 to 3/4 community-acquired but 1/2 pts had been hospitalized in prior 30 days. CXR: 60–80% segmental, 40% bilateral infiltrates, 10–50% cavities. Only 9% bacteremic respond to rx but relapse recurs in 1/3. Mortality 40% (*JAID 5:76, 1994; Ibid, 19:417, 1994; JAIDS 7:823, 1994; AIDS 9:1251, 1995*). Risk with advanced HIV, central venous & urinary caths, ↓ WBCs, prior antibiotics & steroids (*Chest 117:1017, 2000*).
	Legionella sp. 77% community-acquired. Risk in AIDS 42x ↑ (*AriM 154:2417, 1994*). Nosocomial Legionella pneumophila pneumonia uncommon but reported in several small series (*CID 27:97, 1998*). 83% developed respiratory failure with 22% mortality in 18 Spanish pts (*Med Clin 123:582, 2004*).
Selected other HIV-associated pneumonias Aerobic Gram-negative bacilli [TMP/SMX resistance ↑ markedly from 1988 to 1995 in HIV+ pts (*IJID 180:1809, 1999*)]	HIV infection/disease not reported to alter the prevalence or course of nosocomial, usually ventilator-acquired, Gram-negative bacillary pneumonia. M. avium may be acquired from hot water systems (*Ln 343:1137, 1994*) but does not cause pneumonia.
Influenza virus, A or B (common in outbreaks)	No evidence that influenza in general is more severe in HIV-infected patients. 1 study demonstrated ↑ morbidity & mortality from influenza in women <65yrs of age with certain chronic medical conditions including HIV; annual excess mortality 2/10,000 (*JAMA 281:901, 1999*).
Mycoplasma pneumonia uncommon but may cause "flu-like illness"	M. pneumoniae may be less severe in HIV-infected pts & prolonged secretion of organism & relapsing infection reported as in other immunosuppressed pts. Serology of little value for dx (*AIDS 12:751, 1998*).
Chlamydia pneumoniae	Reported to cause 2.5% of pulmonary infections in 1 Italian study, 2/159 in Atlanta (*AIDS 16:85, 2002*). May be cause of severe diffuse interstitial pneumonia (*Eur J Clin Microbiol Inf Dis 16:720, 1997*).
Ehrlichiosis (Ehrlichia chaffeensis)	In a case report, pt presented with fever, tachypnea, neutropenia with 17% bands, thrombocytopenia, ↑ hepatic enzymes. Chest x-ray: diffuse bilateral infiltrates. ↓ PaO₂. Patient deteriorated. Diagnosis suspected on last day, optimal antibiotic rx not given (*NEJM 329:1164, 1993*).
Measles	In U.S. 9/11 had pneumonitis; 3 had no rash & 8 had atypical exanthems; mortality 3/11 (*JAMA 267:1237, 1992*). Immunization of HIV+ children recommended, although immune responses may be ↓. Ribavirin aerosol has been used but efficacy not proven (*Ibid*).
Adenovirus	Adenovirus diarrhea important (*see pg76*). Frequently cultured from HIV+ pts but association with respiratory illnesses not clear (*AIDS 12:751, 1998*).
Bordetella bronchiseptica	9 cases reported by 1999; respiratory illness ranged from mild URI to pneumonia. All had prior AIDS-defining illness & 3/9 had close contact with pets (2 dogs, 1 cat) (*CID 28:1095, 1999*).
Human herpesvirus 6 (HHV-6)	HHV-6 infected cells detected in tissues obtained at necropsy in 9/9 pts. In one pt, probably primary cause of fatal pneumonitis. Relevance is that HHV-6 infections may be treatable with ganciclovir & foscarnet (*Ln 343:577, 1994*).
Varicella	7/12 pts with advanced HIV hospitalized for chickenpox developed pneumonia with typical diffuse reticulonodular infiltrates; 3 died (43%) despite acyclovir rx (*Int J Inf Dis 6:6, 2002*).

See pg102 for abbreviations & footnotes

TABLE 11A (37)

CLINICAL SYNDROME, ETIOLOGY, EPIDEMIOLOGY	CLINICAL PRESENTATION, DIAGNOSTIC TESTS, COURSE

Lung/Pneumonia/CD4 <200/mm³/Etiology of community-acquired pneumonia (continued)

CD4 <200/mm³

Pneumocystis jirovecii (carinii)* (PCP pneumonia) (see review: NEJM 350:24, 2004). Still common cause of pneumonia in U.S., 30% of 160 pts (AIDS 16:85, 2002) & death in those not receiving HAART (CID 36:1030, 2003). Less common in Africa except children: 51/105 admitted for severe pneumonia in S. Africa (AIDS 16:105, 2002; CID 34:1251, 2002; Int J Infect Dis Feb2, 2006). Cause of 26% of Zambian children deaths (Ln 360:985, 2002). 48% of HIV-infec infants <1yr in Botswana (PIDJ 22:43, 2003). PCP also found in adults: 30% of HIV-infec adults with neg. AFB smears were pos. by nested PCR for PCP in Ethiopia (AIDS 17:435, 2003) & 9/27 (33%) BAL specimens pos. in Tunisians (Tunis Med 80:29, 2002). In 1 report from China, demonstrated only by primary symptoms had PCP... (Respir J 5:419, 2000) & frequency in industrialized nations... (CID 36:70, 2003). Single study demonstrated by π3 %, 1/n individuals n ≥34 Zambian children receiving Co-trimoxazole; role of PCP in mortality not known (Cochrane Database Syst Rev Jan25, CD003508, 2006). AIDS 16:85, 2002.

Clinical: Dry cough, fever, progressive dyspnea of 1-wks duration
Laboratory: CD4: 1st episode mean CD4 79/mm³, med. 36/mm³; 2nd episode mean CD4 79/mm³, med. 10/mm³, med. 36/mm³

Arterial blood gas— ↓ pO₂ (<70 mmHg in 80% patients); pulmonary function tests—restrictive type defect with ↓ vital capacity & ↓ total lung capacity. Diffusion abnormalities common; single breath diffusing capacity for CO <80% of predicted (90% sensitivity) but only 25% specificity). ↓ PaO₂ with exercise may be of particular value.

Chest x-ray: 5-10% have normal chest x-ray (in these pts, CO diffusing capacity, ↓ PaO₂, with exercise may be of particular value.

Predicting etiologies of community-acquired pneumonia

Dx (OR=Odds Ratio)	Bact Pn (94) %	OR	PCP (101) %	OR	TBC (37) %	OR
Fever >7 days	11%	1.0	34%	4.3¹	54%	9.9¹
Cough >7 days	20%	1.0	50%	3.9¹	51%	4.2¹
Yellow-green sputum	54%	2.8¹	30%	1.0	30%	1.0
DOE	43%	1.5	81%	9.0¹	32%	1.0
Weight loss	23%	1.0	44%	2.2¹	68%	6.8¹
Night sweats	23%	1.0	46%	2.7¹	54%	3.9¹
Tachycardia	39%	1.8	39%	1.4	32%	1.0
Abn auscultation	57%	2.8¹	22%	1.0	49%	1.6
LDH >400	29%	1.0	62%	4.0¹	43%	1.9
pO₂	36%	1.8	66%	6.0¹	24%	1.0
Interstitial infiltrate	17%	1.3	69%	14.5¹	14%	1.0
Lobar infiltrate	54%	59¹	22%	1.0	32%	24.8¹

OR: 95% CI does not include 1.0 when indicated by ¹

Most common: **diffuse bilateral symmetrical fine heterogeneous reticular infiltrates**

Less common: Unilateral/focal distribution of same quality infiltrates or focal alveolar consolidation (especially upper lobe in patients on aerosolized pentamidine prophylaxis) or an interstitial pattern with fine nodular infiltrates in military lesions or focal nodules without cavitation, thick-walled cysts or pneumatoceles or pneumothorax, may produce pleural effusion (Chest 122:886, 2002).
Rare: pleural effusion &/or intrathoracic adenopathy.

After 4 days TMP/SMX, there is commonly an ↑ infiltrate resembling pulmonary edema. This complication is significantly ↓ when corticosteroid is used with TMP/SMX in pts with low pO₂ (see Table 12, pg126).
Sputum, induced: ↓ sensitivity when P. jirovecii (carinii)—sensitivity 77%, negative predictive value 64%; use of fluorescent antibody technique markedly improves detection over that with Giemsa stain (Eur Resp J 20:982, 2002). Also effective in non-AIDS immunosuppressed pts (CID 37:1380, 2003).

With HAART, incidence of PCP was dramatically ↓ (Chest 118:704, 2000). Use of HAART (either before or during hospitalization) ↓ mortality from 63% to 26% (p=0.03) in 58 ICU pts at San Francisco General Hospital (AIDS 17:73, 2003). HAART did not influence PCP mortality in another study in NYC (J IntensiveCare Med 20:327, 2005). Still accounts for 24% of hospitalization in Miami (Int J Infect Dis 10:47, 2006). Most cases (67%) now occur in pts with previously undiagnosed HIV (Scand J Infect Dis 37: 482, 2005) or in those supposedly taking PCP prophylaxis while receiving TMP/SMX prophylaxis less likely to fail than other regimens. Still common initial presentation for HIV, especially in elderly (CID 30:55, 2000)

Geographical clustering of cases reported (Am J Resp CCU 162:1617, 2000), but evidence for person-to-person transmission weak (AIDS 16:1821, 2002). Recently acquired infection more common cause of disease than previously thought (JAMA 286:2950, 2001).

Bronchoalveolar lavage (BAL): most common initiation of rx if BAL not timely available. Treatment for several days does not ↓ diagnostic sensitivity. Detection of P. jirovecii (carinii)—sensitivity 85-89%. Addition of real time PCR ↑ sensitivity to 100% & specificity to 84.9% (J Med Microbiol 53:603, 2004). Many now use empiric rx without bronchoscopy for typical clinical presentation (CID 37:1549, 2003).
Transbronchial biopsy: detection of P. jirovecii—sensitivity 88-97%. Rarely found on transbronchial biopsy if not found on BAL. PCR on respiratory secretions may ↑ sensitivity but false + still a problem (CID 30:141, 2000).

Response: With effective rx, improvement is expected in 7-10 days. Mutations in dihydropteroate synthase gene (essential for folate pathway) found in 20% of PCP isolates: In one study assoc. with ↓ survival (hazard ratio for death 3.1) (Ln 354:1347, 1999) but no correlation with either response to TMP/SMX rx or survival in others (Ln 358:545, 2001; AIDS 19:801, 2005). In 2002, 80% of HIV+ pts tested had DHFR mutations, while only 7% of clinical specimens had sulfa drug mutations not common (JID 189:1684, 2004). 13% in South Africa (CID 39:1047, 2004). DHFR mutations also arise under TMP/SMX pressure (AAC 48:4301, 2004) (also see EID 10:1721, 2004).
Pneumothorax is a common complication of PCP pneumonia & is associated with a high mortality (CID 23:624, 1996). Permanent ↓ in pulmonary function (↓ FEV, FVC, & FEV/FVC) & ↓ diffusion to CO reported (Am J Resp Crit Care Med 162: 612, 2000). **May coexist with TBc** (CID 32:289, 2001).
Disease process may blossom (pO2 & ↑ pulmonary infiltrates) with robust response to HAART **reconstitution**. Biopsy of lung infiltrate neg. for organisms but strongly pos. for PCP DNA (CID 35:491, 2002; BMC Int Dis 4:57, 2004).

See pg102 for abbreviations & footnotes

TABLE 11A (38)

CLINICAL SYNDROME, ETIOLOGY, EPIDEMIOLOGY	CLINICAL PRESENTATION, DIAGNOSTIC TESTS, COURSE
Lung/Pneumonia/CD4 <200/mm³ (continued)	
Kaposi's sarcoma (KS)[18] (continued) DNA sequences of a herpesvirus, HHV-8, have been identified in >90% of AIDS-associated Kaposi's sarcoma & in classic endemic African, Mediterranean KS, suggesting a role in pathogenesis of KS (NEJM 332:1181, 1995; AIDS 17:215, 2003))	**Clinical:** Usually but not always associated with cutaneous &/or mucosal KS. Present with cough (92%), dyspnea (82%) & fever (67%); less likely than pts with concurrent OI to have temp >38.3 & RR >20 breaths/min. Symptoms prolonged (>2 mos) in 18% (AJRCCM 153:1385, 1996) X-ray: Findings are somewhat distinctive: **coarse, poorly defined nodular densities throughout the lungs with concomitant coarse linear densities in the perihilar regions.** Nodules increase slowly in size, rapid ↑ suggests hemorrhage. Pleural effusions common (up to 50%). Hilar adenopathy rare (<10%). **Dx:** Bronchoscopy will usually show typical violaceous endobronchial lesions. **Rx:** Table 18. May respond to antiretroviral rx.
Lymphoma: HHV-8 also identified in body cavity lymphomas — see above	Lymphomas associated with advanced HIV infection are becoming increasingly common, are usually non-Hodgkin B cell type, with extranodal involvement the rule. Thoracic involvement in 1/4 & either reticulo-nodular interstitial infiltrates or alveolar consolidation in 25%.
Lymphoid interstitial pneumonia (LIP) (children) (Chest 112:2150, 2002)	A disease of unknown etiology which may present with shortness of breath in children with HIV infection (see Table 8E) X-ray: Resembles PCP with diffuse or focal, fine to medium reticular interstitial infiltrate. Findings gradually worsen over mos. Dx: Lung biopsy is necessary for dx; shows an accumulation of lymphocytes & plasma cells in interstitial areas. Rx: Corticosteroids may be beneficial.
CD4 <100/mm³ (For ATS statement on fungal infection in HIV+ persons, see Am J Resp Crit Care Med 152:816, 1995)	
Pulmonary alveolar proteinosis found on lung biopsy in 2 HIV+ pts (Pathol/Res Pract 200:699, 2004) Nocardiosis (Nocardia asteroides) Uncommon, 43 cases reported (Med 71:128, 1992). CD4 <200/mm³.	Fever, malaise, cough, weight loss. Chest x-ray: 83% abnormal, cavitation 62%, lobar consolidation 52%, pleural effusion 33%, reticulonodular infiltrates 33%. Lab: Blood cultures rarely +. May mimic TBc (J/Postgrad Med 47:30, 2001; S Afr J Surg 42:17, 2004).
Cryptococcosis (Cryptococcus neoformans) (common) Most common cause of death (44%) in HIV+ South African gold miners (CID 34:1251, 2002). See Meningitis C. neoformans is a ubiquitous soil fungus which usually affects the CNS (see Meningitis) in patients with CD4 <100/mm³. Pneumonia more common in HIV-neg. (J Med Microbiol 53:935, 2004)	Site of entry is usually the lungs & pneumonia has been reported. X-ray: Variable pattern; single (CID 23:810, 1996) or multiple well-defined nodules with or without cavitation or diffuse reticular infiltrates &/or hilar/mediastinal adenopathy. Occasionally a reticulonodular pattern or isolated pleural effusion may occur. Dx: Isolation of C. neoformans from respiratory secretions or blood cultures (Med Mycol 38:77, 2000). Serum CRAG may be positive. Rx: Table 12, pg121.
Coccidioidomycosis (Coccidioides immitis) (common—endemic areas) (see CID 41:1174 & 1217, 2005) Risk factors include Afro-American race & ↑ level of immunosuppression (oral-esophageal candidiasis) Rx with HAART &/or azole rx ↓ risk (JID 181:1428, 2000) A common reactivation or primary infection in patients from "cocci belt" (southwest U.S.) with CD4 <150/mm³. In HIV-negative individuals, annual incidence of symptomatic infection is 0.43%; in HIV+ individuals 25% developed symptomatic PCP (AJM 94:235, 1993). 15% pts had simultaneous PCP (Med 69:384, 1990).	**Presentation is similar to histoplasmosis—fever, chills, night sweats & weight loss; severe shortness of breath is common.** X-ray: Diffuse bilateral reticulonodular infiltrate (65%) similar to histoplasmosis or focal pulmonary infiltrate (14%) or normal (16%) (CID 23:563, 1996) Dx: Complement fixation antibody tests are frequently positive (68%), dx is established by identification of large spherules of C. immitis in sputum, BAL, biopsy or on culture. Rx: Table 12, pg120

See pg102 for abbreviations & footnotes

TABLE 11A (39)

CLINICAL SYNDROME, ETIOLOGY, EPIDEMIOLOGY	CLINICAL PRESENTATION, DIAGNOSTIC TESTS, COURSE
Lung/Pneumonia/CD4 <100/mm³ *(continued)*	
Histoplasmosis (Histoplasma capsulatum) (common—endemic areas) *(see CID 24:1195, 1997)* A common reactivation infection when CD4 <200/mm³ in pts with geographical history of having been in the "histo belts" (Ohio-Mississippi River Valley, southeastern U.S., St. Lawrence River Valley, Central America & other areas in Latin America) *(JCP 4:300, 1995)*. Annual incidence in Missouri 4.7% in HIV-infected.	Usually presents with nonspecific systemic complaints: fever, weight loss, night sweats, but lungs commonly involved with shortness of breath. Hepatosplenomegaly & rarely focal cutaneous pustules or ulcers commonly presenting findings. Pts may also present with "septic shock" including DIC. CD4 count <150. X-ray: Commonly shows diffuse, bilateral poorly defined small (1–2 mm) nodular infiltrates with or without hilar mediastinal adenopathy. Dx: Identification of H capsulatum in WBC on peripheral blood smear or bone marrow (PAS or silver stain) & culture (about 90% are positive). If suspected & disseminated not positive, biopsy lymph node, liver, lung or lesions. About 80% will have + immunodiffusion or complement fixation test for antibodies. Measurement of H. capsulatum antigen in urine +in 95% AIDS pts with disseminated histo, test useful in following rx & relapse *(CID 19(S1):S19, 1994)*. (Available at MiraVista Diagnostics, 1-866-647-2847). However, cross-reactivity with paracocci, blastomyces, cocci, & penicillium has been detected *(AJRCCM 170:1169, 1997)*. Rx: *Table 12, pg122.*
Blastomycosis (uncommon)	Uncommon; largest series is 15 cases *(AnIM 116:847, 1992)*. CD4 <200/mm³. Pulmonary (7 cases) & dyspnea, 2 chest pain, CXR 3 local, 3 diffuse reticulonodular. BAL cultures +. Disseminated (8 cases) CNS involvement (5 cases), multiple organs (6 cases). Rx: *Table 12, pg118.*
Paracoccidioidomycosis (South America)	Reported in Brazil *(Pathol Res Pract 199:811, 2003)*. 12 cases reported from Brazil. 10 had lymphadenopathy, 7 with interstitial lung disease, 6 with papule-nodular skin lesions with central ulceration, & 5 with ulcerative lesions of the mouth *(J Infect 51:248,2005)*.
Mycobacterium kansasii (may also occur at higher CD4 counts)	Clinical: Fever 78%, cough 57%, weight loss 45%, dyspnea 31%, night sweats 31%, looks like typical tuberculosis. X-ray: Infiltrates "atypical"; alveolar, interstitial or diffuse parenchymal or pleural effusion. Upper lobe cavities, have extrapulmonary dissemination. Cavitation more common at ↓ CD4 counts, hilar adenopathy with dissemination more common in ↓ CD4 counts *(Am J Resp Crit Care Med 160:10, 1999; Eur J Clin Microbial Inf Dis 18:582, 1999)*. Mortality rate 53% in 1 series of 127 pts, pts on HAART did better *(AJRCCM 170:793, 2004)*.
Mycobacterium genavense	Usually presents with fever, weight loss, diarrhea, abdominal pain, hepatosplenomegaly, anemia, pancytopenia, & occ. painful cutaneous nodules *(Ann Int Med 128:409, 1998)*.
Penicillium marneffei	Primarily presents as fever, anemia, weight loss & skin lesions (70%) with lymphadenopathy but 1/2 have cough & organism cultured from lung in 15%. Pulmonary infiltrates (densities, abscesses & cavities) have been seen. Essentially all cases from SE Asia. Dx by isolation from skin, blood or bone marrow *(CID 23:125, 1996)*. Rx: *Table 12, pg123.*
Rhodococcus equi (uncommon) 3% of pts with Rhodococcus equi infection may present with slowly progressive mass lesion which cavitates *(Rev Inf Dis 13:1391, 1991)*. Has tendency to relapse, may require surgery & long-term suppressive rx. One-half of pts thought to have TB: had rhodococcus in Uganda *(J Int 41:227, 2000)*. Also reported from Thailand, confused with TB *(J Int Chemother 6:229, 2000)*.	Rx: Pg114. HAART helps rx *(AIDS 16:509, 2002)*.
Toxoplasma gondii (uncommon)	Rare in U.S. In France represents up to 5% of cases of suspected PCP. Febrile illness, minimal cough, ± dyspnea. Reported to be associated with ARDS *(CID 19:169, 1994)*. Chest x-ray: Diffuse interstitial or diffuse coarse nodular (resembles PCP). Pleural effusion in 2/6 patients. Lab: ↑ transaminase, ↑ LDH. Sputum: BAL + for T. gondii *(CID 23:1249, 1996)*. Rx: *Table 12, pg126.*

See pg102 for abbreviations & footnotes

TABLE 11A (40)

CLINICAL SYNDROME, ETIOLOGY, EPIDEMIOLOGY	CLINICAL PRESENTATION, DIAGNOSTIC TESTS, COURSE
Lung/Pneumonia (continued)	
CD4 <50/mm³	
Aspergillosis (uncommon) Aspergillus spp. are commonly isolated from respiratory sites (4%), but invasive aspergillosis developed in only 15% of colonized patients, more common in pts with AIDS & associated neutropenia (CID 14:141, 1992; ibid., 19(S1):S41, 1994; Mycoses 41:453, 1998).	33 patients reported in one series, 64% had an episode of infectious pneumonia ≤ 1 year before. CD4 <50/mm³. All were febrile, cough 97%, dyspnea 80%, chest pain 20%, hemoptysis 17%, 21% CNS signs. Chest x-ray: cavities 42% (most upper lobe), bilateral interstitial infiltrates 54%, pleural effusion 15%. Despite rx, mean time to death was 8wks (AJM 95:177, 1993). Rx: Table 12, pg117.
M. avium (pulmonary findings **uncommon** but systemic symptoms without pos. blood cultures will occur in up to _ of all pts with AIDS in developed countries)	CD4 usually ≤50/mm³, marked ↓ with HAART (1.4 to 0.2/100 pt yrs) (Am J Resp Crit Care Med 162: 865, 2000) (see Table 12, pg111, & above, Fever of unknown origin). Rx: Table 12, pg111. X-ray: When lungs involved, heterogenous interstitial infiltrates with or without hilar lymphadenopathy. Following institution of highly active antiretroviral rx, pts with MAC infection have developed unusual systemic & pulmonary syndromes: painful generalized lymphadenopathy-like scrofula, massive abdominal & thoracic adenopathy with pulmonary infiltrates, fever, leucocytosis, & cutaneous nodules (Ln 351:252, 1998).
Cytomegalovirus (CMV) (uncommon) **CMV pneumonitis in HIV+ pts is rare but 90% of pts have evidence of CMV in the lungs at autopsy.** (See Sem Resp Inf 14:353, 1999)	Viral cultures of BAL fluid are frequently positive. CMV has been isolated from 30% of pts with PCP & associated with ↑ mortality (AJM 78:429, 1985), but rx with ganciclovir does not appear to affect outcome (NEJM 314:801, 1986). Consider lung bx when CMV cultured from elsewhere, fever, cough & dyspnea, persistent interstitial/alveolar infiltrates (Abst 158, 3rd CRV, 1996). Syndrome of ↑ dyspnea (over 1–3mos), interstitial infiltrates, hypoxemia, hemolytic anemia, siderophages on BAL reported (CID 22:616, 1996). Would rx if biopsy revealed interstitial inflammation with CMV inclusions & no other pathogens. Lung cancer appears to be ↑ with HAART (AIDS 17:371, 2003).
Pulmonary nodules (1 or more on CT scan)	Common condition (87/242 HIV+ pts had pulmonary nodules). 57 had OI: bact. pulmonary nodules in 30, TB in 14. If had fever. cough & nodule < 1 cm = bact. pulmonary nodules likely. If homeless, had weight loss, & adenopathy on CT = TB likely (Chest 117:1023, 2000). M. bovis reported (CID 39:e53, 2004). **Cavitary lesions:** PCP uncommon manifestation of common disease. Frequent: aspergillosis, R. equi, M. tuberculosis (in earlier HIV infection), bacterial pneumonia (P. aeruginosa, N. asteroides, R. equi). Unusual: crypto, coccidio, histo (CID 22:671, 1996; CID 22:81, 1996), & Pseudallescheria boydii. Definitive dx essential: BAL & transbronchial bx. A sarcoid-like response to HAART with non-caseating granulomatous appearing like diffuse interstitial micro-nodular lesions on chest x-ray has been reported (Am J Resp Crit Care Med 158:2009, 1999). Lung cancer appears to be ↑ with HAART (AIDS 17:371, 2003). Following HAART & ↑ CD4 (immune reconstitution) pts may develop hilar adenopathy with MAC, M. Tbc, crypto & other pathogens. Clinically useful predictors of etiology in 110 HIV+ pts: • Cough + necrosis of nodes = mycobacteria (51) • ≤7 days symptoms, dyspnea, airway disease = bacterial pneumonia (26) • >7 days symptoms, no cough or pulmonary nodules = lymphoma (2) 'Sarcoid' diagnosed several months following HAART in 9 cases in France, possibly representing immune reconstitution disease (CID 38:418, 2004).
Mass lesion ± necrosis (abscess) Histoplasmosis, coccidioidomycosis, cryptococcosis, anaerobes, S. aureus, M. kansasii, Rhodococcus equi (Tsukamurella reported, J Infect 49:17, 2004), Mycobacterium tuberculosis, Pneumocystis jiroveci (carinii), lymphoma, Kaposi's sarcoma, aspergillus, MAC, Nocardia asteroides, P. aeruginosa, CMV (AIDS Pt Care Stds 15:353, 2001).	
Hilar &/or mediastinal adenopathy Mycobacterium tuberculosis, Mycobacterium avium-intracellulare Fungal: Histoplasmosis, coccidioidomycosis, cryptococcosis, blastomycosis Lymphoma, Kaposi's sarcoma	In 45 pts with HIV & intrathoracic lymphadenopathy, 22 had infections (17 from mycobacterial disease & 5 from 'bacterial pulmonary nodules') & 17 had tumors (7 lymphomas followed by lung cancer, germ cell tumor, KS). CD4 in tumor vs. infection (314 vs 62). Cavitary lesions = infection (CID 38:418, 2004).

See pg102 for abbreviations & footnotes

TABLE 11A (41)

CLINICAL SYNDROME, ETIOLOGY, EPIDEMIOLOGY	CLINICAL PRESENTATION, DIAGNOSTIC TESTS, COURSE
Lung (continued)	

Pleural effusion (Sex Trans Infect 76:722, 2000)
Infections (66–70%):
  Bacterial pneumonia   31–57%
  P. jiroveci (carinii) pneumonia   15%
  M. tuberculosis   8–16%
  Others (each <5%). Septic embolism, aspergillosis,
  C. neoformans, MAC, nocardia—PCP rarely
	Incidence in 222 pts was 27% (AnIM 118:856, 1993). Large effusions & bilateral associated with Kaposi's sarcoma & lymphoma (South Med J 92:400, 1999). Tuberculosis ↑ likely when associated with miliary nodules or mediastinal adenopathy.

Non-Infectious (31%). (see Curr HIV Res 1:385, 2003)
  KS   19%
  Hypoalbuminemia   10–40%
  Heart failure   5%
  Others: Kaposi's sarcoma (10% in 1 series), non-Hodgkin
  lymphoma (18% in 1 series), atelectasis, uremia, ARDS,
  pulmonary emboli (4%)
	Carcinomatous lymphangitis presented with acute respiratory failure in 2 HIV-infected individuals; both had bronchogenic carcinoma (Intensive Care Med 30:1956, 2004).

Pneumothorax
  P. jiroveci (carinii) pneumonia (more common with aerosolized pentamidine)
  Pulmonary eosinophilia (Loeffler's syndrome)
	Occurred in 2% of a large series of patients (AnIM 114:455, 1991). Has high mortality rate if associated with PCP (CID 23:624, 1996; Lancet ID 4:120, 2004). Can be caused by drugs commonly used in HIV+ pts: sulfonamides, dapsone, penicillin (Ln 343:860, 1994).

Lymph Nodes	
Generalized lymphadenopathy (applies to lymphadenopathy without an obvious primary source) Etiologies: acute HIV infection, TBc, atypical mycobacteria, histoplasmosis, coccidioidomycosis, lymphoma, Kaposi's sarcoma, syphilis, Epstein-Barr virus, toxoplasma, tularemia, sarcoid, CMV, & Castelmian's disease (AIDS 10:61, 1996)	History & physical exam direct evaluation. If nodes fluctuant, aspirate & base rx on Gram & acid-fast stains. Pts receiving HAART may demonstrate fever & generalized lymphadenopathy from MAC infection following ↑ CD4 cells, **Immune reconstitution** (Ln 351:252, 1998) (Table 11B). Percutaneous ultrasound-guided fine needle aspiration effective in abd. adenopathy in AIDS pts in Thailand (J Med Assoc Thai 87:400, 2004).
Musculoskeletal System (see Skeletal Radiol 33:311, 2004; AIDS Reader 14:175, 183, 2004; Curr Opin Rheumatol 18:88, 2006)	
Pyomyositis (Am J Med 117:420, 2004) Staphylococcal; aerobic Gm-neg. bacilli (uncommon) (CID 22:372, 1996) Immune reconstitution with HAART produced pyomyositis & cutaneous abscesses from M. avium (CID 38:461, 2004).	May follow exercise, local trauma or injections. Swelling in muscular area, localized pain & fever. ESR usually ↑. Erythema often absent, can be indolent. ↑ bilateral in HIV. WBC may be normal & blood cultures usually negative (AJM 90:595, 1991).
Osteomyelitis (Brit J Rheum 31:381, 1992) S. aureus, Strep. species, enterobacteriaceae, M. kansasii, H. capsulatum, nocardia	Sinus tract cultures may give misleading results regarding etiology of osteomyelitis—bone biopsy necessary to establish dx.
Septic arthritis	Septic arthritis has a similar course in HIV+ & non-HIV pts (Rheumatol 38:139, 1999). M. kansasii ↑ in AIDS (CID 29:1455, 1999).

See pg 102 for abbreviations & footnotes

TABLE 11A (42)

CLINICAL SYNDROME, ETIOLOGY, EPIDEMIOLOGY	CLINICAL PRESENTATION, DIAGNOSTIC TESTS, COURSE
Musculoskeletal System *(continued)*	
Osteonecrosis (a vascular necrosis) was found in 15/339 (14%) asymptomatic HIV+ pts (*Ann Int Med* 137:17, 2002, *J AIDS* 25:19, 2000). osteoporosis, & osteopenia, assoc. with advanced HIV & traditional risk factors (↓ body mass, weight loss, steroid use, & smoking) but not ART (CID 36:482, 2003). Bone density in 1 in 84 HIV+ women vs HIV-neg age-matched controls: osteopenia 54% vs 30% control (p 0.004). Bone density did not differ according to HAART exposure (*AIDS* 18:475, 2004). Above confirmed in men (*J Bone Miner Res* 19:402, 2003). However, in 51 pts on HAART ↓ in bone density correlated with ↑ central obesity & glucose intolerance (post-load hyperglycemia) (*JCEM* 89:1200, 2004).	Evaluate for osteonecrosis in pt with persistent groin & hip pain. In 1 study of 25 HIV+ pts, 22 had other risk factors: ↑ lipids 32%, alcoholism 28%, pancreatitis 16%, corticosteroid rx 12%, hypercoagulable state 12%—4/25 receiving megestrol acetate. Multiple joints involved in 72%. Assoc (not cause) with HAART but results conflicting. In 1st prospective study of incidence of avascular necrosis found: they had more severe immunosuppression & ↑ body mass index than 260 HIV-infected controls (*AIDS Res Hum Retrovir* 20:909, 2004). In a prospective multicenter randomized open-label study, alendronate 70mg qw + Vit. D 500 intl units q24h & calcium 1000mg q24h improved lumbar bone mineral density & minimized femoral bone mineral density decrease after 52wks vs Vit. D & calcium alone in 41 HIV+ persons on HAART (*HIV Clin Trials* 5:269, 2004).
Arthritis, polyarticular	Typically, non-bacterial urethritis 7-14 days after sexual exposure. Asymmetric polyarticular arthritis involving large joints of legs, including toes, develops over several weeks. Typically resolves in 3-4mos but ~50% have recurrences. HLA B27 uncommon in Africans but reactive spondyloarthropathies still common in HIV+ persons (*Curr Opin Rheum* 12:281, 2000).
Reiter's syndrome: urethritis or cervicitis, conjunctivitis, arthritis, & mucocutaneous lesions (circinate balanitis, keratoderma blennorrhagica). For review of rheumatic diseases, see Semin Arth Rheum 30:47, 2000.Reiter's syndrome occurs in 0.5–10% of HIV+ patients, 75% are HLA B-27 positive (*Rheumatol Int* 9:137, 1989).	Lab: Synovial fluid typically is translucent, 2000–100,000 cells/μl, >50% PMNs, culture negative, glucose <50mg/dl lower than blood glucose.Rx: Since often assoc. with C. trachomatis, empirical rx for chlamydia (see Table 12, pg106) is appropriate. In non-HIV+ patients, methotrexate or folic acid antagonists have been used; they should not be used in HIV+ pts.
Psoriatic arthritis	Psoriasis noted in 1–5% HIV+ population. Frequency of arthritis unknown. Rx with infliximab reported in several cases (*Br J Dermatol* 150:784, 2004).
"Lightning pain" syndrome	Severely painful acute attack of arthralgia or myalgia lasts a few hours to a few days. Often requires narcotics for relief. Clinical exam normal. Cause unknown; no sequelae (*Med J Aust* 158:114, 1993).
Rheumatoid arthritis	Virtually never occurs in pts with HIV. Several pts with rheumatoid-factor positive RA have gone into remission after infection with HIV.
Arthritis, oligoarticular	Usually asymmetrical, lower limbs. HLA B27 negative. Synovial fluid: low WBC with PMNs (*Med J Aust* 158: 114, 1993). HIV-associated arthritis occurred in 7.8% of 270 pts at various stages of HIV. Course was acute, of short duration (2 wks), without recurrences or erosive changes (*J Rheumatol* 26:1158, 1999). A similar aseptic inflammatory arthritis reported from Congo: 83 pts (80% polyarthritis, 20% oligo), asymmetrical & non-erosive, knees 84%, ankles 59%, great toes 23%, wrists 41%, elbows 29%, small joints of hands 23%. All responded to NSAIDs in 4–8 wks (*Joint Bone Spine* 71:309, 2004).
Myopathy (progressive proximal muscle weakness)	Proximal muscle weakness, ↑ creatinine kinase levels. Muscle biopsy: 1/2 had inflammatory infiltrates, 1/2 pts rx with ↓ responded to prednisone (*AJM* 113:492, 1990; *Neurol* 53:241, 1999).
HIV-1 associated myopathy (see *Curr Neurol Neurosci* Rev 4:62, 2004)	
Drug-associated myopathy: zidovudine (ZDV), ddI & ddC (*AIDS* 12:2425, 1996); may be assoc. with d4T, lactic acidosis & mitochondrial toxicity (*AIDS* 18:1403, 2004)	Proximal muscle weakness & atrophy (legs >arms, "saggy butt" syndrome) occurred in 5/86 pts (6%) rx with ZDV >6mos (mean 45wks). Creatinine kinase ↑ (average 777 units/L).Muscle biopsy: "Ragged red fibers" on histology, abnormal mitochondria on EM. Improves with discontinuation of ZDV, recurs with rechallenge. ddC also causes a selective loss of mitochondrial DNA in vitro (*Ln* 337:508, 1991).
	Now reported with most NRTIs (*Ln* 354:1084, 1999).
Polymyositis—also reported from IRIS (*Clin Exp Rheumatol* 22:651, 2004, *Sex Trans Inf* 80:315, 2004)	A dermatomyositis-like disease has been described in AIDS (*Rheum Dis Clin* NA 17:117, 1991; *AnM* 159:1812, 1999).

See pg102 for abbreviations & footnotes

TABLE 11A (43)

CLINICAL SYNDROME, ETIOLOGY, EPIDEMIOLOGY	CLINICAL PRESENTATION, DIAGNOSTIC TESTS, COURSE
Pancreatitis (see above Endocrine System/Pancreas) 52/86 asymptomatic HIV+ pts had at least 1 ↑ amylase or lipase in serum; risk factors were ddI, ddC or IV TMP/SMX. No associated clinical pancreatitis (Am J Gastro 94:1248, 1999). 44 cases: usual major causes—alcohol 39%, gallstones 2%; drugs: pentamidine 27%, ddI 9%, TMP/SMX 5%, 3TC esp. in children; opportunistic infections: CMV 5%, MAC 2%, other 9% (AJM 98:243, 1995). 334/920 HIV+ Italian pts had at least 1 pancreatic lab abnormality (36.3%) in an observational case-controlled study. The 128 who had highest & most prolonged abnormalities were related to ddI. d4T, 3TC, pentamidine, TMP/SMX, anti-TBc Rx, ETOH, OIs, liver or biliary disease. PI-based HAART & ↑ triglycerides. No difference in risk factors seen between symptomatic (32 pts) & asymptomatic (96). After withdrawal of inciting agent, gatexate &/or octreotide appeared to be of benefit (Eur J Med Res 9:557, 2004). Pancreatitis 2° to NRTIs may be ↑ in older pts (Expert Rev Anti-Infect Ther 2:733, 2004). Tenofovir + ddI assoc. with pancreatitis in 6 cases (2.7%) (An Pharmacother 38:1660, 2004) & reduction in ddI dose recommended (Lancet 364:65, 2004). Pts rx for both Hep C & HIV receiving ribavirin & ddI ± d4T at risk for mitochondrial toxicity including pancreatitis (CID 38:e79, 2004). Also reported in 1° HIV infection (South Med J 97:393, 2004).	Pancreatitis due to ddI can be fatal (0.35%). In pts with history of pancreatitis, 8/27 pts on ddI developed pancreatitis. Pancreatitis occurs in <1% on ddC. In patients with a history of pancreatitis, 8/27 developed pancreatitis of ↑ amylase. All NRTIs implicated & likely due to mitochondrial toxicity (L/AIDS 37:S30, 2004). IV pentamidine is associated with pancreatic islet cell damage (hypoglycemia with later diabetes mellitus).
Peritoneal Disease	
Ascites, sudden onset	Symptoms & signs of underlying process.

Transudative ascitic fluid (<3 gm protein/100 ml)
    Concomitant hepatic cirrhosis (alcoholic), congestive heart failure, inferior vena cava obstruction, Budd-Chiari syndrome, hypoalbuminemia, vasculitis, hep B or C
  Exudative ascitic fluid (>3gm protein/100ml) (>500 cells/mm suggests infection, neoplasm)
    Tuberculosis, lymphoma, cytomegalovirus, nocardia (S Afr J Surg 42:17, 2004), strongyloides (Acta Cytol 48:211, 2004)
	Collect large volume (500–1000ml). centrifuge; may reveal AFB on smear
	Biopsy: Etiology most often found on biopsy. Elevated adenosine deaminase (10X ↑ vs cirrhosis or malignancy) found in TBc peritonitis (Eur J Gastro 11:337, 1999).

Renal (see Am J Neph 24:511, 2004 for dialysis issues; for kidney transplantation, Scand J Inf Dis 36:680, 2004) **Proteinuria & azotemia** (screen for proteinuria semi-annually (AJM 164:333, 2004). 14% black & 6% white pts in U.S. dying from AIDS have renal disease AIDS, 10% overall have renal failure (Curr Inf Dis Rep 4:448, 2002). Proteinuria & ↑ serum creatinine were risk factors for progression to AIDS & death (RR 2.5) in >400 HIV+ (J AIDS 32:203, 2003; CID 3:1199, 2004). **HIV-associated nephropathy (glomerulosclerosis) (HIVAN)** (AnIM 139:214, 2003—excellent review). Prevalence 12% in HIV+ African-Americans in Galveston, TX (Am J Neph 19:655, 1999; Am J Kidney Dis 35:884, 2000). 85% pts are black. In 3,926 HIV+ pts, incidence HIVAN 8/1000 person yrs in untreated disease. those with AIDS, HAART, ↓ risk of HIVAN by 60% & no pt developed HIVAN if HAART started before AIDS developed (AIDS 18:541, 2004).	Renal bx: Focal glomerulosclerosis with mesangial deposits of C3 & IgM, tubular ectasia & tubulo-interstitial disease. Course: Death in 3–6mos. even with dialysis. 60mg prednisone for 1mo. followed by 2mos. taper ↓ serum creatinine, ↓ proteinuria, & preserved renal function at 6mos. in 7/13 pts vs. O/8 control (Kidney Int 58:1253, 2000). HAART Rx improves outcome of HIV-assoc. nephropathy but not other renal diseases found in HIV+ pts (AnIM 139:214, 2003; AIDS Reader 14:443, 2004, Kidney Int 66:145, 2004). ⟶

See pg102 & abbreviations & footnotes

TABLE 11A (44)

CLINICAL SYNDROME, ETIOLOGY, EPIDEMIOLOGY	CLINICAL PRESENTATION, DIAGNOSTIC TESTS, COURSE
Renal *(continued)*	
HIV-associated IgA nephropathy More frequent than HIV glomerulosclerosis. Majority of pts are white.	Microscopic hematuria, minimal proteinuria, ↑ serum IgA. Progression of disease is slow. Thought to be immune complex disease (*NEJM 327:729, 1992*).
Nephrotoxic drugs pentamidine, foscarnet, aminoglycosides, amphotericin B, tenofovir	Causes renal tubular damage (*J Scand J Infect Dis 36:369, 627, 2004; CID 42:283, 2006*).
Hemorrhagic cystitis	Hem. cystitis caused by adenovirus reported (*Am J Hematol 63: 32, 2000*).
Urolithiasis: Renal colic occurred in 27/155 pts rx with PIs (*CID 39:248, 2004*)	24 HIV+ pts with nephrolithiasis: 14 on indinavir but only 4 (28%) had indinavir-containing stones. Others contained Ca oxalate, ammonia acid urate & uric acid. Abnormalities included hypocitraturia (5), hypomagnesuria (4), hypercalciuria (3), supersaturation of Ca oxylate (3), & hyperuricosuria (2) (*J Urol 169:475, 2003*).
Immune reconstitution syndrome (IRIS)	Inflammatory response following 8 wks of HAART in pt with miliary TB with AFB urinary shedding, developed acute renal failure (*CID 38:e32, 2004*).
Sepsis/Bacteremia (M. tuberculosis, non-typhi salmonella & S. pneumo were most common causes in Nairobi, Kenya (*CID 33:248, 2001*)	
Disseminated pneumococcal disease	30–85% of pts with pneumococcal pneumonia have bacteremia. Rate of S. pneumoniae bacteremia is 100-fold ↑ in HIV+ pts. It often occurs in early stage HIV disease. 86% of serotypes are included in current vaccine (*Am J Epidem 138:909, 1993*). Outcome of rx has been good, although rare relapsing infections reported (*CID 14: 1050, 1992*). In addition, S. pneumoniae may cause soft tissue infections (*JID 163:897, 1991*) (*See pg89*) *CID 24:1195, 1997*
Disseminated histoplasmosis may mimic sepsis syndrome	See pg89
Haemophilus influenzae bacteremia Causes include those seen in the non-HIV+ patient, especially the febrile neutropenic patient: enterobacteriaceae, Pseudomonas sp., Staph. aureus, Staph. epidermidis	Nasopharyngeal carriage rates for Staph. aureus in HIV+ 44% vs 23% in hospital personnel; rates of Staph aureus bacteremia ↑ (*Europ J Clin Micro:(1): 1985, 1992*). Nosocomial bacteremia still common in HAART era (*J: 45/1000 pt days*) (*CID 34:677, 2002*).
Recurrent bacteremia Non-typhi salmonella, especially S. typhimurium (outside of U.S.; Salmonella typhi) (*Trop Doct 34:198, 2004*)	In U.S., 20-fold ↑ in risk in HIV+ individuals (*Rev Inf Dis 9:925, 1987*). With CD4 >200/mm³ clinical presentation & response to rx similar to HIV-negative individuals. With CD4 <200/mm³, diarrhea is a less prominent symptom. 1-16% relapse within several months (*AIM 151:381, 1991*).
Mycobacterium avium-intracellulare (MAC)	See pg94
Bartonella henselae, B. quintana	See pg86&100
Rhodococcus equi	See pg93
Sinuses, paranasal (*Rhinol 39:136, 2001*) **Sinusitis:** microbial flora similar to HIV-negative (S. pneumoniae, H. influenzae, M. catarrhalis) plus other Gram-positives (Staph. epidermidis, P. acnes), aerobic Gram-negatives (Pseudomonas aeruginosa), fungi (aspergillus, rhizopus (mucor)). Alternaria alternata, H. capsulatum) (*CID 24:1178, 1997*). Rarely parasites (microsporidium, cryptosporidium, CMV, & mycobacteria (*CID 25:267, 1997*). Sinusitis occurs in 1/3 to 2/3 of adults with AIDS (*Ear, Nose, Throat J 69:460, 1990*).	Sinusitis may be part of acquired atopy in AIDS (*JID 167:283, 1993*). 2/3 pts are symptomatic (fever, nasal congestion, discharge). X-ray: 79% had air fluid level, usually more than one sinus. Despite rx, 60% pts had recurrent or persistent infection (*AIM 93:163, 1992*). Antral puncture required for accurate cultures & indicated if rx against common pathogens fails (*CID 16:404, 1993*). Think fungal if facial pain or headache out of proportion to clinical or x-ray finding. If CD4<50 & ANC <1000, incident course & subtle x-ray findings of invasion. Most common fungus Aspergillus fumigatus (*Otolaryng Clin NA 33:335, 2000*).

See pg102 for abbreviations & footnotes

TABLE 11A (45)

CLINICAL SYNDROME, ETIOLOGY, EPIDEMIOLOGY	CLINICAL PRESENTATION, DIAGNOSTIC TESTS, COURSE
Skin/Hair[11]	
HIV-associated pruritus (see *Am J Clin Dermat 4:177, 2003*) Etiology: Skin infections or infestations; papulosquamous disorders; photodermatitis; xerosis; drug reactions; rarely lymphoproliferative disorders.	One of the most common symptoms in pts with HIV. Workup with careful exam of skin, nails, hair & mucous membranes to establish primary dermatological diagnosis; biopsy skin if necessary. HAART may improve idiopathic HIV pts but some may flare with immune reconstitution.
Eosinophilic folliculitis (resembles Ofuji's disease); marked pruritus, discrete, erythematous, follicular papers on trunk, head, neck, proximal extremities. 90% above nipple line. Eos ↑ & IgE ↑. (*Mayo Clin Proc 70:677:1089, 1995*). Rx: Itraconazole 200mg po q24h improves ~75% pts (fluconazole of no benefit) (*Arch Derm 131:358, 1995*). Isotretinoin 0.75-1.0μg/kg/day may also benefit (*Arch Derm 131:1047, 1995*). Metronidazole 250mg po tid x 3 wks works in some (*Acta Derm Venereol 81:66, 2001*). Immune reaction to sebum. Difficult to differentiate from infective folliculitis; tx is useful (*Br J Dermatol 141:3, 1999*). In large study of 878 HIV-infec women, HAART ↓ folliculitis (*CID 38:579, 2004*).	
Maculopapular lesions	
Acute retroviral syndrome	Lesions 5–10mm diam symmetrical, esp. on face on trunk. (may involve palms & soles), erythematous, non-pruritic. Stevens-Johnson syndrome (*CID 19:798, 1994*), see pg55. Constitutional "mono-like" symptoms;" fever (87%), skin rash (68%). Mean duration of symptoms/signs 21 days (*CID 17:59, 1993*).
	Erythematous, urticarial papules.
Insect bites—axilla, groin, fingerweb; fleas—lower legs; mosquitoes—arms & legs	
Most common cause of pruritic papular eruption in Africa: 86/102 pts from the Academic Alliance Clinic, Mulago Hospital & Reachout Clinic, Uganda had biopsy findings characteristic of arthropod bites. These lesions assoc. with ↑ peripheral eosinophilia counts & ↓ CD4 counts (*JAMA 292:2614, 2004*).	
Drugs: Common cause of rash (esp. TMP/SMX & nevirapine) HIV+ pts have ↑ frequency of skin reactions to most drugs.	When pts were initiated in 1,251 NRTI-experienced pts with ~<50 CD4 cells, 66 (5.3%) developed rash; risk factors: sex (female) & high CD4 count at HAART (HIV Med 5:334, 2004). On the other hand, overall HAART assoc. with ↓ of dermatologic manifestations (*CID 38:579, 2004*).
Molluscum contagiosum More common in young women (*CID 38:579, 2004*)	Occurs in 8–15% AIDS pts. 2–5mm pearly flesh-colored papules, often with central umbilication on face, anogenital region. Disseminated cryptococcosis, P. marneffei, granuloma annulare (*J Am Acad Dermatol 49:S184, 2003*) may mimic.
Syphilis, secondary.	See above. Genital Tract.
Candidiasis (47% of AIDS pts had mucocutaneous candidal infections in 1 series)	Adults: diaper-rash type rash involving trunk & extremities. Adults: red, hemorrhagic maculopapular lesions.
Cryptococcosis	Common. Widespread skin-colored, dome-shaped translucent papules 1–4mm in diameter. Resemble Molluscum contagiosum.
Histoplasmosis	Slightly pink 2–6mm cutaneous papules to larger reddish plaques & multiple shallow crusted ulcerations (*J Drug Dermatol 2:189, 2003*).
Mycobacterial infections: M. tuberculosis, M. avium-intracellulare, M. kansasii, M. marinum, M. haemophilum, M. genavense (see pg93)	Vary from acneiform plaques, pustules or indurated verrucous plaques to ulcerative nodular lesions. See pg89. A case report of painful vesiculopustular rash secondary to hypersensitivity reaction to M. tbc antigen (tuberculide) (*Ln 347:372, 1996*).
Mycobacterium leprae	Clinical presentation of borderline leprosy similar in HIV+ & HIV−, but rx for neuritis less successful in HIV+ (*Lep Rev 63:134, 1992*).
Penicillium marneffei (See *CID 23:125, 1996; 24:1080, 1997*)	Clinically present with fever, weight loss, small umbilicated maculopapular skin lesions (2/3 pts) hepatosplenomegaly, adenopathy. Almost all pts lived or travelled in Southeast Asia (*J AIDS 6:466, 1993; CID 15:744, 1992*).
Cutaneous Pneumocystis jiroveci (carinii)	Rare but reported with underlying PCP. More common if pt on aerosolized pentamidine. Typically verrucous, translucent papules anywhere on body.

See pg102 for abbreviations & footnotes

TABLE 11A (46)

CLINICAL SYNDROME, ETIOLOGY, EPIDEMIOLOGY	CLINICAL PRESENTATION, DIAGNOSTIC TESTS, COURSE
Skin/Hair[11]: Maculopapular lesions (continued)	
Human papillomavirus (warts, condyloma acuminatum)	Diffuse flat & filiform lesions, often in unusual sites. See GI & Genital Tract, above.
Kaposi's sarcoma (CD4: mean 87/mm³; median 37/mm³)	Early lesions are round or irregular pinkish-red to violaceous macules to papules, usually non-tender. Often symmetrical along skin tension lines. (See below).
	Chronic recurrent eruption of papules & nodules that undergo spontaneous regression. Usually
Lymphoid papulosis (LyP)	benign with minority progressing to lymphoma. May resemble pityriasis but histologically resembles
Rare cutaneous lymphoproliferative disorder (AIDS Pt Care STDs 18:563, 2004)	lymphoma (Anaplastic T-cell or HD).
Nodular, verrucous, &/or ulcerative lesions	
Mycobacterial infections	See above
Bacillary angiomatosis (Reference: CID 22:794, 1996)	Friable vascular papules, cellulitis, plaques & subcutaneous nodules, usually tender. May be confused with KS. Etiology: Bartonella henselae & B. quintana. May be isolated from blood (5–15 days incubation of lysis centrifugation cultures on blood agar, 5% CO₂) & identified with Warthin Starry stain. See pg86 & pg100.
Acanthamoeba, disseminated	Rare (NEJM 331:85, 1994)
Sporotrichosis	Uncommon, but reported
Cryptococcosis	As above
Histoplasmosis	As above
Kaposi's sarcoma. Kaposi-associated herpesvirus (KSHV) now called HHV 8 is found in biopsy samples & blood mononuclear cells of pts with AIDS-related or classical KS (Ln 346:799, 1995).	Skin usually 1st site of presentation. Lesions palpable, firm, non-tender nodules. Early lesions may resemble ecchymoses. Typically violaceous, hyperpigmented, involving head, neck. Later become confluent, form large tumor masses & occur throughout the body. Up to 40% GI involvement. Oral lesions may precede skin lesions. In 107 Brazilian pts with KS, 61.6% demonstrated complete response to HAART, 23% partial response & 15.4% progressed. None receiving Pts progressed (Int J Dermatol 43:643, 2004).
Non-Hodgkins lymphoma	Skin involved in 15% of pts with non-Hodgkin lymphoma. Lesions are usually papules or nodules.
Mycobacterium avium-intracellulare (MAI/MAC)	Fever & extensive cutaneous nodules (granulomas or focal necrosies) have been reported in pts infected with MAC who responded to HAART with **immune reconstitution** (↑ CD4 counts & ↓ viral load). Steroids may be useful (x-59 Conf Retrovir 3:167, 1998, Abst. 726) (Table 11B).
Leishmania	May produce a wide spectrum of localized cutaneous, mucosal or diffuse lesions (An Trop
4% of cutaneous lesions in India (Indian J Path Micro 45:293, 2002)	Med Parasitol 97:S107, 2003). Most lesions are small, papular with ulceration but with HIV may widely disseminate with hundreds of lesions (Am J Trop Med Hyg 7:558, 2004).
Vesicular bullous or pustular lesions	
Herpes simplex virus	Grouped vesicles on erythematous base, rapidly evolve into ulcerations or fissures. May persist as chronic large ulcerative lesions, esp. in perianal area.
Varicella-zoster virus: Common in HIV+ pts & frequently precedes AIDS. 10–20%, frequency overall (Int J Dermatol 39:192, 2000; J Clin Epid 54:522, 2001; Am J Med Sci 321:372, 2001)	Grouped vesicles on erythematous base. May be verrucous in chronic form may persist as hyperkeratotic lesions. Dermatomal distribution. May be multidermatomal.
Cytomegalovirus	Small reddish-purple macules that ulcerate. May present with non-healing perianal ulceration.
Staphylococcal impetigo	Erythematous crusted papules, may be pruritic on face, trunk, groin.
"typical scabies"	Extremely pruritic, papular & vesicular lesions characterized by linear or serpentine burrows most commonly on hands, wrists, elbows, ankles. Average number of mites is 11.
Stevens-Johnson syndrome	Most often drug-related: TMP/SMX, fluconazole, ddl, anti-TBc drugs. 1 case reported with acute HIV infection (CID 19:798, 1994).

See pg102 for abbreviations & footnotes

TABLE 11A (47)

CLINICAL SYNDROME, ETIOLOGY, EPIDEMIOLOGY	CLINICAL PRESENTATION, DIAGNOSTIC TESTS, COURSE
Skin/Hair"/Vesicular bullous or pustular lesions (continued)	
Porphyria cutanea tarda	Association with HIV described but the co-occurrence may reflect coexistence of risk factors, esp. alcohol use, Hep C, rather than causal association (CID 20:348, 1995). Lesions especially over sun-exposed areas.
Papulosquamous lesions	
Seborrheic dermatitis	Occurs in 20-80% HIV+ individuals, dandruff to patches & plaques of erythema with indistinct margins & yellowish scale on "hairy" areas. Malassezia furfur may be causative agent (CID 22:S128, 1996).
Xerotic eczema (dry-skin syndrome), ↑ with ↓ CD4 counts (CID 38:579, 2004)	Occurs in 5-20% HIV+ individuals. Often severely pruritic & resistant to antihistamines.
Dermatophytosis (T. rubrum most common, then T. mentagrophytes & E. floccosum)	Occurs in 20-35% HIV+ individuals. Widespread, often severe with scaly red pruritic papules & plaques.
Tinea versicolor	Patchy areas of fine scale & hypopigmentation. CD4 often >300/mm³. Usually resistant to topical agents.
Psoriasis	Presents as (1) discrete plaques or (2) a diffuse dermatitis often associated with palmoplantar keratoderma. Distribution may be atypical: groin, axilla & scalp rather than elbows & knees. Common nail changes & psoriatic arthritis (JRD 17:914, 1996).
Crusted (Norwegian) scabies	**Highly contagious** to close contacts (health care workers). Characterized by erythema, hyperkeratosis & crusting. Pruritus is typically present but hyperkeratotic, crusted form may be absent. Burrows usually not seen. Gross nail thickening & subungual debris common. Alopecia, hyperpigmentation, pyoderma & eosinophilia may occur. Dx is suspected on demonstration of heavy mite burden (1000s) on scraping vs a few in typical scabies. Combination rx with topical benzyl benzoate & ivermectin po x1 effective in severe crusted scabies in one series of 39 pts (Br J Dermatol 142:969, 2000). Ivermectin may also be of value topically (Fundam Clin Pharmacol 17:217, 2003).
Occurs in 1.3-5% HIV+ individuals. A marker for HIV or HTLV-1 infection in Brazil & India (AIDS 16:1292, 2002). Found in 13/109 CSWs in Nigeria—all had HIV infection (Afr J Med Sci 31:243, 2002).	
Folliculitis	
Staphylococcal folliculitis	An uncommon presentation is violaceous plaques (up to 10cm) in groin, axilla & scalp.
Eosinophilic folliculitis	See above. Skin, eosinophilic folliculitis.
Skin discoloration (reddish-brown, occ. black or bluish)	Seen in 75-100% of pts on clofazimine, but also think Addison's disease, toxoplasmosis, etc. (J Derm 31:756, 2004).
Pressure ulcers (PUs)	Aggressive preventive strategies should be implemented.
Incidence 2.3/100 hospital admissions: ↑ with female sex, length of hospital stay (1.06/100 pt days), advanced HIV. Mortality 50% with PU vs 7.2% without PU with attributed mortality of 42.8.	
Hair disease Diffuse thinning, premature graying, elongated eyelashes. In African-Americans peculiar straightening of previously curly hair has been observed in advanced HIV (JRD 17:914, 1996).	
Nail disease	
Onychomycosis	
Longitudinal pigmented nail bands	
Splenomegaly	Seen in almost 1/2 on ZDV, more common in dark-skinned patients, occurs within 4-8wks of starting rx.
23% of 70 consecutive HIV+ pts were found to have splenomegaly on physical exam & 66% by ultrasound. Pts with liver disease were more likely to have it (RR=1.84, p<0.001). Splenomegaly was not a clinical event during a 1-yr follow-up or with developing AIDS in a 6-yr follow-up (CID 30: 943, 2000).	**Massive splenomegaly: think leishmaniasis!**

See pg102 for abbreviations & footnotes

TABLE 11A (4B)

CLINICAL SYNDROME, ETIOLOGY, EPIDEMIOLOGY	CLINICAL PRESENTATION, DIAGNOSTIC TESTS, COURSE
Systemic, wasting syndromes "Slim" disease (enteropathic AIDS), rule out: Cryptosporidium & other causes of chronic diarrhea Mycobacterium avium-intracellulare complex (MAC) Mycobacterium tuberculosis Histoplasma capsulatum Kaposi's sarcoma Non-Hodgkin lymphoma	Weight loss is common (29% in one series). Causes: opportunistic infections (47%), psychosocial factors (17%), drug-associated (7%), unexplained (29%). In Africa, most common symptom of AIDS is slim disease: weight loss (often >30% body weight), chronic fever, intermittent watery diarrhea without blood or mucus [to have parasites (cryptosporidium, Strongyloides stercoralis, I. belli Ethiop Med J 43:93, 2005). Many die without an apparent OI. Treatment unsuccessful. Nutritional deficiencies were found in 86% of 125 HIV-infected IVDUs & could account for unexplained weight loss (J AIDS & Human Retro 16:272, 1997). Rapid weight loss (>4 kg in <4 mos.) is generally associated by anorexia & is often due to a secondary infection; slower weight loss (>4 kg in >4 mos.) is often due to GI disease with diarrhea, less marked weight loss may be due to ↓ caloric intake (NEJM 333:123, 1995). Usually reversed with HAART response/Assoc. with ↓ survival in South Africa (S Afr Med J 91:583, 2001).

Abbreviations: 2° = secondary; **abn** = abnormal; **AFB** = acid-fast bacilli; **AM/CL** = amoxicillin clavulanate; **ARDS** = adult respiratory distress syndrome; **ATS** = American Thoracic Society; **BAL** = bronchoalveolar lavage; **bc** = blood culture; **CD4** = T helper lymphocytes; **CNS** = central nervous system; **CPK** = serum creatine phosphokinase; **CRAG** = cryptococcal antigen; **CSF** = cerebrospinal fluid; **CT** = computed tomographic scan; **CXR** = chest x-ray; **DIC** = disseminated intravascular coagulopathy; **DOE** = dyspnea on exertion; **DTR** = deep tendon reflex; **dx** = diagnosis; **Echo** = echocardiogram; **EIA** = enzyme immunoassay; **EMG** = electromyogram; **ERCP** = endoscopic retrograde cholangiopancreatography; **ESR** = erythrocyte sedimentation rate; **FTA/ABS** = fluorescent treponemal antibody-absorbed test; **hx** = history; **G6PD** = glucose-6-phosphate dehydrogenase; **HAART** = highly active antiretroviral therapy; **IDU** = injection drug user; **IL-2** = interleukin-2; **INH** = isoniazid; **ITP** = idiopathic thrombocytopenic purpura; **KOH** = potassium hydroxide; **LFTs** = liver function tests; **LP** = lumbar puncture; **LV** = left ventricular;
MAC = Mycobacterium avium-intracellulare complex; **MHA-TP** = microhemagglutination-T. pallidum; **M. tbc** = Mycobacterium tuberculosis;
MRI = magnetic resonance imaging; **NSAIDs** = non-steroidal anti-inflammatory drugs & salicylates; **PAS** = periodic acid Schiff stain; **PCP** = Pneumocystis jiroveci (carinii) pneumonia; **PCR** = polymerase chain reaction; **PI** = protease inhibitor; **PMN** = polymorphonuclear neutrophilic leucocytes; **RPR** = rapid plasma reagin test; **RTI** = reverse transcriptase inhibitor; **rx** = treatment; **SIADH** = syndrome of inappropriate antidiuretic hormone secretion; **TMP/SMX** = trimethoprim/sulfamethoxazole; **UTI** = urinary tract infection; **VDRL** = a reaginic antibody test (Venereal Disease Research Lab.); **ZDV** = zidovudine

1. These summaries have been extensively used the 6th Edition of *The Medical Mgmt of AIDS*, edited by Merle A. Sande & Paul A. Volberding, W.B. Saunders & Co., 1999. See Table 12 for details of treatment/disease entity. 2. Adapted from R.W. Price, Chapter 14, *ibid.*; 3. J.S. Greenspan, D. Greenspan, J.R. Winkler, Chapter 11, *ibid.*; 4. Adapted from J.P. Cello, Chapter 13, *ibid.*; 5. Adapted from R.W. Goodgame, *AnIM* 124:429, 1996; J.G. Bartlett, et al., *CID* 15:726, 1992; J.P. Cello, *Medical Mgmt of AIDS*, 6th Ed. 1999; J. Hambleton, Chapter 16, *ibid.*; J.P. Dowelko, *Blood Rev* 7:121, 1993; T.H.F. Chambers, Chapter 23, *Medical Mgmt of AIDS, 6th Ed.* 1999; 8. J.D. Stansell, L. Huang, H. Masur, Chapter 20, *ibid.*; 9. P. Goodman, *ibid.*; 10. L.O. Kaplan, D.W. Northfelt, Chapter 28, *ibid.*; 11. T.C. Berger, Chapter 11, *ibid.*; Also ref.: Ln 348:659, 1996

See pg102 for abbreviations & footnotes

TABLE 11B: IMMUNE RECONSTITUTION & NOVEL SYNDROMES ASSOCIATED WITH HAART

As noted in Table 6A, the use of Highly Active Antiretroviral Therapy (HAART) has led to a marked improvement in the control of HIV infections & significant reduction in mortality from AIDS wherever it has been employed (AnIM 135:19, 2001). In addition, HAART has led to reconstitution of the immune deficiencies in the majority of patients receiving this therapy. As a result of this, the incidence of opportunistic infections & AIDS-defining illnesses has also declined. This has been noted most dramatically in multi-center studies of treatment of AIDS-associated opportunistic infections, as the rate of accrual of patients in these studies has declined markedly in the past several years. The incidence of certain other infections including invasive S. pneumoniae has also declined in the US since the advent of HAART (JID 191:2038, 2005). In addition to the direct antiretroviral effects of HAART, a number of novel clinical syndromes have been seen as well. Among the syndromes associated with HAART are adverse effects due to protease inhibitors & other components of HAART, new syndromes associated with immune reconstitution, & the clinical effects of HAART on opportunistic disorders.

1. **Adverse effects due to drugs used in HAART**
   Many of the most important adverse events directly related to the agents used in HAART (such as renal lithiasis due to indinavir, gastrointestinal events related to ritonavir & other protease inhibitors) are detailed in Table 6B. In addition, a number of unusual syndromes (not necessarily related to a specific agent, but to classes of agents used in HAART) have been described in the past several years. Included among these syndromes (some of which may cause serious morbidity or even death) are lactic acidosis, abnormalities in glucose metabolism, disorders of lipid metabolism, lipodystrophy syndromes such as lipoatrophy & lipohypertrophy, osteopenia & possibly aseptic necrosis of the hip. These complications are covered in detail in Table 6C.

2. **New syndromes associated with immune reconstitution**
   Patients receiving HAART have reduced plasma HIV-1 viral load & increased CD4 T-lymphocyte counts. Despite this, there are reports of development of AIDS-defining events, particularly in the first several months after initiation of therapy (JAMA 282:2220, 1999). It is unclear at this point as to whether this is related to a delay in restoration of immune function or the fact that HAART may actually promote clinical development &/or expression of such infections as well as AIDS-related malignant disease. More commonly, however, one sees a variety of inflammatory reactions associated with immune reconstitution (Med 81:213, 2002; JAC 51:1, 2003). This syndrome is often termed the **immune reconstitution inflammatory syndrome (IRIS)** & occurs in up to 25% of patients with an underlying opportunistic infection after initiation of HAART (JAC 57:157, 2006). For instance, in patients with disseminated MAC disease, elevations in CD4 cells & associated immune reconstitution may be coupled with the development of painful generalized lymphadenopathy resembling scrofula. Massive mesenteric adenopathy with severe abdominal pain & thoracic adenopathy associated with pulmonary infiltrates & endobronchial proliferative lesions have also been described (JID 179:329, 1999; JID 180:76, 1999; AIDS 13:177, 1999). These patients are often systemically ill with fever, leukocytosis & malaise sufficient to require hospital admission (Ln 351:252, 1998). We have seen one patient with disseminated MAC disease who developed a symptomatic brain abscess due to MAC after initiating HAART. The resultant brisk granulomatous response & macrophage activation may lead to increased levels of 1,25 hydroxy vitamin D & hypercalcemia. One of the authors has observed 5 cases of hypercalcemia in this setting.

   "Paradoxical reactions" (hectic fevers, lymphadenopathy, worsening chest film) have also been described in patients with HIV and tuberculosis receiving concomitant therapy for both diseases (AJRCCM 158:157, 1998). The development of symptomatic cytomegalovirus retinitis shortly after initiation of HAART is likely a manifestation of the same phenomenon. Flares in hepatitis in patients chronically infected with hepatitis B & C viruses are likely also the result of improvement in immune status (Ln 349:996, 1997). Note that this syndrome must be distinguished from the mild hepatotoxicity associated with drugs used to treat HAART. The symptoms of the immune reconstitution syndromes usually subside spontaneously with continued therapy for the underlying disease or with the use of nonsteroidal anti-inflammatory agents. Occasionally reactions may be severe enough to be life-threatening & may require corticosteroid therapy (CID 38:1159, 2004). A summary of the clinical manifestations of specific opportunistic infections in HIV-1 infected patients receiving & not receiving HAART is given below (adapted from AnIM 133:447, 2000):

3. **Selected effects of HAART on opportunistic infections or other complications of HIV infection** (also see Table 11A for individual OIs)

Opportunistic Infection	Common Clinical Presentation	Presentation After Highly Active Antiretroviral Therapy (HAART)
Castleman disease	Fever, lymphadenopathy	Clinical recovery with resolution of lymphadenopathy (J Inf 40:90, 2000). However, late relapse (fatal) after initial response described in 5 patients despite immune reconstitution (CID 35:880, 2002)
Cryptococcus neoformans	Meningitis usually indolent, cerebrospinal fluid leukocytosis uncommon	Overt meningitis, marked cerebrospinal fluid leukocytosis
Cryptosporidiosis, microsporidiosis	Diarrhea	Clinical microbiological resolution associated with significant reduction in viral load (Ln 351: 256, 1998)
Cytomegalovirus	Retinitis, vitreitis, uveitis uncommon	Atypical (non-retinitis) manifestations of CMV, including pneumonitis, pseudotumoral colitis, adenitis & symptoms of viremia (Ln 351:228, 1998). Immune recovery uveitis (JAMA 282:1633, 1999; Eur J Clin Micro Inf Dis 22:114, 2003)
Hepatitis B (chronic)	Asymptomatic or nonspecific symptoms	Acute flare of clinical hepatitis 5–12wks after beginning HAART. Usually resolves without change in therapy. There is a description of reappearance of e-antigen in a patient with a 5-yr history of e-antigen positive hepatitis B (Ln 349:996, 1997).

TABLE 11B (2)

Opportunistic Infection	Common Clinical Presentation	Presentation After Highly Active Antiretroviral Therapy (HAART)
Hepatitis C (chronic)	Asymptomatic	Acute hepatitis, cirrhosis or HCV-associated disorder such as cryoglobulinemia within 1-9 months after initiation of HAART (JID 181:2033, 2000) HCV seropositivity may be associated with smaller CD4 recovery on HAART (Ln 356:1800, 2000). Both ↑ & ↓ in HCV DNA levels have been described following HAART & overall outcomes no yet known (CID 35: 873, 2002).
Herpes simplex (ano-genital)	Painful ulcerated lesions	Recrudescence of recurrent episodes of ano-genital lesions (CID 42:418, 2006)
Herpes zoster	May be severe accompanied by complications	Mild presentation, uncomplicated. May see increased incidence of zoster after initiation of HAART, possibly due to ↑ CD8 cells (Am J Med 110:605, 2001).
HIV-1 associated nephropathy	Impaired renal function	Reversal of pathology & recovery of function (Ln 352:783, 1998)
HIV-associated non-Hodgkin's lymphoma	Typical Stage I-IV lymphoma	Improved clinical outcome & survival (CID 37:1556 2003)
Kaposi's sarcoma	Skin lesions, disseminated disease, oral lesions	Regression of lesions coincident with significant reduction in viral load (AIDS 11:161, 1997; Ln 357:1411, 2001; J AIDS 31:384, 2002; JAC 51:1095, 2003). Laryngeal obstruction from mucosal edema is rare complication of HAART (CID 34: 231, 2002).
Lymphoepithelial parotid cysts	Parotid cysts	Resolution on antiretroviral therapy (AnIM 128:455,1998)
Molluscum contagiosum	Disseminated skin lesions	Resolution of severe disease coincident with 10-fold increase in CD4 cells (CID 24:1023, 1997)
Mycobacterium avium complex	Disseminated disease, weight loss, diarrhea, mycobacteremia	Focal lymphadenitis, granulomatous masses, endobronchial proliferative lesions, abdominal lymphadenopathy & pain (see above for more details), clearance of bacteremia without antimyco-bacterial therapy (CID 26:758, 1998), development of cavitation in pulmonary nodules (CID 27:1542, 1998). Immune reconstitution lymphadenitis may occur despite azithromycin prophylaxis (CID 34:371, 2002; CID 42:418, 2006). Intraabdominal disease results in greater morbidity than peripheral lymphadenitis (CID 41:1483, 2005).
Oral candidiasis	White plaques on oral & pharyngeal mucosa (thrush)	Clinical resolution of oral candidiasis without anti-fungal therapy. This is independent of immune reconstitution & may be a direct effect of PIs (JID 185:188, 2002).
Oral warts	Relatively rare oral lesions	Marked ↑ in oral warts which are progressive & recur after removal (Ln 357:1411, 2001; CID 34:641, 2002)
Chronic parvovirus B-19 infection	Anemia; AIDS wasting syndrome; encephalitis	Anecdotal case reports of response in patients with each syndrome receiving HAART (The AIDS Reade 8:21, 1998; CID 36:1191, 2003). Case report of development of parvovirus B-19 encephalitis in 1 patient on HAART (CID 36:1191, 2003).
Progressive multifocal leukoencephalopathy	Neurologic deficits, MRI demonstration of hypodensities without contrast enhancement	Neurologic deficits; neurologic deficits with enhancing lesions on MRI, frequently with peripheral enhancement (AIDS 13:1426, 1999); long-term, see remission of neurologic symptoms & improvement of radiographic findings (Ln 349:850, 1997) & increased survival in approx. 50% of cases (CID 36:1047, 2003; JID 180:621, 1999). Fatal, paradoxical worsening of PML (non-responsive to steroids) has also been described in pts shortly after initiation of HAART (CID 35:1250, 2002)
Pulmonary tuberculosis	Pulmonary infiltrates	Fever, lymphadenopathy, worsening pulmonary infiltrates
Systemic lupus erythematosus	Incidence of SLE decreased in immuno-suppressed AIDS pts	Anecdotal reports of new onset of SLE & flares of preexisting SLE following HAART (J Rheum 27:11, 2000)
Tegumentary leishmaniasis	No lesions or few erythematous papules	Worsening of prior lesions or development of disseminated lesions (JID 192:1819, 2005)
Visceral leishmaniasis	Fever, hepatosplenomegaly	Long-term remission (J Inf 40:94, 2000); development of post-kala-azar dermal leishmaniasis (J Inf 40:199, 2000). Decreased incidence of VL seen in France after HAART in 1996 (JID 186:1366, 2002).

TABLE 11B (3)

4. **Effect on incidence of AIDS-related opportunistic infections** The immune reconstitution associated with HAART has clearly led to a striking decline in the incidence of AIDS-related opportunistic infections, although the spectrum of these diseases, in general, has not been altered *(CID 27:1379, 1998)*. The incidence is highest immediately after starting HAART & declines progressively after that *(JAMA 282: 2220, 1999)*. The decreased incidence is also manifest by a striking decline in enrollment of patients into NIH-sponsored treatment protocols for opportunistic infections. Recent studies suggest that in patients receiving HAART, diarrhea is more likely due to therapy itself than to any of the formerly frequent opportunistic pathogens that cause diarrhea *(CID 28:701, 1999)*. A retrospective study has also suggested a significant decrease in incidence of cardiac involvement, especially pericarditis, arrhythmias & dilated cardiomyopathy in patients receiving HAART *(J Inf 40:282, 2000)*.

5. **Discontinuation of prophylaxis for opportunistic infections** *(Also see Table 10)* Data have now accumulated that it is possible to stop primary prophylaxis for MAI, PCP, & toxoplasmosis in patients with sustained responses (CD4 cell counts >100–200) to HAART [*Ln 353:1293, 1999; NEJM 340:1301, 1999; MMWR 51(RR-8):1, 2002*]. It is also now possible to stop secondary prophylaxis for PCP, MAI [especially in patients who received at least 1 year of macrolide-based therapy *(JID 187:1046, 2003)*], toxoplasmosis, cryptococcosis, & CMV retinitis in patients with sustained CD4 cell responses [*JAMA 282:1633, 1999; Ln 353:1293, 1999; NEJM 342:1460, 2000; MMWR 51(RR-8):1, 2002; CID 36:645, 2003*]. Although it may be possible to stop secondary prophylaxis for other opportunistic infections including varicella zoster virus, Histoplasma capsulatum, & Coccidioides immitis, further data are necessary to ascertain that this is safe *(J Inf 41:18, 2000; NEJM 342:1416, 2000; MMWR 51:RR-8, 2002)*. Rare instances of recurrence of MAI infection following immune reconstitution & cessation of therapy for disseminated MAI have been described *(Eur J CMID 20:199, 2001)*. The same may be true for patients in whom secondary prophylaxis for PCP is discontinued *(CID 36:645, 2003)*. It appears that discontinuation of PCP prophylaxis is not associated with increase in community-acquired pneumonia in patients with sustained CD4 cell count increase to >200 *(CID 36:917, 2003)*.

6. **Infectivity** Although one might expect that effective suppression of viral load might decrease the chance of transmission of HIV from patients responding to HAART, a serious note of caution is injected by data showing that in HIV-1 infected men on HAART (& no detectable plasma viral RNA), the virus may persist in seminal cells & semen & may be capable of sexual transmission *(NEJM 339:1803, 1998)*. Although a recent report suggests that people on HAART are more likely to develop a sexually transmitted disease, an epidemiological marker for unsafe sex *(Ln 357:432, 2001)*, the increased prevalence of unsafe sex in this setting is likely related to the perception that the subjects are at low risk of transmitting HIV & not to the administration of HAART *(JAMA 292:224, 2004)*.

TABLE 12: TREATMENT OF SPECIFIC INFECTIONS/MICROORGANISMS IN HIV+/AIDS PATIENTS

CAUSATIVE AGENT/DISEASE	MODIFYING CIRCUMSTANCES	SUGGESTED REGIMENS		COMMENTS
		PRIMARY	ALTERNATIVE	
BACTERIAL INFECTIONS				
Bartonella				
Cat-scratch disease—immunocompetent patient—lymphadenopathy Axillary/ epitrochlear nodes 46%, neck 26%, inguinal 17%	Etiology: Bartonella henselae Ref: PIDJ 23:1161, 2004	**Azithro:** Adults (>45.5kg): 500mg po x1, then 250mg/day x4d Children (<45.5kg): liquid azithro po 10mg/kg x1, then 5mg/kg/day x4d Treatment controversial—see Comment	No rx: resolves in 2-6mos. Needle aspiration relieves pain in suppurative nodes. Avoid surgical I&D. Rev.: AAC 48:1921, 2004	**Clinical:** 10% nodes suppurate. Atypical presentation in <5%, i.e., lung nodules, liver/spleen lesions, Parinaud's oculoglandular syndrome (CID 28:1156, 1999). CNS manifestations in 2% (encephalitis, peripheral neuropathy, retinitis, FUO). **Dx:** Cat exposure. Positive IFA serology. Rarely biopsy. **Rx:** 1 prospective randomized blinded study, used azithro (PIDJ 17:447, 1998), faster ↓ node size with azithro
Bacillary angiomatosis; Peliosis hepatis—patients with AIDS	Etiology: B. henselae, B. quintana	**Clarithro** 500mg q12h or **clarithro ER** 1gm q24h) or (**azithro** 250mg q24h) or **CIP** 500-750mg q12h), po x8wks	**Erythro** 500mg q6h po or **doxy** 100mg q12h po) x8wks. If severe, combine **doxy** with **RIF** 300mg po q12h)	**Dx:** Positive antibody. Blood cultures: use lysis centrifugation or blind subculture onto chocolate agar after 7–14d of incubation. Blood PCR good if available.
Endocarditis (see Table 11A, p.62) Ref.: AAC 48:1921, 2004	Etiology: B. henselae, B. quintana	**Optimal rx evolving. Retrospective & open prospective trials support: Gentamicin** 3mg/kg IV q24h x min 14 d + **doxy** 100mg po q12h x4-6wks Surgery—Over 1/2 pts require valve surgery, relation to cure unclear.		
Trench fever For suppression in AIDS patients	B. quintana	**Doxy** 100mg po q12h x4wks + **Erythro** 250-500mg po q6h (see Comments)	**Claritho, azithro,** or **CIP** in above doses	Suppression until CD4 T-lymphocyte count above 200/mm3
Campylobacter jejuni Fever in 53-83%, bloody stools ~37%	CAUTION: See Comment on quinolone resistance	**CIP** 500mg po q12h or **azithro** 500mg po q24h x3d.	**Erythromycin stearate** 500mg po q6h x5d	↑ worldwide resistance to FQs varies from 10% (USA) to 84% (Thailand) (JAC 47:2358, 2003). Erythro resistance rarely reported (CID 37:731, 2003). 15% of Guillain-Barre follows campylobacter (CID 37:307, 2003). Reactive arthritis occurs.
Chlamydia trachomatis (non-gonococcal or postgonococcal urethritis, cervicitis) Refs: MMWR 51:RR-6, 2002; NEJM 349:2424, 2003	NOTE: Assume concomitant GC. **Evaluate & rx sexual partners.**	**Doxycycline** 100mg po q12h x7 days OR **Azithro** 1 gm po (single dose) **In pregnancy: erythro** base 500mg po q6h x7 days OR amox 500mg po q8h x7-10d OR **azithro** 1gm po x1	**Erythro** 500mg po q6h x7d OR **Ofloxacin** 300mg po q12h x7d OR **Levo** 500mg po q24h x7 days OR **amoxicillin** 500mg po q8h x7 days OR erythro ethylsuccinate 800mg po q6h x7d)	**Diagnosis:** Nucleic acid amplification test on urine, urethral swab, or cervical swab (MMWR 51(RR-15):1–39, 2002). **Doxy & FQ not recommended in pregnancy.** Clarithro active in vitro vs C. trachomatis, but not FDA-approved for STDs. **For recurrent or persistent disease:** either metro 2gm po x1 + (either erythro base 500mg po q6h x7d or erythro ethylsuccinate 800mg po q6h x7d)
Clostridium difficile toxin-mediated diarrhea (Ln D 5:549, 2005)	See Sanford Guide to Antimicrobial Therapy for more detail	**Metronidazole** 500mg po q8h or 250mg po q6h x10–14d. If severe use **vanco** 125mg po q6h x14d (CID 40:1586, 1591 & 1598, 2005)	**Vancomycin** 125mg po q6h x14d	Avoid anti-motility agents. **Relapse occurs in 10-20% of patients;** use vanco + RIF 300mg po q12h x7–14d for relapse. Isolate patient.
Granuloma inguinale (Calymmatobacterium granulomatis or donovanosis)		**Doxycycline** 100mg po q12h x minimum of 3-4wks or (**TMP/SMX** 1 DS tablet (160mg TMP) po q12h x21d	(**Erythro** 500mg po q6h x21d (can be used in pregnancy)) or **CIP** 750mg po q12h x3wks) or **azithro** 1gm po q week x3wks	Rare in U.S. Should see clinical response after 1wk. Rx until all lesions healed—may require 4wks of rx. Rx failure/relapse seen with doxy & TMP/SMX. FQ & chloro reported efficacious (CID 25:24, 1997)
Haemophilus ducreyi (chancroid)	Painful genital ulcer(s)	**Ceftriaxone** 250mg IM (single dose) or **azithro** 1gm po single dose	**CIP** 500mg po q12h x3d OR **Erythro** 500mg po q6h x7d	In HIV+ pts, failures reported with single dose azithro, may require usual regimen (0.5gm po, then 250mg po q24h x4d) (CID 35(Suppl.2):S135, 2002

TABLE 12 (2)

CAUSATIVE AGENT/DISEASE	MODIFYING CIRCUMSTANCES	SUGGESTED REGIMENS		COMMENTS
		PRIMARY	**ALTERNATIVE**	
BACTERIAL INFECTIONS *(continued)*				
Listeriosis Ref.: CID 24:1, 1997	Bacteremia, meningitis, focal infections	**Ampicillin** 2gm IV q4h ± **gentamicin** IV 2mg/kg load dose, then 1.7mg/kg q8h.	If pen allergic: **TMP/SMX** 20mg/kg/day TMP (component) IV divided q6-8h dosage	Some evidence suggests synergy with ampicillin + an aminoglycoside (gentamicin). Duration of rx 2-4wks. **(Cephalosporins not active vs L. monocytogenes)**
Lymphogranuloma Venereum Etiology: C. trachomatis, serovars		**Doxycycline** 100mg po q12h	**Erythro** 500mg po q6h x21d	Dx based on serology, biopsy contraindicated. Rectal LGV may need ...
Mycobacterium tuberculosis: Treatment of latent infection (LTBI) [previously known as preventive treatment, infection without disease (pos tuberculin test)] or **HIV+ pt with anergy & high risk for tuberculosis** (AnIM 119: 185, 1993). HIV+ pts with anergy need prophylaxis only if exposed to active TB (NEJM 337: 315, 1997) or if they fall into a group at high risk for TBc (e.g. HIV-infected IV drug abusers) (AIDS 13: 2069, 1999). Therefore use of anergy testing in conjunction with tuberculin testing is no longer recommended for routine screening programs for TB among HIV-infected pts in U.S. (MMWR 46(RR-15):1, 1997; JAMA 283:2003, 2000)		**INH** 5mg/kg/day (max. 300mg/day) po + **pyridoxine** (B6) 25-50 mg po x6mo (See Comment). For children, see Table 9F, pg47. **If INH not possible, options:** **RIF**** 600mg po q24h OR **RFB**** 300mg po q24h x4 mos.	If compliance problem: INH by DOT 15mg/kg 2x/wk x9mos + RIF also ↓ risk of TB (NEJM 337:801, 1997). 2mo regimens of RIF + PZA or RFB + PZA also shown to be effective (AIDS 13:1549, 1999). **However, there are recent descriptions of severe & fatal hepatitis in immunocompetent pts on RIF + PZA** (MMWR 52:735, 2003)	For pts given ddC+ INH, suggest 50mg pyridoxine/day. Duration of preventive rx unclear: recommendations range from 2-12mos. Ugandan study suggests 6mos of INH or 3mos of INH + RIF + PZA also shown to be effective (AIDS 13:1549, 1999). **However, there are recent descriptions of severe & fatal hepatitis in immunocompetent pts on RIF + PZA** (MMWR 52:735, 2003; CID 39:561, 2004). The risk appears lower in HIV+ patients (CID 39:561, 2004). Therefore, regimen is no longer rec for LTBI (MMWR 52:735, 2003; CID 39:484, 2004). Resistant TBc occurred in INH + pts given INH + RIF by DOT —presum. due to malabsorption (NEJM 332:336, 1995; AJM 127:286, 1997; CID 25:1044, 1997), although 1 study failed to detect direct effect on bioavailability of antimycobacterial drugs in pts with AIDS + diarrhea (CID 25: 104, 1997). INH prophylaxis reported to ↓ progression of HIV (Lancet 342:268, 1993). Late "failures" of INH prophylaxis usually due to reinfection, not primary failure of regimen (CID 34:386, 2002).
	INH-resistant (or adverse reaction to INH), RIF-sensitive organisms likely	**RIF** 600 mg po q24h or **RFB** 300 mg po q24h x4 mos.	Efficacy of all regimens unproven. ♂ **PZA** 25-30mg/kg/day to max. of 2gm/day + **ETB** 15-25mg/kg/day po x12mos.	
For more details, see USPHS recommendations (AnIM 137 No. 5 (Suppl, Part 2), 2002; CID 37:1686, 2003; NEJM 350:2060, 2004; NEJM 293:2776, 2005)	INH- & RIF-resistant organisms likely		**PZA** 25mg/kg/day to max of 2gm/day + **CIP** 750mg q12h or **oflox** 400mg q12h or **levoflox** 500mg/day po, x6-12mos.	If ETB used in dose above 15mg/kg/day, monitor pt for retrobulbar neuritis. (Visual acuity & red/green color test. ≥10% loss considered significant.) **Consultation recommended.**
Treatment, active tuberculosis in HIV-neg pts who are HIV+ & have active TBc are bacteremic (AIDS 13: 2193, 1999). 10-20% of HIV+ pts who are ...	**General principles TBc therapy in pts co-infected with HIV:** • Rx of TBc in pts with HIV infec. should follow same principles as for persons without HIV. • Presence of active TBc requires immed. initiation of rx. • In antiretroviral-naive pts, delay of HAART for 4-8wks after initiation of HAART. Further delay could be detrimental (JID 190: 1670, 2004). • Directly observed therapy strongly recommended for HIV/TB co-infected • Rifampin/rifabutin-based regimens should be given at least 3x weekly in pts with CD4 <100/mm³ • Once weekly rifapentine not recommended in HIV-infected pts. • Despite drug interactions, rifamycin should be included in pts receiving HAART, with dosage adjustment as necessary. • Paradoxical reaction should be treated with continuation of rx for TBc & HIV, along with use of NSAIDs. • In severe cases of paradoxical reaction, some suggest use of high-dose prednisone. (www.aidsinfo.nih.gov)			

* See end of section for options regarding concomitant use of protease inhibitors & RIF or RFB.

** Tuberculin test. The standard is the Mantoux test 5 TU (intermediate) PPD in 0.1 ml diluent stabilized with Tween 80. Read at 48-72hrs, measuring the maximum diameter of induration (not erythema). A reaction of ≥5mm is defined as + in pt. For HIV+ pts who have received BCG ≥10mm is cutoff (Brit Med J 304:1231, 1992). See also Table 23 for details of PPD testing.
NOTE: All dosage recommendations are for adults (unless otherwise indicated) & assume normal renal function.

TABLE 12 (3)

CAUSATIVE AGENT/DISEASE	MODIFYING CIRCUMSTANCES	PRIMARY			ALTERNATIVE			COMMENTS

SUGGESTED REGIMENS (in vitro susceptibility known)[3]

BACTERIAL INFECTIONS/Mycobacterium tuberculosis (continued)

		INITIAL PHASE[1]		CONTINUATION PHASE OF THERAPY			

SEE COMMENTS FOR DOSAGE

Regimen	Drugs	Interval/Doses (min. duration)[2]	Regimen	Drugs	Interval/Doses (min. duration)[2,3]	Range of Total Doses (min. duration)[2,3]
1	INH RIF PZA ETB	7d/wk x56 doses (8wk) or 5d/wk x40 doses (8wk)[4]	1a	INH/RIF	7d/wk x126 doses (18wk) or 5d/wk x90 doses	182–130 (26wk)
			1b	INH/RIF	2x/wk x36 doses (18wk)[4]	92–76 (26wk)
			1c[5]	INF/RPF	1x/wk x18 doses (18wk)	74–58 (26wk)
2	INH RIF PZA ETB	7d/wk x14 doses (2wk), then 2x/wk x12 doses (6wk) or 5d/wk x10 doses (2wk) then 2x/wk x12 doses (6wk)[4]	2a	INH/RIF	2x/wk x36 doses (18wk)	62–58 (26wk)
			2b[5]	INH/RFP	1x/wk x18 doses (18wk)	44–40 (26wk)
3	INH RIF PZA ETB	3d/wk x24 doses (8wk)	3a	INH/RIF	3x/wk x54 doses (18 wk)	78 (26wk)
4	INH RIF ETB	7d/wk x56 doses (8wk) or 5d/wk x40 doses (8wk)[4]	4a	INH/RIF	7d/wk x217 doses (31wk) or 5d/wk x155 doses (31wk)[4]	273–195 (39wk)
			4b	INH/RIF	2x/wk x62 doses (31 wk)	118–102 (39wk)

Dose in mg/kg (max. daily dose)

Regimen[*]	INH	RIF	PZA	ETB	SM	RFB
Daily						
Child	10–20 (300)	10–20 (600)	15–30 (2000)	15–25 (1600)	20–40 (1000)	10–20 (300)
Adult	5 (300)	10 (600)	15–30 (2000)	15–25 (1600)	15 (1000)	5 (300)
2x/wk (DOT)						
Child	20–40 (900)	10–20 (600)	50–70 (4000)	50 (4000)	25–30 (1500)	10–20 (300)
Adult	15 (900)	10 (600)	50–70 (4000)	50 (4000)	25–30 (1500)	5 (300)
3x/wk (DOT)						
Child	20–40 (900)	10–20 (600)	50–70 (3000)	25–30 (2000)	25–30 (1500)	NA
Adult	15 (900)	10 (600)	50–70 (3000)	25–30 (2000)	25–30 (1500)	NA

Second-line anti-TB agents can be dosed as follows to facilitate DOT:
Cycloserine 500–750mg po q24h (5x/wk)
Ethionamide 500–750mg po q24h (5x/wk)
Kanamycin or capreomycin 15mg/kg IM/IV q24h (3–5x/wk)
CIP 750mg po q24h (5x/wk)
Ofloxacin 600–800mg po q24h (5x/wk)
Levofloxacin 750mg po q24h (5x/wk) (CID 21:1245, 1995)

NOTE:
1. Clinical & microbiologic response same as in HIV-neg patient, although there is considerable variability among currently available studies (CID 32:623, 2001)
2. Post-treatment long-term suppression not necessary for drug-susceptible strains
3. Short course (6mo) therapy, including 2x weekly DOT regimens in HIV+ pts clearly shown effective in U.S. & Africa (AIDS 13:1899 & 1543, 1999). However, because **of possibility of dev resistance to rifampin in pts with low CD4 cell counts who receive weekly or biweekly doses of rifabutin,** it is recommended that such pts receive daily (or at least 3x-weekly) doses of RFB for initiation & continuation phase of TBc (MMWR 51:214, 2002; CID 41:83, 2005). Low serum levels of RIF & ETB noted in HIV+ patients. Where practical, therapeutic monitoring may be useful (CID 41:1638, 2005)

CAUSATIVE AGENT/DISEASE — Isolation essential! (See Table 11, pg40.) Older observations on infectivity of susceptible & resistant M. tbc before & after (Am Rev Resp Dis 85:511, 1962) may not be applicable to MDR M. tbc or to the HIV+ individual. Extended isolation may be appropriate.

MODIFYING CIRCUMSTANCES — Rate of INH resistance known to be <4% (drug-susceptible organisms)

General references on therapeutic options: CID 28:130, 1999; NEJM 340: 367, 1999; J Resp Dis 21:9, 2000; BMJ 325:1282, 2002; MMWR 52(RR-11):1, 2003; MMWR 53(RR-15):1, 2004; CID 40 (Suppl.1):S1, 2005

[**] See end of section for options regarding concomitant use of protease inhibitors & **RIF** or **RFB**

[*] All dosage recommendations are for adults (unless otherwise indicated) & assume normal renal function.

NOTE: All dosage recommendations are for adults (unless otherwise indicated) & assume normal renal function.

TABLE 12 (4)

Treatment, active tuberculosis (continued). Review of therapy for MDR TB: *JAC 54:593, 2004; Med Lett 2:83, 2004*

MODIFYING CIRCUMSTANCES	SUGGESTED REGIMENS	DUR OF TREATMENT (MO.)	SPECIFIC COMMENTS	COMMENTS
INH (± SM) resistance	**RIF, PZA, ETB** (an **FO** to strengthen the regimen for pts with extensive disease)	6	In Brit Medical Research Council trials, 6mos regimens have yielded ≥95% success rates despite resistance to INH if 4 drugs were used in the initial phase & RIF + ETB or SM was used throughout (*ARRD 133:423, 1986*). Add'l studies suggested results were best if PZA also used throughout 6mos (*ARRD 136:1339, 1987*). FQs not employed in BMRC studies, but may strengthen regimen for pts with extensive disease. INH should be stopped.	NOTE: FQ resistance may be seen in pts previously treated with FQ (*CID 37:1448, 2003*). Moxifloxacin, gatifloxacin, levofloxacin have enhanced activity compared with ciprofloxacin against M. tuberculosis (*AAC 46:1022, 2002; AAC 47: 2442, 2003; AAC 47:3117, 2003; JAC 53:441, 2004; AAC 48:780, 2004*). Linezolid has excellent in vitro activity, including MDR strains (*AAC 47:416, 2003*).
Resistance to INH & RIF (± SM)	**FO, PZA, ETB, IA,** ± alternative agent[*]	18–24	In cases of INH resistance [see *MMWR 52(RR-11):1, 2003 for add'l discussion*]. In such cases, extended rx is needed to ↓ the risk of relapses. In cases of failure & acquired drug resistance, or with extensive disease, the use of an additional agent (alternative agents) may be prudent to ↓ the risk of failure & additional acquired drug resistance. Resectional therapy may be appropriate. Surgical intervention may be considered. Survival ↑ in pts receiving active FQ & surgical intervention (*AJRCCM 169:1103, 2004*).	
Resistance to INH, RIF (± SM), & ETB or PZA	**FO** (**ETB** or **PZA** if active), **IA,** & 2 alternative agents[*]	24	Use the first-line agents to which there is susceptibility. Add 2 or more alternative agents in pts receiving active drug.	
Resistance to RIF	**INH, ETB, FO,** supplemented with **PZA** for the first 2 mos (an IA may be included for the first 2–3mos. for pts with extensive disease	12–18	Daily & 3x/wk regimens of INH, PZA, & SM given for 9mos were effective in a BMRC trial (*ARRD 115:727, 1977*). However, extended duration of rx may not be feasible. It is not known if ETB would be as effective as SM in these regimens. An all-oral regimen x12–18mos. should be effective. But for more extensive disease &/or to shorten duration (e.g., to 12mos.), an IA may be added in the initial 2mos.	

INITIAL & CONTINUATION THERAPY			COMMENTS
INH 300mg + **RFB** (see below for doses) + **PZA** 25mg/kg + **ETB** 15mg/kg q24h x2 mos., then **INH** + **RFB** x4mos. (up to 7mos.)			Adapted from *MMWR 49:185, 2000; AJRCCM 162:7, 2001)* Rifamycins induce cytochrome CYP450 enzymes (RIF > rifapentine > RFB), & reduce serum levels of concomitantly administered Pls. Conversely, Pls (ritonavir > amprenavir > indinavir > nelfinavir > saquinavir) inhibit CYP450 & cause ↑ in serum levels of RIF & RFB. If dose of RFB is not reduced, toxicity ↑. RFB/Pl combinations are therapeutically effective (*CID 30:779, 2000*). For detailed discussion of drug interactions in rx of TB in HIV-infected pts, see *CID 28:419, 1999*. Based on new data, MMWR now recommends against use of RIF for rx of active TB in pts on regimens containing efavirenz or ritonavir. **RIF should not be administered with ritonavir + saquinavir because drug-induced hepatitis with marked transaminase elevations has been observed in healthy volunteers receiving this regimen** (*Roche; www.fda.gov*). RFB can also be used with efavirenz but the dose should be ↑ to 450–600mg/day with efavirenz & ↓ to 150 or 3x/wk with ritonavir. (*CID 41:1343, 2005*). No dose modification of RFB with saquinavir (softgel) as single agent (*MMWR 49: 185, 2000*). RFB has no effect on nelfinavir levels at nelfinavir dose of 1250mg po q12h (*Can JID 10:218, 1999*).

Conco-mitant protease inhibitor (PI) therapy requires dose modification	PI Regimen	PI Dose	RFB Dose	ALT. REGIMEN
	Nelfinavir, indinavir or amprenavir	Nelfinavir 1200mg q12h Indinavir—consider ↑ to 1000mg q8h Amprenavir 1200mg q12h	150mg q24h or 300mg intermittently	**INH + SM + PZA** x2mos., then **INH + SM + PZA** x7mos. May be prolonged to 12mos. in pts with delayed response. May be used with any PI regimen.
	Saquinavir	300mg q24h or intermittently		
	Ritonavir	150 mg 2x/wk	No change	
	Lopinavir/ritonavir	150 mg 2x/wk	No change	

[1] In order of preference.   [2] When DOT is used, drugs may be given 5 days/wk & the necessary number of doses adjusted accordingly. Although there are no studies that compare 5 with 7 daily doses, extensive experience indicates that this would be an effective practice.   [3] Patients with cavitation on initial chest x-ray & positive cultures at completion of 2mos of rx should receive a 7-month (31 wk; either 217 doses [daily] or 62 doses [2x/wk]) continuation phase.   [4] 5-day a wk administration is always given by DOT.   [5] Not recommended for HIV-infected pts with CD4 cell counts <100 cells/μl.   [6] Options 1c & 2b should be used only in HIV-neg. pts who have felt x-ray & who do not have cavitation on initial chest x-ray. For pts started on this regimen & found to have a pos. culture from the 2-mo specimen, rx should be extended an extra 3 months.   [7] Options 4a & 4b should be considered only when options ↑–3 cannot be given.   *Alternative agents* = ethionamide, cycloserine, p-aminosalicylic acid, clarithromycin, AMCl, linezolid.   * *Modified from MMWR 52(RR-11):1, 2003.* See also *IDCP 11:329, 2002.*

NOTE: All dosage recommendations are for adults (unless otherwise indicated) & assume normal renal function.

TABLE 12 (5)

CAUSATIVE AGENT/DISEASE	MODIFYING CIRCUMSTANCES	SUGGESTED REGIMENS — PRIMARY	SUGGESTED REGIMENS — ALTERNATIVE	COMMENTS
BACTERIAL INFECTIONS (continued)				
Mycobacterium avium-intracellulare complex (MAC or MAI)	**Primary prophylaxis**— Pt's CD4 count <50–100/mm³ NOTE: Prophylaxis may be discontinued in pts with sustained ↑ in CD4 cells of ≥100/mm³ on HAART (AnIM 133:493, 2000; NEJM 342:1085, 2000)	Azithro 1200mg po weekly OR Clarithro 500mg po q12h	RBF 300mg po q24h OR Azithro 1200mg po weekly + RIF 300mg po q24h	RFB reduces MAC infection rate by 55% (no survival benefit), clarithro by 68% (30% survival benefit), azithro by 59% (NEJM 335:384 & 428, 1996; NEJM 335:392, 1996). RFB more effective than either alone but not as well tolerated (NEJM 335:392, 1996). Many drug-drug interactions, see Table 16B. RFB ↑ metabolism of ZDV with 32% ↓ in AUC. Clarithro ↑ blood levels of non-sedating antihistamines with attendant risk of arrhythmias. Drug-resistant MAI disease seen in 29–58% of pts in whom disease develops while taking clarithro prophylaxis & in 11% of those on azithro but has not been observed with RFB prophylaxis (J Inf 38:6, 1999). Clarithro resistance more likely to be seen in pts with extremely low CD4 counts at initiation (CID 27:807, 1998). Need to be sure no active M. tbc. RFB used for prophylaxis may promote selection of (rifamycin)-resistant M. tbc (NEJM 335:384 & 428, 1996).
	Treatment: Either presumptive dx or after positive culture of blood, bone marrow, or other usually sterile body fluids, e.g., liver	Clarithro 500mg po q12h or azithro 600mg po q24h + ETB 15–25mg/kg/day + RFB 300 mg po q24h * **Higher doses of clari (1000mg q12h) may be associated with ↑ mortality** (CID 29:125, 1999)	Clarithro or azithro + ETB (Clarithro or azithro + one or more of: CIP 750mg po q12h Oflox 400mg po q12h Amikacin 7.5–15mg/kg IV q24h In pts receiving protease inhibitors can use (clarithro 500mg q12h (or azithro 600mg q24h) + ETB 15–25mg/kg/day] if the pt has not had previous prophylaxis with a neomacrolide (Johns Hopkins AIDS Report 9:2, 1997).	Median time to neg blood culture: clarithro + ETB 4.4wks vs clarithro + RFB >16wks. At 16wks, clearance of bacteremia seen in 37.5% of clarithro- & 85.7% of clarithro-treated pts (CID 27:1278, 1998). More recent study suggests similar clearance rates for azithro (46%) vs clarithro (56%) at 24wks when combined with ETB (CID 31:1245, 2000). Azithro 250mg q24h not effective but azithro 600mg po q24h as effective and ↓ yields fewer adverse effects (AAC 43:2869, 1999). Addition of RFB to clarithro + ETB ↓ emergence of resistance to clari, ↓ relapse rate, & improves survival (CID 37:1234, 2003). Data on clofazimine difficult to assess. Earlier study suggested adding CLO of no value (CID 25:621, 1997). More recent study suggests it may be as effective as RFB in 3 drug regimens containing clari & ETB (CID 29:125, 1999) although it may not be as effective as RFB at preventing clari resistance (CID 28:136, 1999. Thus, pending more data, we still do not recommend CLO for MAI in HIV+ pts. Drug toxicity: With clarithro, 23% pts had to stop drug 2° to dose-limiting adverse reaction (AnIM 121:905, 1994). Combo of clarithro, ETB & RFB led to uveitis & pseudojaundice (NEJM 330:438, 1994); result is reduction in max. dose of RFB to 300mg.
	Chronic post-treatment suppression—secondary prophylaxis	Always necessary (Clarithro or azithro) + ETB (lower dose to 15mg/kg/day) (Dosage above)	Clarithro or azithro or RFB (dosage above)	Treatment failure rate is high. Reasons: drug toxicity, development of drug resistance, & inadequate serum levels. Serum levels of clarithro ↓ in pts also given RIF or RFB (JID 171:747, 1995). 1 pt not responding to initial regimen after 2–4wks, add 1 or more drugs. Several anecdotal reports of pts not responding to usual primary regimen who gained weight & became afebrile with dexamethasone 2–4mg/day po (AAC 38: 2215, 1994; CID 26:682, 1998). Recurrences almost universal without chronic suppression. In pts with good response to HAART (robust CD4 ↑) it is possible to discontinue chronic suppression (JID 178:1446, 1998; NEJM 340:1301, 1999) (see Table 11B).

NOTE: All dosage recommendations are for adults (unless otherwise indicated) & assume normal renal function.

TABLE 12 (6)

CAUSATIVE AGENT/DISEASE	MODIFYING CIRCUMSTANCES	SUGGESTED REGIMENS PRIMARY	SUGGESTED REGIMENS ALTERNATIVE	COMMENTS
BACTERIAL INFECTIONS (continued)				
Mycobacterium celatum	Treatment; optimal regimen not defined		Easily confused with M. xenopi & MAC. May be susceptible to clarithro, FQ (Clin Microbiol Inf 3:582, 1997). Suggested treatment like MAI but may be resistant to RIF (J Inf 38:157, 1999). Most reported cases received 3 or 4 drugs—usually **clari + ETB + CIP + RFB** (EID 9:399, 2003).	Isolated from blood of patients with AIDS (CID 24:140 & 144, 1997). Usually resistant to INH, RIF, PZA, capreomycin (JCM 33:137, 1995; CID 24:140, 1997).
Mycobacterium chelonae, ssp. abscessus, chelonae	Treatment. Surgery is important adjunct to therapy (CID 24:1147, 1997).	**Clarithro** 500mg po q12h x6mos (AnIM 119:482, 1993; CID 24:1147, 1997; EJCMID 19:43, 2000). **Azithro** may also be effective. For serious, disseminated infections add **tobramycin + IMP** (CID 15:716, 2002).		M. abscessus susceptible in vitro to clarithro (95%), clofazimine, amikacin (70%) & cefoxitin (70%). Clarithro-resistant strains described (JCM 39:2745, 2001). M. chelonae susceptible in vitro to clarithro, tobramycin (100%), amikacin (80%), IMP (60%), clarithrox, gatifloxacin, linezolid, moxifloxacin (AJRCCM 156:S1, 1997; AAC 46:3283, 2002).
Mycobacterium fortuitum	Treatment	Optimal regimen not defined. **Amikacin + cefoxitin + probenecid** 2–6wks, then po TMP/SMX, or doxycycline 2–6mos (J Inf Dis 152:50, 1985). Surgical excision of infected areas. Nail salon-acquired skin infections in immunocompetent pts have responded to 4–6mos. of minocycline or doxycycline or CIP (CID 38:38, 2004).		Resistant to all standard anti-Tbc drugs. Sensitive in vitro to cefoxitin, imipenem, amikacin, TMP/SMX, CIP, oflox. May be resistant to RFB, azithro, variably susceptible to clarithro, gatifloxacin, linezolid (JAC 39:567, 1997). Usually responds to 6–12mos of oral rx with 2 drugs to which it is susceptible (AJRCCM 156:S1, 1997; AAC 46:3283, 2002; CMR 15:716, 2002).
Mycobacterium genavense	Treatment	Regimens used include ≥2 drugs: **ETB, RIF, RFB, clofazimine, clarithro.** In animal model, clarithro & RFB (& to lesser extent amikacin & ETB) shown effective in reducing bacterial counts; CIP not effective (JAC 42:483, 1998).		Clinical: CD4 <50. Symptoms of fever, weight loss, diarrhea. Lab: growth in BACTEC vials slow (mean 42 days). Subcultures grow only on Middlebrook 7H11 agar containing 2 mcg/ml mycobactin J—growth still insufficient for in vitro sensitivity testing (Lancet 340:76, 1992; AnIM 117:586, 1992). Survival 1 from 81 to 263 days in pts rx for at least 1 month with ≥2 drugs (Arch Int Med 155:400, 1995).
Mycobacterium gordonae	Treatment	Regimen(s) not defined, but consider **RIF + ETB + kanamycin** or **CIP** (J Inf 38:157, 1999).		In vitro: sensitive to ETB, RIF, clarithro, CIP, clarithro, linezolid (AAC 47:1736, 2003). Resistant to INH (CID 14:1229, 1992). Surgical excision.
Mycobacterium haemophilum	Treatment	Regimen(s) not defined. **clarithro + RFB** effective (AAC 39:2316, 1995). Combo of **CIP + RFB + clarithro** reported effective but clinical experience limited (CMR 9:435, 1996). Surgical debridement may be nec. (CID 26:505, 1998).		Clinical: Ulcerating skin lesions, synovitis, osteomyelitis. Lab: Requires supplemented media to isolate. Sensitive in vitro to: CIP, cycloserine, RFB. Over _ resistant to: INH, RIF, ETB, PZA (AnIM 120:118, 1994).
Mycobacterium kansasii	Treatment	**RIF** (600mg po q24h) + **ETB** (25 mg/kg x 2 mos, then 15 mg/kg/day) + **INH** (300 mg po q24h) for 15–18mos (AnIM 120:945, 1994).	If RIF-resistant, use **INH** 900mg po q24h + **pyridoxine** 50mg po q24h + **RFB** 25→15 mg/kg/day po + **sulfamethoxazole** 1gm po q8h. Rx until culture negative x12–15mos. **Clarithro** or **RFB + ETB** also effective in small study (CID 37:1178, 2003).	If organism resistant to (≥1mg/ml) INH, discontinue INH. Rifampin, clarithro, azithro, ETB effective alone or in combo in athymic mice (JAC 42:417, 2001). Highly susceptible to linezolid in vitro (AAC 47:1736, 2003). If HIV+ pt taking protease inhibitor, sub either clarithro (500mg bid) or RFB (150mg/d) for RIF (AJRCCM 156:S1, 1997). Because of variable susceptibility to INH, some sub clarithro – 750mg q24h for INH. Resistance to clarithro reported (DMID 31:369, 1998) but most strains susceptible to clarithro as well as moxifloxacin (JAC 55:950, 2005) & levofloxacin (AAC 48:4562, 2004). Prog related to level of immunosuppression (CID 37:584, 2003).

NOTE: All dosage recommendations are for adults (unless otherwise indicated) & assume normal renal function.

TABLE 12 (7)

CAUSATIVE AGENT/DISEASE	MODIFYING CIRCUMSTANCES	SUGGESTED REGIMENS PRIMARY	ALTERNATIVE	COMMENTS
BACTERIAL INFECTIONS (continued)				
Mycobacterium marinum	Treatment	(RIF + ETB) or doxycycline or minocycline or TMP/SMX or clarithro for at least 12wks (Arch Int Med 147:817, 1986; AJRCCM 156:S1, 1997). Surgical excision.		Sensitive in vitro to clarithro, reported effective in 2 pts (1 HIV+ who failed on other regimens) (CID 18:664, 1994). Resistant to INH & PZA (AJRCCM 156:S1, 1997). Susceptible in vitro to linezolid, CIP, gatifloxacin, moxifloxacin also show moderate in vitro activity (AAC 46:1114, 2002).
Mycobacterium scrofulaceum	Treatment	Although regimens not defined, clarithro + clofazimine with or without ETB. Surgical excision		In vitro resistant to INH, RIF, ETB, PZA, amikacin, CIP (CID 20:549, 1995).
Mycobacterium simiae	Treatment	Regimen(s) not defined. If true infection, start 4 drugs as for disseminated MAI. Anecdotal reports of response in pts on HAART who received clarithro, ETB & CIP (J Int 41:143, 2000).		
Mycobacterium ulcerans (Buruli ulcer)	Treatment	[RIF + AMK (7.5mg/kg IM bid)] or [ETB + TMP/SMX (160/800mg po tid)] for 4–6wks. Surgical excision.		Susceptible in vitro to RIF, strep, CLO, clarithro, CIP, oflox, amikacin (AAC 42:2070, 1998; JAC 45:231, 2000; AAC 46:3193, 2002). Monotherapy with RIF selects resistant mutants in mice (AAC 47:1228, 2003). RIF + Strep effective in small study (AAC 49:3182, 2005). Treatment generally disappointing—see review, Ln 354:1013, 1999. RIF + dapsone only slightly better (82% improved) than placebo (76%) in small study (JID 6:80, 2002).
Mycobacterium xenopi	Treatment (NOTE: Recent study suggests no need to treat in most pts with HIV (CID 37:1250, 2003)	Regimen(s) not defined (CID 24:226 & 233, 1997). INH + RIF + ETB suggested but no clinical trials available (Clin Chest Med 17:697, 1996). Not always susceptible to these agents in vitro (CID 25:206, 1997). Macrolide + (RIF or RFB) + ETB ± SM also recommended (AJRCCM 156:S1, 1997) or RIF + INH + ETB (Resp Med 97:439, 2003); but recent study suggests no need to treat in most pts with HIV (CID 37:1250, 2003)		In vitro: sensitive to clarithro (Antimic Ag Chemo 36:2841, 1992) & RFB (JAC 39:567, 1997) & many standard antimyco-bacterial drugs. Clarithro-containing regimens more effective than RIF/INH/ETB in mice (AAC 45:3229, 2001). FQs, linezolid also active.
Neisseria gonorrhoeae (gonococcus) Ref.: MMWR 51(RR-6):1, 2002	Gonorrhea: urethritis, conjunctivitis, proctitis; mucopurulent cervicitis; epididymo-orchitis (sexually acquired); for disseminated disease, see *Sanford Guide to Antimicrobial Therapy*	[(**Ceftriaxone** 125mg IM x1) or (**cefixime** 400mg po x 1) (cefpodoxime 400mg po x1) or **CIP** 500mg po x1) or **oflox** 400mg po x1) or (**levo** 250mg po x1) or (**gati** 400mg po x1)] **PLUS** [(**Azithro** 1gm po x1) or (**doxy** 100mg po x2/day x7d)] **Evaluate & rx sex partner** No quinolones for men who have sex with men or GC acquired in Hawaii, US West Coast or England.		**Treat for both GC & C. trachomatis.** Other alternatives for **GC**: Spectinomycin 2gm IM x1 Other single-dose cephalosporins: ceftizoxime 500mg IM, cefotaxime 500mg IM, cefoxitin 1gm IM, (cefotetan 2gm IM + probenecid 1gm po). Azithro 1gm po x1 effective for chlamydia but need 2gm po x1 for GC; not recommended for GC due to GI side-effects & expense. FQ resistance refs.: MMWR 53:335, 2004; CID 38:649, 2004; EID 11:1009, 2005.

NOTE: All dosage recommendations are for adults (unless otherwise indicated) & assume normal renal function.

TABLE 12 (8)

CAUSATIVE AGENT/DISEASE	MODIFYING CIRCUMSTANCES	SUGGESTED REGIMENS		COMMENTS
		PRIMARY	ALTERNATIVE	
BACTERIAL INFECTIONS *(continued)*				
Pelvic inflammatory disease (PID), salpingitis, tubo-ovarian abscess. Etiology polymicrobic: gonococcus, C. trachomatis, bacteroides, enterobacteriaceae, streptococci, myco-plasma. *Ref: MMWR 51:RR-6, 2002*	Outpatient (limit to pts with temp <38°C, WBC <11,000/mm³, minimal evidence of peritonitis, active bowel sounds & able to tolerate oral nourishment)	**Outpatient rx:** [(Ofloxo 400mg po q12h or **levo** 500mg po q24h) ± **metro** 500mg po q12h)] **OR** (**ceftriaxone** 250mg IM x 1 + **metro** 500mg po q12h; then **doxy** 100mg po q12h). Treat for 14 days.	**Inpatient regimens:** [(**Cefotetan** 2gm IV q12h or **cefoxitin** 2gm IV q6h) ± **doxy** 100mg IV/po q12h] **OR** (**Clinda** 900mg IV q8h + (**gentamicin** 1.5mg/kg q8h or single daily dosing), then **doxy** 100mg po q12h x14d **Remember: Evaluate & treat sex partner.**	Alternative parenteral regimens: 1. Ofloxo 400mg IV q12h + metro 500mg IV q8h 2. AM/SB 3gm IV q6h + doxy 100mg IV/po q12h 3. CIP 200mg IV q12h + doxy 100mg IV/po q12h + metro 500mg IV q8h **Remember: Evaluate & treat sex partner.**
Prostatitis—Review: *AJM 106:327, 1999*				
Acute	N. gonorrhoeae	Ofloxo 400mg po x1, then 300mg po q12h x10d OR (**ceftriaxone** 250mg IM x1, then **doxy** 100mg po q12h x10d)		Ofloxo effective vs gonococci & C. trachomatis & penetrates prostate. In AIDS pts. prostate may be focus on Cryptococcus neoformans.
≤35 years of age	C. trachomatis			
>35 years of age	Enterobacteriaceae (coliforms)	**FQ** (dosage: see Epididymo-orchitis, >35 yrs, above) or **TMP/SMX** 1 DS tablet 160mg TMP, 800mg SMX po q12h x10d	Treat as acute urinary infection, 14d (not single dose regimen). Some authorities recommend 3-4wk rx *(IDCP 4:325, 1995)*.	
Chronic bacterial	Enterobacteriaceae (80%), enterococci (15%), P. aeruginosa	**FQ** (CIP 500mg po q12h x4wks, OR levo 500mg po q24h x4wks)—see Comment	**TMP/SMX-DS** 1 tab po q12h x1-3mos.	With rx failures, consider infected prostatic calculi.
Chronic prostatitis/chronic pain syndrome (New NIH classification, *JAMA 282:236, 1999)*	The most common pro-statitis syndrome, etiology is unknown; molecular data suggest infectious etiology *(Clin Micro Rev 11:604, 1998)*	**Doxy** 100 mg po q12h x14 days	**Erythro base** 500mg po q6h x14d	Pt has sx of prostatitis, cells in prostatic secretions, but routine cultures negative. Chlamydia, ureaplasma suspected. Pt has sx of prostatitis but negative cultures & no cells in prostatic secretions. Review: *JAC 46:157, 2000*
	α-adrenergic blocking agents are controversial *(AnIM 133:367, 2000).*			
Rhodococcus equi (Corynebacterium equi)	Pulmonary	[Erythro (0.5gm IV q6h) or IMP (0.5gm IV q8h)] + RIF 600mg po q24h for at least 2wks	CIP 750mg po q12h ≥2wks. CIP-resistant strains SE Asia *(CID 27:370, 1998)*	3/4 pts have positive blood cultures *(Medicine 73:119, 1994)*. Prolonged oral suppressive therapy (macrolide + RIF) indicated since relapses are frequent. Vancomycin active in vitro & rx success in pt who relapsed after erythro + RIF *(IDCP 7:480, 1998)*. Linezolid active in vitro.
Salmonella sp. Fever in 71–91% Bloody stool 34%	**Bacteremia, recurrent** For typhoid fever, see *Sanford Guide to Antimicrobial Therapy*	CIP 500mg po q12h x 5-7d. If re-lapse occurs, CIP 500mg po q12h indefinitely. % resistant to FQs *(Ln 363:1285, 2004)*	**Azithro** 1gm po & then 500mg po q24h x6d *(AAC 43:1441, 1999)*—for uncomplicated non-bacteremic	Ceftriaxone, cefotaxime usually active. Often resistant to TMP/SMX & chloro. Ceftriaxone & FQ resistance in SE Asia *(Ln 363:1285, 2004)*.
Shigellosis Fever in 58% Bloody stool 51%	Treatment Acute	CIP 500mg po q12h x3d or **azithro** 500mg po x1, then 250mg/day x4d	(**TMP/SMX-DS** q12h po x3d) or (**azithro** 500mg po q24h indefinitely	In immunocompromised children & adults, treat for 7-10 days.
	Recurrent in AIDS pts	CIP 500mg po q12h indefinitely	CIP 750mg po q24h [perhaps 750mg po q24h] indefinitely	

NOTE: All dosage recommendations are for adults (unless otherwise indicated) & assume normal renal function.

TABLE 12 (9)

CAUSATIVE AGENT/DISEASE	MODIFYING CIRCUMSTANCES	SUGGESTED REGIMENS		COMMENTS
		PRIMARY	ALTERNATIVE	
BACTERIAL INFECTIONS: (continued)				
Staphylococcus aureus: methicillin/oxacillin/ erythro susceptible (MSSA)	Treatment: Folliculitis/ furunculosis/ subcutaneous abscess in "skin poppers" Bacteremia &/or endocarditis	Dicloxacillin 500mg po q6h for 7–14d. If refractory/recurrent, add **RIF** 600mg po q24h or 300mg po q12h	**Erythro** 500mg po q6h for 7–14d or **Mupirocin** (Bactroban), apply to affected area q8h for 5d (if infection not disseminated)	**Hot packs & drainage of equal import to antimicrobic therapy.**
		PRSP [**naficillin** or **oxacillin** 2gm IV q4h x4wks]) + **gentamicin** 1mg/kg IV q8h x3–5d]	**Cefazolin** 2gm IV q8h x4–6wks) + (gentamicin 1mg/kg IV q8h x3–5d)	In IV drug users with right-sided endocarditis, 2wks rx with nafcillin/gentamicin is usually adequate (AnIM 109:619, 1988).
	Suppression: Recurrent infections (most likely pt is a nasal carrier)	**Dicloxacillin** 500mg po q6h + (**RIF** 600mg po q24h or 300mg po q12h) x10d	**Dicloxacillin** 500mg po q6h + **Mupirocin** (Bactroban), apply to nasal vestibule q8h x5d	Culture nasal vestibule to determine if nasal carrier. Mupirocin effective vs both MSSA & MRSA.
Staphylococcus aureus: methicillin/oxacillin resistant (MRSA) Community acquired (CA) or hospital (ventilator) acquired (HA) **Need culture & susceptibility data** **NOTE:** If erythro-resistant, assume clinda resistance pending results of in vitro "D" test.	Furunculosis/ subcutaneous abscess in skin poppers	Hot packs, incision & drainage most important If CA-MRSA: **TMP/SMX-DS** 2 tabs po q12h ± **RIF** 300mg po q12h x7–14d. Clinda, minocycline, & sometimes FQs active in vitro	If HA-MRSA: usually need linezolid to all oral drugs except linezolid. Try not to use linezolid if I&D will suffice. **Linezolid** 600mg po q12h.	In children, if abscess >5cm in diameter, antimicrobic therapy lessened probability of infectious complications (PIDJ 23:123, 2004). High dose of TMP/SMX-DS due to high concentrations of thymidine in abscess (antagonizes TMP/SMX). Worry about overuse of linezolid if hot packs & I&D will suffice.
	Hospital (ventilator)-acquired pneumonia	**Vanco** 1gm IV q12h x2–4d & then linezolid 600mg IV/po q12h x7–21d	**Linezolid** 600mg IV/po q12h x7–21d. **Quinu/dalayto** 7.5mg/kg IV q8h x7–21d.	In retrospective analysis of controlled clinical trials, linezolid appears superior to vanco for VAP (Chest 124:1789, 2003). Risk of selecting linezolid-resistant MRSA mutants may be lessened by starting with vanco (Editor's opinion without data).
	Bacteremia/ endocarditis	**Vanco** 30mg/kg/day IV in 2 div. doses (check levels if >2gm/day) x4–6wks.	Fails/intolerant to vanco: success (CID 38:521, 2004 & J Infection 47:164, 2003) & failure (CID 35:1018, 2002) reported with linezolid 600mg IV/po q12h.	In retrospective analysis of rifampin did not shorten duration of bacteremia (AnIM 115:674, 1991). For MRSA, addition of rifampin did not shorten duration of bacteremia (AnIM 115:674, 1991). **Daptomycin as effective as vanco for right-sided endocarditis.** Isolated reports of success with quinu/dalayto. Isolated reports of success with quinu/dalayto. followed by linezolid (J Chemother 14:526, 2002) or quinu/dalayto + vanco (Scand J Int Dis 34:122, 2002).
Streptococcus pneumoniae Pneumonia—culture & in vitro susceptibility results available Ref.: CID 37:1405, 2003)	Susceptible or intermediate resistance to pen G in vitro	**Ceftriaxone** Over age 60—1gm IV q24h Under age 60—2gm IV q24h OR **Penicillin G** 2 million units IV q4h OR **Ampicillin** 2gm IV q6h OR **Levo** 750mg IV q24h or **gati** 400mg IV q24h or **moxi** 400mg IV q24h	**Erythro** 500mg IV/po q6h OR **Azithro** 500mg IV/dev q24h OR **Clindamycin** 600mg IV q8h	The prevalence of high-level pen G-resistant S. pneumo varies by region: average is 18%. **Resistant strains** are often cross-resistant to erythro, azithro (80%), clarithro (80%) & ceftriaxone (22%). U.S. isolates may or may not be clindamycin-susceptible. β-lactam/β-lactamase inhibitor combinations are not effective, as mechanism of resistance is target change, not β-lactamase production. Physicians warned about both hypo- & hyperglycemia in association with Gatifloxacin.
	High-level resistance to pen G in vitro	**Vancomycin** 1gm IV q12h OR if oral therapy: **Telithro** 800mg po q24h or **Gemi** 320mg po q24h		

NOTE: All dosage recommendations are for adults (unless otherwise indicated) & assume normal renal function.

TABLE 12 (10)

CAUSATIVE AGENT/DISEASE	MODIFYING CIRCUMSTANCES	SUGGESTED REGIMENS		COMMENTS
		PRIMARY	ALTERNATIVE	
BACTERIAL INFECTIONS (continued)				
Meningitis—culture & in vitro susceptibility results available Ref. on steroid use: *NEJM 347:1549 & 1613, 2002* General ref: *CID 39:1267, 2004*	Susceptible to pen G in vitro	**(Aq. pen G** 4 million units IV q4h OR **ceftriaxone** 2 gm IV q12h OR **ampicillin** 2 gm IV q4h) + **dexamethasone—See Comment** **(Vancomycin** 15mg/kg IV q6 (see Comment) + **ceftriaxone** 2gm IV q12h) + **dexamethasone—See Comment**	For severe penicillin allergy (IgE-mediated anaphylaxis, angioneurotic edema): **Vanco** 15mg/kg IV q6–12h + **RIF** (600mg/day po/IV) **Meropenem** may work—**1gm** IV q8h. Severe penicillin allergy: **Vanco** 500–750mg IV q8h + **RIF** 600mg po/IV q24h	**Adjunctive dexamethasone, 1st dose 15–20min. prior to, or concomitant with, 1st dose of antibiotic.** Dose: 0.4mg/kg IV q12h x2d. (1) In children, steroids do **not** reduce CSF penetration of vanco. (2) In adults, unclear if steroids ↓ vanco CSF penetration. If steroids used, add RIF 600mg/day IV or po. **Vanco dosage.** Due to low/erratic CSF penetration, recommended dosage in children of 15mg/kg q6h is double usual dose; in adults, a max. dose of 2–3gm of vanco/day suggested, i.e. 500–700mg IV q8h.
Syphilis (Treponema pallidum) Recommendations are for pts with normal CD4 T-lymphocyte counts. In AIDS pts, clinical course may be atypical. Higher doses/ longer periods of rx may be required—see *Ln ID 4:456, 2004; MMWR 53:RR-15, 2004.*	Primary (chancre), secondary (rash, mucositis, lymphadenopathy), & early latent (<1 year)	**Benzathine penicillin G** 2.4 mUnits IM x1 Dose for children: 50,000 units/kg IM up to max. of 2.4 mUnits	**Doxycycline** 100mg po q12h x14 d **or Tetracycline** 500mg po q6h x14 d **or Ceftriaxone** 1gm IM/IV q24h x8–10d For failures of initial rx, re-treat with benzathine penicillin G 2.4 mUnits IM weekly x3.	If early latent, do CSF VDRL to exclude neurosyphilis. For all stages, penicillin best drug. If penicillin allergy, skin test if available or desensitize & treat with penicillin. Erythro not acceptable alternative agent (*CID 20:387, 1995*); use doxycycline if unable to desensitize. Limited data on efficacy of alternative regimens. Need baseline titered VDRL (RPR) & repeat titered serology at 3, 6, 12, 24mos. Repeat rx if (1) persistent clinical signs, (2) titer ↑ 4-fold or fails to decrease 4-fold (2 titers). Even with recommended rx, serologic relapse frequent. (*AnJ Med 99:55, 1995*).
	Late latent: >1 year duration & neg. CSF exam	**Benzathine penicillin G** 2.4 mUnits IM q wkly x3wks	**Doxycycline** 100mg po q12h x28d **or Tetracycline** 500mg po q6h x28d	**CSF exam mandatory in late latent stage in HIV+ patients.**
Streptococcus pneumoniae	Neurosyphilis or optic neuritis	**Pen G** 3–4 mUnits q4h IV x10–14d	**(Procaine pen G** 2.4 mUnits IM q24h x10–14d + **probenecid** 0.5gm po q6h) both x10–14d—*See Comment*	**Ceftriaxone** 2gm q24h (IV or IM) x14d. 23% failure rate reported (*AJM 93:481, 1992*). For penicillin allergy: either desensitize to penicillin or obtain infectious diseases consultation. **Serologic criteria for response to rx: 4-fold or greater ↓ in VDRL titer over 6–12mos.** (*CID 28(Suppl.1):S21, 1999*).

NOTE: All dosage recommendations are for adults (unless otherwise indicated) & assume normal renal function.

TABLE 12 [11]

TYPE OF INFECTION/ORGANISM/ SITE OF INFECTION	SUGGESTED REGIMENS		COMMENTS
	PRIMARY	ALTERNATIVE	
FUNGAL INFECTIONS			
Aspergillosis (See Chest 114:251, 1999) **Invasive, pulmonary (IPA) or extrapulmonary:** (See COID 18:314, 2005) Post-transplantation & post-chemotherapy in neutropenic pts (PMN <500 per mm³) but may also present with neutrophil recovery (Mycopathologia 159:181, 2005). Most common pneumonia in transplant recipients. Have a late (≥100 days) complication in allogeneic bone marrow & liver transplantation: median 36 days, but **overall mortality rates vary from 78–94%** (in above dosages) + **caspo** (dosage below) are currently preferred initial treatment in many bone marrow transplant units, esp. in pts receiving high 2003). May complicate COPD when corticosteroids used (Clin Micro Inf 11:427, 2005). **Typical x-ray/CT lung lesions** (halo sign, cavitation, or mycotic lung sequestration) have 90% positive predictive value for invasive pulmonary aspergillosis in pts with hematologic malignancies (CID 31:859, 2000). An immunologic test that detects circulating galactomannan is available for dx of invasive aspergillosis. A recent article reviews the strengths & weaknesses of the test (CID 41(Suppl. 6):S381, 2005).	**Voriconazole** 6mg per kg IV q12h on day 1, then either (4mg per kg IV q12h) or (200mg po q12h for body weight ≥40kg, but 100mg po q12h for body weight <40kg) **OR** **Lipid-based ampho B** may be as effective & less nephrotoxic than standard ampho B but much more expensive (see footnote³ for dosage) Some authorities now prefer lipid-based ampho B over standard ampho B as initial rx (CID 32: 415, 2003). **OR** **Ampho B** (see footnote³ pg109): Rapid increase to 1mg per kg (1–1.25mg per kg if neutropenic) IV q24h: Total dose of 2–2.5gm rec. by some but data to support this lacking, **OR Combination rx: Vori** (in above dosages) + **caspo** (dosage below) are currently preferred initial treatment in many bone marrow transplant units, esp. in pts receiving high doses of corticosteroids (Abstracts in Heme & Onc 8:11, 2005) **Alternative: Caspofungin** 70mg IV on day 1, then 50mg IV q24h (reduce to 35mg with moderate hepatic insufficiency). For all regimens: If response good may switch to oral **vori** after 2–3wks.	**Voriconazole** more effective than ampho B in randomized trial of 277 immunosuppressed pts with IPA. 53% responded vs 32% rx with ampho B. Overall survival better (71 vs 58%) (NEJM 347: 408, 2002). Appears particularly advantageous in cerebral aspergillosis (Eur J Neurol 9:748, 2002) & as salvage therapy in pts with refractory infection. (In one trial of 81 pts, 13 of 31 pts survived with vori alone. Vori reported satisfactory results in 11/20 pts with bone involvement (18 for salvage), follow-up average of 3 mos. (CID 40:1141, 2005). **Ampho B overall success rate 34–42%** (CID 32:358, 2001) in pulmonary aspergillosis in pts rx ≥14 days. Success dependent on underlying disease: 83% heart/kidney transplants, 54% neutropenic leukemia pts, 33% bone marrow transplant, 20% liver transplant (CID 23: 608, 1996). 44% of 398 pts receiving **ampho B lipid complex (ABLC)** were cured or improved & 21% stabilized; most failed to respond to prior antifungal rx (CID 40:S392, 2005). **A. terreus infections particularly resistant to ampho B: in 83 cases, 73.4% mortality with ampho B rx vs 55.8% with voriconazole rx (p <0.01)** (CID 39:192, 2004). **Use vori!** **Caspofungin:** Among 83 pts with IPA included in primary (MITT) analysis, 37 (45%) had favorable response following salvage rx with caspo monotherapy. In pts receiving >7 days of caspo monotherapy, 56% (37/66) responded favorably (CID 39:1563, 2004). Response in compassionate use program 44% (J Inf 50:196, 2005). Minimal toxicity reported (Transpl Int Dis 1:25, 2002). **Micafungin:** 57% clinical response in an open-label study of "deep-seated" infections (Scand J Inf Dis 36:372, 2004). **Combo therapy:** To date no controlled pt trials, they're needed (CID 39:803, 2004). No antagonism between triazoles (vori & itra), echinocandins (caspo), & ampho B. Synergy demonstrated vs aspergillus in vitro &/or animal models between triazoles & caspo (AAC 47:1416, 2003) & ampho B plus caspo (AAC 46:2564, 2002; JID 187:1834, 2003). Some failures to show synergy (JAC 56:166, 2005). In retrospective evaluation of bone marrow transplant pts with IPA who failed ampho B, **vori + caspo** superior to **vori** alone (CID 39:797, 2004). No controlled trials conducted in HIV/AIDS pts with invasive aspergillosis (See 2005 Sanford Guide to Antimicrobial Therapy, Table 11A, & MMWR 53/RR-15/98, 2004).

³ **Dosages: ABLC** 5mg per kg per day IV over 2 hrs; **ABCC 3–4** mg per kg per day IV given over 1–2hrs; **liposomal Ampho B** 3–5mg per kg per day IV given over 1–2hrs.
NOTE: All dosage recommendations are for adults (unless otherwise indicated) **& assume normal renal function.**

TABLE 12 (12)

TYPE OF INFECTION/ORGANISM/ SITE OF INFECTION	SUGGESTED REGIMENS		COMMENTS
	PRIMARY	**ALTERNATIVE**	
Blastomycosis (CID 30:679, 2000)	**Ampho B** 0.7–1mg/kg IV until evidence of response, then **itraconazole** 200mg po q24h if pt not critically ill or does not have CNS involvement	Limited data with lipid preparations of ampho B & fluconazole in HIV+ pts.	Ampho B cumulative dose >1gm results in cure without relapse in 70–91% of pts (CID 22:S102, 1996). In HIV+ pt, itraconazole is drug of choice (Am J Med 93:489, 1992). Experience in HIV+ pts is limited, hence more traditional regimen is recommended. Should give with food or acidic cola to increase absorption.

Candidiasis. Oral, esophageal & vaginal candidiasis is a major manifestation of advanced HIV & represents one of the most common AIDS-defining diagnoses (JID 188:118, 2003). Candida is also a common cause of nosocomial bloodstream infection. A decrease in C. albicans & increase in non-albicans species show ↓ susceptibility to antifungal agents (esp. fluconazole). These changes have predominantly affected immunocompromised pts in environments where antifungal prophylaxis (esp. fluconazole) is widely used (JAC 49 (Suppl.1):3, 2002; PIDJ 23:635 & 687, 2004). In vitro susceptibility testing to antifungal drugs to date has not undergone rigorous in vivo validation studies, & clinical outcomes are often more dependent on host factors (Am J Med 1:12:380, 2002). Yet, it seems prudent to use susceptibility profiles to help select empiric antifungal therapy. The table summarizes current published reports of frequency of candida isolates, & interpretation as to whether a drug is clinically effective (**S = susceptible**), may require dose escalation (**S-DD = susceptible with dose escalation**), or is likely to be ineffective (**R = resistant**) (Ln 359:1135, 2002). **S-I = less activity in vitro but clinically effective**; only rare failures reported (IDSA Guidelines, 2004; CID 38:161, 2004). In vitro testing for caspo not standardized in clinical studies of candida infections. MIC of caspo did not correlate with treatment outcome following caspofungin therapy (AAC 49:3616, 2005).

	% of Candida Isolates	Risk Factors	% Sensitive In Vitro						Rx if species known
			Fluconazole	Itraconazole	Voriconazole	Ampho B	Caspo-fungin	Micafungin/ Anidulafungin	
C. albicans	41–65	HIV/AIDS, surgery	97% (S)	93% (S)	99% (S)	>95% (S)	S	S	Flu,** caspo, or ampho B
C. glabrata	10–15	Heme malignancies, azole prophylaxis	85–90% (S-DD)	50% (R)	92% (S-I)	>95% (S-I)	S	S	Caspo, ampho B, or vori
C. parapsilosis	15–24	Azole prophylaxis, neonates, foreign bodies	99% (S)	4% (S-DD)	99% (S)	>95% (S)	S-I	S-I	Flu, caspo, or ampho B
C. tropicalis	5–10	Neutropenia	98% (S)	58% (S)	99% (S)	>95% (S)	S	S	Flu, caspo, or ampho B
C. krusei	2–10	Heme malignancies, azole prophylaxis	5% (R)	69% (R)	99% (S-I)	>95% (S-I)	S	S	Caspo, ampho B, or vori
C. guilliermondi	1	Azole prophylaxis, previous ampho rx	>95% (S)	? (S)	>95% (S)	(R)	S-I	S	Flu, caspo, or vori
C. lusitaniae	1	Previous ampho rx	>95% (S)	? (S)	>95% (S)	(R)	S	S	Flu, caspo, or vori

** If patient had prior heavy basal exposure, use ampho B or caspo (CID 35:1073, 2002; 36:1497, 2003)

* Hydration before & after infusion with 500 cc saline has been shown to reduce renal toxicity.
NOTE: All dosage recommendations are for adults (unless otherwise indicated) & assume normal renal function.

TABLE 12 (13)

TYPE OF INFECTION/ORGANISM/ SITE OF INFECTION	SUGGESTED REGIMENS		COMMENTS
	PRIMARY	ALTERNATIVE	
FUNGAL INFECTIONS/Candidiasis *(continued)*			
Bloodstream: clinically stable with or without venous catheter *(IDSA Guidelines: CID 38:161, 2004)*			
All positive blood cultures require therapy!	Fluconazole 6mg/kg/day or 400mg IV or po q24h x7d then po for 14d after last + blood culture **OR**	Voriconazole: **loading dose 6mg/kg q12h x1d IV, then maintenance dose 3mg/kg q12h IV** for serious candida infections.	Observational studies suggest flu & ampho B are similarly effective in neutropenic pts *(IDSA Guidelines, 2003)*
• Remove & replace venous catheter ("not over a wire")! if possible *(CID 34:591 & 600, 2002; 36:1221, 2003)*, esp. in non-neutropenic; mortality 21% vs 4% if catheter not removed.	Caspofungin 70mg IV on day 1 followed by 50mg IV q24h (reduce to 35mg IV q24h with moderate hepatic insufficiency). Would use in place of flu in those heavily pretreated with azoles i.e., flu or itra prophylaxis) **OR**		A randomized study (277 pts, 10% were neutropenic) found caspofungin equivalent to ampho B (0.6–1 mg/kg/day) for invasive candidiasis. For candidemia 71.7% rx with caspo vs 62.8% with ampho B had successful outcomes but caspo had significantly less toxicity *(NEJM 347:2020, 2002).*
• Ophthalmologic exam recommended for all pts with candidemia.	Micafungin 50mg IV q24h for C. albicans, 100mg IV q24h for non-albicans candida **OR**		Preliminary data from a randomized double-blind study (n=245) suggests anidulafungin may be superior to flu for invasive candidiasis. Global
• Treat for 2 wks after pos. blood culture & resolution of signs & symptoms of infection	Anidulafungin 200mg IV times 1, then 100mg IV q24h (no dosage adjustments for renal or hepatic insufficiency)		response (clinical + micro) at end of IV rx, 75.6% rx with anidula vs 60.2% with flu had successful outcomes. Tolerability was comparable *(ICAAC 2005; IDSA 2005, #259).*
	Ampho B 0.6mg per kg IV q24h, total dose 5–7mg per kg or lipid-based ampho B*		
Bloodstream: unstable, deteriorating ± neutropenia OR stable disseminated (pulmonary, eye, hepatosplenic) *(IDSA Guidelines: CID 38:161, 2004)* For endophthalmitis, see pg69	Ampho B 0.8–1mg/kg/day IV ± 5FC 37.5* mg/kg po q6h or **lipid-based ampho B** (ABLC) 5mg/kg/day **OR**	Voriconazole: loading dose 6mg/kg IV q12h x1d, then maintenance dose 3mg/kg IV q12h for serious candida infections.	In a randomized trial of 219 pts with non-neutropenic candidemia, fluconazole (800mg/day) + ampho B (0.7mg/kg/day for the 1st 5 days) was superior to flu alone: Primary analysis, success rate on day 30 was 69% vs 57% (p=.08) respectively, overall success rate 69% vs 56% (p=.043) & clearance of
	Fluconazole 400–800mg/day (or >6 mg/kg/day) IV q24h. If start ampho B, switch to fluconazole 400mg po q24h x14d after last positive blood culture, resolution of neutropenia & disappearance of signs/ symptoms of candidal infection **OR**	**or** Caspofungin 70mg IV on day 1 followed by 50mg IV q24h (reduce to 35mg IV q24h with moderate hepatic insufficiency)	fungemia 94% vs 83% (p=.02). The flu alone group was slightly sicker (APACHE 15.0 vs 16.8, p<.001) & renal toxicity in combination greater (23% vs 3%, p<.001). Given difficulty with interpretation of this study, the editors would reserve combination of flu + ampho B for only the sickest candidemic patient.
	Combination of fluconazole 800mg/day + ampho B 0.7mg/kg/day for first 5–6d, then switch to flu 400mg/day po		Voriconazole may have a role in this clinical setting *(Euro Con Clin Micro & Inf Dis 2002, Abst. 237; IDSA 2002, Abst. 352)*

---

* ABLC or liposomal ampho B recommended for pts intolerant of or refractory to ampho B, i.e., failure of 500 mg of ampho B, initial renal insufficiency (creatinine >2.5 mg per dL or CrCl <25 mL per min), a sig. ↑ in serum Cr (to >2.5 mg per dL for adults or 1.5 mg per dL for children) or severe ampho administration-related toxicity *(CID 26:1383, 1998)*. Since efficacy similar & toxicity less, some now recommend lipid-based preps in place of ampho B as initial rx *(CID 32:415, 2003)*.

* Some experts reduce dose of 5FC to 25mg/kg q6h.

NOTE: All dosage recommendations are for adults (unless otherwise indicated) & assume normal renal function.

TABLE 12 (14)

TYPE OF INFECTION/ORGANISM/ SITE OF INFECTION	SUGGESTED REGIMENS		COMMENTS
	PRIMARY	ALTERNATIVE	
FUNGAL INFECTIONS (continued)			
Stomatitis, esophagitis Oral colonization with candida correlates with HIV RNA levels in plasma & with CD4 counts (JID 180:534, 1999). HAART has resulted in dramatic ↓ in prevalence of oropharyngeal & esophageal candidiasis & ↓ in refractory disease. See MMWR 53(RR-15):97, 2004	**Oropharyngeal**, initial episodes (7–14d rx): • **Fluconazole** 100mg po q24h; or • **Itraconazole** oral solution 200mg po q24h; or • **clotrimazole** troches 10mg po 5x/day; or • **nystatin** flavored pastilles 4–5x/day	**Fluconazole-refractory oropharyngeal:** • **Itra** oral solution ≥200mg po q24h; or • **ampho B** suspension 100mg/ml^ous 1ml po q6h; or • **ampho B** 0.3mg/kg IV q24h	**Fluconazole-refractory disease remains uncommon** (4% in ACTG 816) & is seen in pts with low CD4 counts (<50/mm³). **Flu** superior to oral suspension of **nystatin** (CID 24:1204, 1997). **Itra** 100mg po q12h x14d achieved clinical response in 41/74 (55%) pts unresponsive to flu (AIDS Res Hum Retrovir 15:1413, 1999). **Ampho B oral suspension** gave 42.6% response rate in 54 pts refractory to flu, but 70% of those relapsed (AIDS 14: 845, 2000). For esophagitis, **caspofungin** as effective as **ampho B** IV but less toxic (CID 33:1529, 2001; AAC 46:451, 2002; J AIDS 31:183, 2002). **Voriconazole** as effective as **fluconazole** for esophagitis (CID 33:1447, 2001). **Micafungin** 100 mg or 150 mg IV per day equal to flu 200 mg per day = flu 200 mg per day (Aliment Pharmacol 21:899, 2005). **Anidulafungin** 100 mg IV day 1 followed by 50 mg po = flu 200 mg per day in day 1 followed by 100 mg per day in 494 pts: cure rate 97% vs 98.8% (CID 39:770, 2004). Pending FDA labeling.
	• flavored pastilles 4–5x/day	**Fluconazole-refractory esophageal:** **Caspofungin** 50mg IV q24h; or • **vori** 200mg po/IV q12h; or • **ampho B** 0.3–0.7mg/kg IV q24h; or • **ampho B lipsomal or lipid complex** 3–5mg/kg IV q24h; or **anidulafungin** 100 mg IV day 1 followed by 50 mg po q day	
	Esophageal (14–21d): • **Flucon** 100mg (up to 400mg) po or IV q24h; or • **itra** oral solution 200mg po q24h; or • **vori** 200mg po q12h; or • **caspofungin** 50mg IV q24h; or •		
Vulvovaginitis Common among healthy young females & unrelated to HIV status.	• Topical **azoles** (clotrimazole, buto, mico, tico, or tercon) x3–7d; or • oral **nystatin** 100,000units/day as vaginal tablet x14d; or • oral **itra** 200mg q12h x1d or 200mg q24h x3d; or • oral **flucon** 150 mg x1 dose	3–5mg/kg IV q24h	
Post-treatment chronic suppression (secondary prophylaxis) for disabling recurrent oral, esophageal disease. Authors would do it sustained CD4 count ↑ (>200/mm³) following HAART	Suppressive rx is generally not recommended unless pts have frequent or severe recurrences. • **Oropharyngeal: fluconazole** or **itraconazole** oral solution may be considered. • **Vulvovaginal:** daily **topical azole** for recurrent cases. • **Esophageal: fluconazole** 100–200mg q24h.		Fluconazole 200mg q24h does reduce risk of candida esophagitis & cryptococcosis (NEJM 332:700, 1995). Disadvantages: Concern of enhanced risk of emergence of fluconazole (azole)-resistant Candida species.
	Chronic or prolonged use of azoles might promote development of resistance.		
Coccidioidomycosis MMWR 53:35, 2004; Med 83:149, 2004) Pulmonary & extrapulmonary (not meningitis). Usually seen in pts with <250 CD4/mm³. Usually involves generalized lymphadenopathy, skin nodules or ulcers, peritonitis, liver abnormalities, & bone/joint involvement.	**Primary prophylaxis:** Not recommended for most pts, consider for pts from endemic area with CD4 <50/µl. Primary **fluconazole** 200mg po q24h; **Alternative itraconazole** 200mg q12h **Acute phase (milder disease):** • **Flucon** 400–800mg po q24h; or • **Itra** 200mg po q12h	**Acute phase (diffuse pulmonary or disseminated disease):** Some specialists add azole to ampho B rx	Lung infection in 80% of pts. Despite rx with ampho B ± subsequent po azole, mortality reported as 60% (CID 23:563, 1996). ↑ number of cases in Arizona since 1990 (250 cases), 600 cases in 1995 (MMWR 45:1069, 1997). Relapses in roughly 25% of pts. See post-rx suppression, below. **Posaconazole**, oral suspension 800 mg po day, successful in 5/6 pts with refractory non-meningeal cocci (CID 40:1770, 2005) & 11/16 cases successful reported overall (Drugs 65:1559, 2005).
	Acute phase (diffuse pulmonary or disseminated disease): • **Ampho B** 0.5–1mg/kg IV q24h; or • **Itra** 200mg q24h; continue until clinical improvement, usually 500–1000mg total dose		

NOTE: All dosage recommendations are for adults (unless otherwise indicated) & assume normal renal function.

TABLE 12 (15)

TYPE OF INFECTION/ORGANISM/ SITE OF INFECTION	SUGGESTED REGIMENS		COMMENTS
	PRIMARY	ALTERNATIVE	

FUNGAL INFECTIONS/Coccidioidomycosis *(continued)*

TYPE OF INFECTION/ORGANISM/ SITE OF INFECTION	PRIMARY	ALTERNATIVE	COMMENTS
Meningitis Occurs in 1/10 to 1/3 of pts with disseminated cocci CSF demonstrates lymphocytic pleocytosis. CSF glucose <50mg/day& ↓ normal to mildly ↑ protein.	**Treatment: Fluconazole** 400–800 mg po q24h	IV amphotericin B as for pulmonary + 0.2–0.5 mg intrathecal (intraventricular via reservoir device) 2–3x/wk	*CID 133:5/00, 1992.* Flu effective in up to 80% of cases. Vori successful in high doses (6 mg/kg IV q12h) followed by oral suppression (400 mg po q12h) (*CID 36:1619, 2003*). & in a pt who failed flu, liposomal ampho B + intrathecal ampho B (*AAC 48:2341, 2004*). Caspofungin also used (*JAC 54:292, 2004*.) & failed in another case (*CID 39:879, 2004*).
	Suppression: Would not dc even with robust response to HAART **Fluconazole** 200 mg/day po as single dose or 200 mg po q12h	**Amphotericin B** 1 mg/kg IV once/ week or **Itraconazole** 200 mg po q12h (not for meningitis; does not penetrate CSF) (*AnIM 120:932, 1994*)	Relapses are common in both HIV+ & HIV– pts (*AnIM 124:305, 1996*). Lifelong suppression indicated.

Cryptococcosis (*CID 30:710, 2000*)			
Cryptococcemia &/or Meningitis **Treatment** (see *CID 30:710, 2000 & Table 11*) ↓ in era of HAART (*Neurol 56:257, 2001; CID 36:789, 2003*), but still common with AIDS at presentation with AIDS & HIV status unknown (*AIDS 18:555, 2004*). Cryptococci in blood may be manifest by positive blood culture or positive test of serum for cryptococcal antigen	**[Ampho B 0.7mg/kg IV q24h + flucytosine** 25mg/kg q6h x2wks] or **Liposomal amphotericin B** 4mg/kg IV q24h + **flucytosine** 25mg/kg po q6h x2wks]	**[Fluconazole** 400–800mg/day po or IV for less severe disease or **Fluconazole** 400–800mg/day po q6h x 4–6wks or **Ampho B** 0.7mg/kg/day IV x2wks]	If normal mental status, >20 cells/mm³ CSF & CSF crypto antigen <1:1024, flucon alone is reasonable (*CID 22:322, 1996*). Serum cryptococcal antigen useful in dx (95% sens.); no help in monitoring therapy. CSF pressure lower with HAART removal (*CID 38:1394, 2004*). If frequent LPs not possible, ventriculoperitoneal shunts an option (*Surg Neurol 63:529 & 531, 2005*). Itraconazole does not penetrate CSF (*CID 22:329, 1996*). Ampho B + 5FC treatment: 29/236 pts died within 1st 2 wks & 62 (26%) by 10wks; only 129 (55%) were alive & culture-neg at 10wks (*CID 28:82, 1999*). In 64 pts, ampho + 5FC ↓ crypto CFUs more rapidly than ampho + flu or combination of all 3 drugs (p <0.001) (*Ln 363:1764, 2004*).
Cryptococcus in blood may be manifest by positive blood culture or positive test of serum for cryptococcal antigen With HAART, symptoms of acute meningitis may return.	**Consolidation therapy:** Fluconazole 400mg po q24h to complete a 10-wk course or until CSF culture sterile, then suppression (see below). Start Highly Active Antiretroviral Therapy (HAART) if possible.		Must monitor 5-FC levels: peak 70–80 mg/L, trough 30–40 mg/L. Higher levels assoc. with bone marrow toxicity. In 163 pts (15 on HAART) survival was 85%, 6 months after discharge from hospital & receiving flucon. Flu may rarely be due to resistant organism (*Clin Micro Inf 9:1477, 2003; JAC 54:563, 2004*). Failure of flu may rarely be due to resistant organism (*JAC 54:563, 2004*). Successful outcomes were observed in 14/29 (48%) subjects with cryptococcal meningitis treated with posaconazole (*JAC 56:745, 2005*).

---

[7] Flucytosine = 5-FC

NOTE: All dosage recommendations are for adults (unless otherwise indicated) & assume normal renal function.

TABLE 12 (16)

TYPE OF INFECTION/ORGANISM/ SITE OF INFECTION	SUGGESTED REGIMENS		COMMENTS
	PRIMARY	ALTERNATIVE	
FUNGAL INFECTIONS/Cryptococcosis (continued)			
Suppression (chronic maintenance therapy) Discontinuation of antifungal rx can be considered among pts who remain asymptomatic, with CD4 >100–200/mm³ for ≥6 months. Some might consider performing a lumbar puncture before discontinuation of maintenance rx.	**Fluconazole** 200mg/day po [If CD4 count rises to >100/mm³ with effective antiretroviral rx, some authorities now recommend dc suppressive rx. See www.hivatis.org. Authors would only dc if CSF culture negative.]	**Itraconazole** 200mg po q12h if flu intolerant or failure	Itraconazole not as effective as fluconazole Not recommended. 13/57 (23%) pts relapsed vs 2/51 (4%) receiving fluconazole (p = 0.006) (CID 28:291, 1999) although at doses of 600mg/day equal to flu as consolidation rx in 35 pts in Thailand (J Med Assoc Thai 86:293, 2003). No recurrences of crypto meningitis in 22 pts who dc flu suppression with >100 CD4 & undetectable VL x3mos. in Thailand (CID 36:1329, 2003) & 1.53 relapses/100 person-yrs in 100 pts in a European study (CID 38:565, 2004). Reappearance of pos. serum CRAG may predict relapse.
Fusariosis Causes infection in eye, skin, sinus & disseminated diseases—increased in transplant patients (CID 34:909, 2002)	**Voriconazole** 6mg/kg IV q12h on day 1, then either (4mg/kg q12h) or (200mg po q12h for body weight ≥40kg, and 100mg po q12h for body weight <40kg)	**Ampho B** 1–1.2mg/kg or **lipid-associated ampho B**	Voriconazole successful in 9/21: 4 eye, 2 bloodstream, 2 sinus & 1 skin (CID 35:909, 2002; 37:311, 2003)
Histoplasmosis (CID 24:1195, 1997; CID 30:688, 2000; CID 32:1215, 2001) Risk factors for death: dyspnea, platelet count <100,000/mm³, & LDH >2x upper limit normal (CID 38:134, 2004). In 1 study suppression was safely dc after 12mos. of antifungal rx & 6mos. of HAART with CD4 >150: 0 relapses after 2yrs followup in 32 pts (CID 38:1485, 2004).	**Primary prophylaxis:** Not recommended for most pts, consider for pts from endemic area with CD4 <150/µL, if used. **Severe disseminated:** **Acute phase** (3–10 days or until clinically improved): • **Ampho B** 0.7mg/kg IV q24h; or **liposomal ampho B** 4mg/kg IV q24h **Continuation phase** (12wks): **itra** 200mg po q12h **Less severe disseminated:** **Itra** 200mg po q8h x3d, then 200 mg po q12h x12wks **Meningitis:** **Ampho B or liposomal ampho B** x12–16wks **Suppression:** Insufficient data to rec. dc with ↑ CD4 from HAART but probably OK—**Itraconazole** 200mg po q24h indefinitely	**Acute phase:** **itra** 400mg IV q24h **Continuation phase:** • **itra** oral solution 200mg po q12h; or • **flucon** 800mg po q24h **Fluconazole** 800mg po q24h **Amphotericin B** 1mg/kg IV weekly or biweekly indefinitely (lifetime)	**Itraconazole** 200 mg po q24h (Table 10). Acute pulmonary histoplasmosis among HIV-1 infected pts with CD4 counts >300/mm³ might require no rx. Liposomal Ampho B superior at 2 weeks vs Ampho B (88% vs 64% clinical success) in 81 patients with a difference in acute toxicity (97% vs 25%) but no difference in mortality after 10 additional weeks of itra in both arms (AnM 137:105, 2002). Itra (ACTG 120) 50/59 (85%) pts responded. Fluconazole fungemia with only 5% toxicity. 1 pt with meningitis failed, 2 failed because of low serum levels. Avoid rifampin, reduces itra serum concentration (AJM 98:336, 1995). Itra best drug for suppression at 200 mg q24h but 3/46 had probable hepatic toxicity (J AIDS & Human Retro 16:100, 1997). Flu less effective than itra & relapses flu resistant (CID 33:1910, 2001). 10–20% relapses with ampho B, 60% with ketoconazole. Itraconazole: 2/42 (5%) pts relapsed with median follow-up 2 yrs (AnIM 118: 610, 1993) & 2/46 with median follow-up 87 wks (J AIDS & HR 16:100, 1997).

NOTE: All dosage recommendations are for adults (unless otherwise indicated) & assume normal renal function.

TABLE 12 (17)

TYPE OF INFECTION/ORGANISM/ SITE OF INFECTION	SUGGESTED REGIMENS		COMMENTS
	PRIMARY	ALTERNATIVE	
FUNGAL INFECTIONS (continued)			
Nocardiosis (N. asteroides & N. brasiliensis): Uncommon in AIDS pts. 0.38% of AIDS pts 0.38% in Spain (Clin Microbiol Inf 9:716, 2003)			
Cutaneous & lymphocutaneous (sporotrichoid)	**TMP/SMX**: 5–10mg/kg/day TMP & 25–50 mg/kg/day SMX in 2–4 div. doses/day, po or IV	**Sulfisoxazole** 2gm po q6h or **minocycline** 100–200mg po q12h	Linezolid 300–600mg po q12h x3–24mos. was successful in 6/6 pts, 4 with disseminated disease of whom 2 had brain abscesses (CID 36:313, 2003)
Pulmonary, disseminated, brain abscess Duration of rx generally 3mos. for immuno-competent host (38%) & 6mos. for immuno-compromised (62% organ transplant, malig-nancy, chronic lung disease, diabetes, ETOH use, steroid rx, & AIDS).	**TMP/SMX**: Initially 15 mg/kg/day of TMP & 75 mg/kg/day of SMX IV or po. div. in 2–4 doses. After 3–4wks, ↓ dose to 10 mg/kg/day TMP in 2–4 doses po. Do serum level (see Comment)	**IMP** 500mg IV q6h) + (**amikacin** 7.5mg/kg IV q12h) x3–4wks & then po regimen	Survival may be improved when sulfa-containing regimen used (Medicine 68:38, 1999). Measure sulfonamide blood levels early to ensure absorption of po rx. Desire peak level of 100–150mcg/ml 2hrs post-dose.
Paracoccidioidomycosis (South American blastomycosis)/P. brasiliensis CID 31:1032, 2000	Itraconazole 200mg/day po x 6mos or **Ketoconazole** 400mg/day po for 6–18mos	**Ampho B** for severe cases 0.4–0.5mg/kg/day IV to total dose of 1.5–2.5gm or **sulfonamides** (dose: see Comment)	Improvement in >90% pts with itra or keto.[MDM] Sulfa: 4–6gm/ day for several weeks, then 500mg/day for 3–5yrs also used (CID 14 (Suppl) S–68, 1992). Low-dose itra (50–100mg/day), keto (200–400mg/day) & sulfadiazine (up to 150mg/day) showed similar clinical responses in 4–6mos. in a randomized study 14/14, 14/14, 13/14 respectively (Med Mycol 40:411, 2002)
Lobomycosis (keloidal blastomycosis)/ P. lobol	Surgical excision, clofazimine or ampho B		
Penicilliosis (Penicillium marneffei) Common disseminated fungal infection in AIDS pts in SE Asia (esp. Thailand & Vietnam) (CID 24:1080, 1997; Int J Inf Dis 3:48, 1998). Most occur when CD4 <50/mm³	**Treatment: Ampho B** 0.6 mg/kg/day x2 wks followed by **Itraconazole** 400 mg/day po for 10 wks followed by 200 mg/day po **indefinitely for HIV-infected pts** (CID 26:1107, 1998). See Comment **Suppression:** Itra 200mg/day po indefinitely	**Itra** 200 mg po q8h x3 days, then 200 mg po q12h x12 wks, then 200 mg po q24h,[†] (IV if unable to take po)	HIV+: **TMP/SMX suppressive rx indefinitely** ↑ (CID 21: 1275, 1995). Terbinafine has good in vitro activity (JCM 40:3824, 2002). Flu not effective (AAC 43:321, 1999). 3rd most common OI in AIDS following TBc & cryptococcal meningitis. May resemble histoplasmosis or TBc (CID 23: 125, 1996). Skin nodules are umbilicated (mimic cryptococcal infection of molluscum contagiosum). Chronic suppression ↓ relapses to 0/36 vs 20/35 placebo over 1yr period (p <0.001) (NEJM 339:1739, 1998).
Phaeohyphomycosis (black molds/ dematiaceous fungi) [See Table 13, pg139] sinuses, skin, brain abscess **Species: Scedosporium prolificans**, Bipolaris, Wangiella, Curvularia, Exophiala, Phialemonium, Scytalidium, Alternaria, & others)	Surgery + **Itraconazole** 400mg/day po, duration not defined, probably 6mos[MDM]	**Voriconazole** has same in vitro activity, but clinical experience limited to date vs S. prolificans (AAC 45:2151, 2001). **Itraconazole + terbinafine** synergistic against S. prolificans (AAC 44:470, 2000). No clinical data but combination could show ↑ toxicity (see Table 13).	Notoriously resistant to antifungal rx including amphotericin & azoles (CID 34:909, 2002). Mortality >80%. Cause of disseminated disease in immunosuppressed pts (3/4), esp. neutropenia [accounted for 10% of mycelial infections post-transplant (CID 37:221, 2003)] & fungal endocarditis, esp. porcine valve. Blood cultures pos in >50%, eosinophilia in 11%.

* **Oral solution preferred to tablets because of ↑ absorption** (see Table 13, pg139)
NOTE: All dosage recommendations are for adults (unless otherwise indicated) & assume normal renal function.

TABLE 12 (18)

TYPE OF INFECTION/ORGANISM/ SITE OF INFECTION	SUGGESTED REGIMENS		COMMENTS
	PRIMARY	ALTERNATIVE	
FUNGAL INFECTIONS (continued)			
Pseudallescheria boydii (Scedosporium apiospermum) (not considered a true dematiaceous mold) (Med 81:333, 2002) Skin, subcutaneous (Madura foot), brain abscess, recurrent meningitis	Voriconazole 6mg/kg IV q12h x 1, then either (4mg/kg IV q12h) or (200mg po q12h for body weight ≥40kg, but 100mg po q12h for body weight <40kg) (PIDJ 21:240, 2002)	Surgery + itraconazole 200mg po q12h until clinically well.[NFDA] (Many species now resistant or refractory to itra) or Miconazole[AUS] 600mg IV q8h	Notoriously resistant to antifungal drugs including amphotericin. In vitro voriconazole more active than itra (J Clin Micro 39: 954, 2001). Case reports of successful rx of disseminated & CNS disease with voriconazole (CID 31:1499 & 673, 2000; Clin Microbiol Inf 9:750, 2003; Eur J Clin Micro Inf Dis 22:408, 2003).
Sporotrichosis (CID 29:231, 1999; CID 30:684, 2000; CID 36:34, 2003; ID Clin N.A. 17:59, 2003)			
Cutaneous/Lymphonodular	Itraconazole 100–200mg/day solution po x3-6mos. (then 200mg po q12h long-term for HIV-infected pts)[NFDA]	Fluconazole 400mg po q24h x6mos or Sat. soln. potassium iodide (SSKI) (1gm of KI in 1ml of H₂O). Start with 5–10 drops q8h, gradually ↑ to 40–50 drops q8h for 3–6mos. Take after meals.	Itra ref: CID 17:210, 1993. Some authorities use ampho B as primary therapy. Ampho B resistant strains reported (AJM 95: 279, 1993). Itra rx for up to 24mos effective in multifocal osteoarticular infection (CID 23: 394, 1996).
Osteoarticular, pulmonary: itraconazole 300mg po q12h x6-12mos., then 200mg po q12h long-term for HIV-infected pts) (IV if unable to take po)			SSKI side-effects: nausea, rash, fever, metallic taste, salivary gland swelling.
Extracutaneous Osteoarticular, pulmonary, disseminated, meningeal		**Disseminated, meningeal: Ampho B** 0.5mg/kg/day to total of 1–2gm, followed by itra 200mg q12h or flu 800mg q24h	

Reference with pediatric dosages: Medical Letter online version: www.medletter.com (August 2004)

CAUSATIVE AGENT/DISEASE	MODIFYING CIRCUMSTANCES	SUGGESTED REGIMENS		COMMENTS
		PRIMARY	ALTERNATIVE	
PARASITIC INFECTIONS. Reference with pediatric dosages: Medical Letter online version: www.medletter.com (August 2004)				
Protozoan—Intestinal				
Blastocystis hominis	Role as pathogen supported by one controlled rx trial: metro vs placebo	Metronidazole 750mg po q8h x10d; alternatives: **Iodoquinol** 650mg po q8h x20d or **TMP/SMX-DS.** 1 po q12h x7d		
Cryptosporidium parvum Rx is unsatisfactory. Ref.: CID 39:504, 2004	Immunocompetent —no HIV: Nitazoxanide 500mg po q12h x3d			Nitazoxanide: Approved in liquid formulation for rx of children & 500 mg tabs for adults. Ref: Med Lett 45:29, 2003. C. hominis assoc. with ↑ in post-infection eye & joint pain, recurrent headache, & dizzy spells (CID 39:504, 2004).
		HIV with immunodeficiency: Nitazoxanide 500mg po q12h x14d in adults (60% response.) No response in HIV+ children.		
Cyclospora cayetanensis		Immunocompetent pts: TMP/SMX-DS 1 po q12h x7d	AIDS pts: TMP/SMX-DS 1 po q6h x10d; then 1 po 3x/wk.	Ref.: CID 23:429, 1996. If sulfa-allergic: CIP 500mg po q12h x7d & then 1 tab po 3x/wk x2 wks.
Entamoeba histolytica Refs.: Ln 361:1025, 2003; NEJM 348:1563, 2003	Asymptomatic cyst passer	Immunocompetent pts: TMP/SMX-DS tab 1 po q12h x7d	Paromomycin (aminocidine in U.K.) 500mg po q8h x7d OR Iodoquinol (Yodoxin) 650 mg po q8h x20 days	Metronidazole not effective vs cysts.
			Diloxanide furoate[AUS] (Furamide) 500 mg po q8h x10 days (Source: Panorama Compound Pharm, 800-247-9767)	

NOTE: All dosage recommendations are for adults (unless otherwise indicated) & assume normal renal function.

TABLE 12 (19)

CAUSATIVE AGENT/DISEASE	MODIFYING CIRCUMSTANCES	SUGGESTED REGIMENS		COMMENTS
PARASITIC INFECTIONS/Protozoan—Intestinal (continued)				
	Patient with diarrhea/ dysentery; mild/moderate disease. Oral rx possible	**Metronidazole** 500–750mg po q8h x10d **or tinidazole** 2gm po q24hr x3d, followed by:	**Ornidazole**[NUS] 500mg po q12h x5d followed by:	Colitis can mimic ulcerative colitis; ameboma can mimic adenocarcinoma of colon. Dx: trophs or cysts in stool. Watch out for non-pathogenic but morphologically identical E. dispar (CID 29:1117, 1999). Antigen detection & PCR better than O&P (Clin Micro Rev. 16:713, 2003)
		Either [**iodoquinol** (was diiododohydroxyquin) 650mg po q8h x20d] or [**paromomycin** 500mg po q8h x7d]		**Serology positive with extraintestinal disease.**
	Extraintestinal infection, e.g., hepatic abscess	**Metronidazole** 750mg IV/po q8h x10d **OR tinidazole** 800mg po q8h x20d followed by **paromomycin** 500mg po q8h x7d		
Giardia lamblia Ref: MMWR 49:55, 2000		**Tinidazole** 2gm po x1 **OR** **Nitazoxanide** 500mg po q12h x3d		**Refractory pts:** (Metro 750mg po + **quinacrine** 100mg po)—both qid/day x3wks). Ref. CID 33:22, 2001. **Nitazoxanide** ref: CID 32:1792, 2001.
Isospora belli		**TMP/SMX-DS** tab 1 po q12h x10d: if AIDS pt, then TMP-SMX-DS q6h x10d & then q12h x3wks	[(**Pyrimethamine** 75mg/day po + **folinic acid** 10mg/day po) x14 days] or **CIP** 500mg po q12h x7d (AnIM 132:885, 2000)	Chronic suppression in AIDS pts. either 1 TMP/SMX-DS tab 3x/wk. OR (pyrimethamine 25mg/day po + folinic acid 5mg/day po)
Microsporidiosis (Ref.: MMWR 53:RR-15, 2004)				
Ocular: Encephalitozoon hellum or cuniculi. Vittaforma corneae or Nosema sp.		**Albendazole** 400mg po q12h x3wks	In HIV+ pts, reports of response of E. corneae, may need keratoplasty. For V. corneae, may need fumagillin eyedrops.	To obtain fumagillin: 1-800-292-6773 or www.leiterrx.com. Dx: Most labs use modified trichrome stain. Need electron micrographs for species identification. FA & PCR methods in development.
Intestinal (diarrhea): Enterocytozoon bieneusi; Encephalitozoon (Septata) intestinalis		**Albendazole** 400mg po q12h x3wks	**Fumagillin** 20mg po q8h reported effective for E. bieneusi (NEJM 346:1963, 2002)	To obtain fumagillin: 800-292-6773 or www.leiterrx.com.
Disseminated: E. hellum, cuniculi or intestinalis; Pleistophora sp. Ref.: NEJM 351:42, 2004		**Albendazole** 400mg po q12h x3wks	No established rx for Pleistophora sp.	For Trachipleistophora sp., try itraconazole + albendazole (NEJM 351:42, 2004)
Protozoan—Extraintestinal				
Babesiosis (B. microti) Refs.: CID 32:1117, 2001)	Treatment. Exchange transfusion if >10% parasitemia & hemolysis	**Atovaquone** 750mg po q12h x7–10d + **azithro** 500mg po x1d, then 250mg/day x7 d (NEJM 343:1454, 2000)	(**Clinda** 600mg po q8h) + (**quinine** 650mg po q8h) x7d. For adults, can give **clinda** IV as 1.2gm q12h.	Long-term suppressive rx in AIDS pts: clindamycin + doxycycline + azithro (2gm po q24h) has been used (CID 22:809, 1996).

NOTE: All dosage recommendations are for adults (unless otherwise indicated) & assume normal renal function.

TABLE 12 (20)

CAUSATIVE AGENT/DISEASE	MODIFYING CIRCUMSTANCES	SUGGESTED REGIMENS		COMMENTS
		PRIMARY	ALTERNATIVE	
PARASITIC INFECTIONS/Protozoan—Extraintestinal *(continued)*				
Pneumocystis carinii pneumonia (PCP) New name: **Pneumocystis jiroveci** (yee-row-vek-ee) Refs: *NEJM* 350:2487, 2004; *CID* 40 (suppl 3), 2005.	**Not acutely ill,** able to take po meds. PaO₂ >70 mmHg	**TMP/SMX-DS,** 2 tabs po q8h x21d) OR (**Dapsone** 100mg po q24h + **TMP** 5mg/kg po q8h x21d)	(**Clinda** (600mg IV or 300-450mg po) q8h + **primaquine** 15mg base po q24h) x21d **OR atovaquone suspension** 750mg po q12h with food x21d	DAP/TMP, TMP/SMX, clinda/prima regimens equally effective. Rash/fever 10% with DAP/TMP, 19% with TMP/SMX, 21% with clinda/prima. Refs.: *CID* 27:191 & 524, 1998
	Acutely ill, po rx not possible. PaO₂ <70 mmHg	**Prednisone** 15-30min. before TMP/ SMX—start with 40mg po q12h x5d, then 40mg po q24h x5d, then 20mg po q24h x11d + **TMP/ SMX** (15mg of TMP component/kg/day) IV div. q6-8h x21d]	**Prednisone** as in primary rx PLUS (**Clinda** 600mg IV q8h) + (**primaquine** 15mg base po q24h) x21d OR **Pentamidine** 4 mg/kg/day IV x21d	**After 21 days of therapy, then chronic suppression in AIDS pts (see next page).** After 21 days of therapy, then chronic suppression (see below). Clinical failure defined as absence of clinical response after 4-8d; then switch to another regimen. Optimal alternative drug is unclear.
		NOTE: Concomitant use of corticosteroids usually reserved for sicker pts with PaO₂ <70 (see below).		
		Can substitute IV prednisone (reduce dose 25%) for po prednisone	**Pentamidine** 300mg IV q24h in 6ml sterile water by aerosol q4wks) OR (**dapsone** 200mg po + **pyrimethamine** 75mg po + **folinic acid** 25mg po all once a week) OR atovaquone 1500mg po q24h with food.	TMP/SMX-DS regimen also provides cross-protection vs toxo & other bacterial infections. Dapsone + pyrimethamine protects vs toxo. Atovaquone refs.: *JID* 180:369, 1999; *NEJM* 339:1889, 1998
	Primary prophylaxis & post-treatment suppression Ref *CID* 40 (suppl 3), 2005	**TMP/SMX-DS,** 1 tab po q24h or 3x/wk) OR (**dapsone** 100mg po q24h) OR (**TMP/SMX-SS,** 1 tab po q24h) DC when CD4 >200 x3 mos.		
Toxoplasma gondii (Ln 363:1965, 2004; MMWR 53:RR-15, 2004; CID 40 (suppl 3), 2005)				
Cerebral toxoplasmosis (Toxoplasma encephalitis)		**Pyrimethamine** (pyri) 200mg x1 po, then 50-75mg/day po] + (**sulfadiazine** 1-1.5gm po q6h) + (**folinic acid** 10-25mg po q24h)	[**Pyri + folinic acid** (as in primary regimen)] plus one of the following: (1) **Clinda** 600mg IV q6h or (2) **atovaquone** 1500mg po b.i.d. or (3) **azithro** 900-1200mg po q24h. All for 6wks.	Use alternative regimen for pts with severe sulfa allergy. If multiple ring-enhancing brain lesions (CT or MRI), ~85-88% do respond to 7-10days of empiric rx; if no response, suggest brain biopsy. IgG Toxo antibody positive in approx. 84% (*NEJM* 327:1643, 1992). **Pyri.** Dose weight based: <60kg, 500mg/day; ≥60kg 75mg/day.
Primary prophylaxis, AIDS pts—IgG toxo antibody + CD4 count <100/μl		**Pyrimethamine** (pyri) 50-75mg po q week) + (**sulfadiazine** 500-1000mg po 4v/day) + (**folinic acid** 10-25mg po q24h) or (**TMP/SMX-DS,** 1 tab po q24h) or (**TMP/SMX-SS,** 1 tab po q24h)		Prophylaxis for pneumocystis also effective vs toxo except when rx with dapsone + pyri. Refs.: *CID* 25(Suppl.3):S299, 1997; *Amer Fam Phys* 56:1387, 1997. (Pyri + sulfa) prevents PCP & toxo; (clinda + pyri) prevents toxo.
Suppression after rx of cerebral toxo. Ref. *CID* 40 (suppl 3), 2005		(**Sulfadiazine** 500-1000mg po q6h] + (**pyri** 25-50mg po q24h) + (**folinic acid** 10-25mg po q24h)	[(**Clinda** 300-450mg po q6-8h) + (**pyri** 25-50mg po q24h) + (**folinic acid** 10-25mg po q24h) or (**atovaquone** 750mg po q6-12h (± **pyri** + folinic acid)]	

NOTE: All dosage recommendations are for adults (unless otherwise indicated) & assume normal renal function.

TABLE 12 (21)

CAUSATIVE AGENT/DISEASE	MODIFYING CIRCUMSTANCES	SUGGESTED REGIMENS		COMMENTS
		PRIMARY	ALTERNATIVE	

PARASITIC INFECTIONS/Protozoan—Extraintestinal *(continued)*

Vaginitis—*MMWR 51:RR-6, 2002 or CID 35(Suppl 2):S135, 2002.*

CAUSATIVE AGENT/DISEASE	MODIFYING CIRCUMSTANCES	PRIMARY	ALTERNATIVE	COMMENTS
Bacterial vaginosis Malodorous vaginal discharge, pH >4.5	Polymicrobic: associated with Gardnerella vaginalis, bacteroides non-fragilis, Mobiluncus, peptococci, Mycoplasma hominis	**Metronidazole** (0.5gm q12h po x7d) or **metronidazole vaginal gel†** (1 applicator intravaginally) 2x/day x5d (avoid in 1st trimester pregnancy)	**Clinda** (0.3gm q12h po x7d) or **2% clinda vaginal cream** 5gm intravaginally at bedtime x7d OR **clinda ovules** 100mg intravaginally at bedtime x3d	Wet prep shows cells covered with organisms "clue" cells. "Fishy" odor when discharge rx with KOH. **Rx of male sex partner not indicated unless balantitis present.** Metronidazole: 2gm po single dose not as effective as 5–7d course (*JAMA 268:92, 1992*). **In pregnancy:** Rx same as non-pregnancy, except avoid clindamycin cream (↑ risk premature birth). **Intravaginal azoles available both OTC & by prescription.**
Candidiasis, vulvovaginal Pruritus thick, cheesy discharge, pH <4.5	Candida albicans 80–90%, C. glabrata, C. tropicalis may be increasing—less suscept. to azoles	**Fluconazole** 150mg single dose po or **itraconazole** 200mg po q12h x1d	**Intravaginal azoles:** Variety of strengths. Regimens vary from 1 dose to 7–14d. Examples: (all end in -azole): butaconz, clotrim, micon, tiocon, tercon.	Other rx for azole-resistant strains: gentian violet, boric acid. With normal CD4 lymphocyte count, usual duration of rx; if AIDS incr. treat for 10–14d. Also see above. *Fungal Infections, Candidiasis.*
Trichomoniasis Copious foamy discharge, pH >4.5	Trichomonas vaginalis	**Metronidazole** (2gm as single dose) (contraindicated in 1st trimester of pregnancy) OR **Tinidazole** 2gm po x1 dose	**For rx failure:** Re-treat with metro 500mg po q12h x7d; if 2nd failure: metro 2gm po q24h x3–5d. If still failure, suggest ID consultation &/or contact CDC: 770-488-4115 or www.cdc.gov/std.	Retreatment often required. Long-term suppressive rx likely to be necessary. **Treat male sexual partners** (**2gm metronidazole po as single dose**).

Nematode infections

CAUSATIVE AGENT/DISEASE	MODIFYING CIRCUMSTANCES	PRIMARY	ALTERNATIVE	COMMENTS
Strongyloides stercoralis (strongyloidiasis)		**Ivermectin** 200mcg/kg po q24h x2d	**Albendazole** 400mg po q12h x2d	

Ectoparasites. Refs.: *CID 36:1355, 2003; Ln 363:889, 2004.* **NOTE: Due to potential neurotoxicity, use lindane products only as last resort.**

CAUSATIVE AGENT/DISEASE	MODIFYING CIRCUMSTANCES	PRIMARY	ALTERNATIVE	COMMENTS
Pediculus humanus corporis (**body lice**)		**Ivermectin** 200mcg po q12h x2d or q24h x2d	7–10d for hyperinfection syndrome	Treat the clothing. Organism lives in, deposits eggs in seams of clothing. Discard clothing; if not possible, treat clothing with 1% malathion powder or 10% DDT powder.
P. humanus var capitis (**head louse nits**) Ref.: Med Lett 47:68, 2005.		**Permethrin,** 1% generic lotion or cream rinse (NIX). Apply to shampooed dry hair for 10min; repeat in one week OR **Ivermectin** 200mcg/kg single dose po in 2 doses 10 days apart; does not affect nits. OR **Malathion 0.5% lotion** (Ovide). Apply for 8–12hrs, then shampoo.		Body louse leaves clothing only for blood meal. Nits in clothing viable for 1 month. **Permethrin:** Success in 78%. Extra nit combing of no benefit. Resistance increasing. No advantage to 5% permethrin. **Malathion:** 98% effective. In alcohol—potentially flammable. Ref. *Ped Derm 21:670, 2004.* Cost: Permethrin 1% $8–9; Malathion 0.5%, $119; Ivermectin $20.
Phthirus pubis (**crabs**)				Treat sex partners if body or pubic lice.

† 1 applicator contains 5 gm of gel with 37.5 mg metronidazole

NOTE: All dosage recommendations are for adults (unless otherwise indicated) & assume normal renal function.

TABLE 12 (22)

CAUSATIVE AGENT/DISEASE	MODIFYING CIRCUMSTANCES	SUGGESTED REGIMENS		COMMENTS
		PRIMARY	ALTERNATIVE	
PARASITIC INFECTIONS/Ectoparasites (continued)				
Sarcoptes scabiei (**scabies**) (mites)				
Immunocompetent patients		**Primary: Permethrin** 5% cream (ELIMITE). Apply entire skin from chin to toes. Leave on 8–10hrs. Repeat in 1wk. Safe for children >2mos. old. Alternatives: **ivermectin** 200mcg/kg po x1 OR **crotamiton** topically q24h x2d		Trim fingernails. Reapply to hands after handwashing. Pruritus may persist x2wks after mites gone. **Do not use lindane in pregnancy or in young children**—absorbed through skin; can use 6–10% precipitated sulfur in petrolatum q24h x5d.
AIDS patients, CD4 <150/mm³ (**Norwegian scabies**—See Comments)		For Norwegian scabies: Permethrin 5% as above on day 1, then 6% sulfur in petrolatum q24h on days 2–7, then repeat x several weeks. **ivermectin** 200mcg/kg po x1 reported effective.		Norwegian scabies in AIDS pts: Extensive, crusted. Can mimic psoriasis. Not pruritic. ELIMITE: 60 gm $18.10. Ivermectin $20. **Highly contagious—isolate!**

TYPE OF INFECTION/ORGANISM/ SITE OF INFECTION		SUGGESTED REGIMENS		COMMENTS
		PRIMARY	ALTERNATIVE	
VIRAL INFECTIONS				
Cytomegalovirus (CMV) Marked ↓ in CMV infections & death from CMV with Highly Active Antiretroviral Rx: there is a progressive ↓ in CMV DNA & most pts actually become neg. after a median time of 13mos (AIDS 13:1203 & 1497, 1999; JID 180:847, 1999; JAC 54:582, 2004; EJCMID 23:550, 2004). Initial rx for CMV infections should include optimization of HAART.		Primary prophylaxis not generally recommended; preemptive rx in pts with ↑ CMV DNA titers in plasma & CD4 < 100/mm³. Recommended by some: **valganciclovir** 900mg po q24h (CID 32:783, 2001). Authors rec. primary prophylaxis be dc if response to HAART is ↑ CD4 >100 for 6mos. (MMWR 53:98, 2004).		Risk for developing CMV disease correlates with quantity of CMV DNA in plasma: +DNAα ↑ 3.4-fold & each log₁₀ ↑ associated with 3.1-fold ↑ in disease (JCI 101:497, 1998; CID 28:758, 1999).
Colitis, esophagitis		**Ganciclovir** as with retinitis except induction period extended for 3–4wks.		No agreement on use of maintenance; may not be necessary except after relapse (AIM 158:957, 1998). Responses less predictable than for retinitis (9/10 effective in 9/10
Dx best by biopsy of ulcer base/edge (Clin Gastro Hepatol 2:564, 2004)			pts (AAC 41:1226, 1997). **Valganciclovir also likely effective.** Switch to oral valganciclovir when po tolerated & when symptoms not severe enough to interfere with absorption.	
CMV of the nervous system: Encephalitis & ventriculitis: Treatment not defined, but should be considered the same as retinitis. Disease may develop while taking ganciclovir as suppressive therapy. [See Herpes 11(Suppl 2):95A, 2004]				
Lumbosacral polyradiculopathy		**Ganciclovir**, as with retinitis. Consider combination of ganciclovir & foscarnet, esp. if prior CMV rx used. Switch to valganciclovir when possible. Suppression continued until CD4 remains >100/mm³ for 6mos.		About 50% will respond (CID 20:747, 1995), survival ↑ (5.4wks to 14.6wks) (CID 27:345, 1998).
Mononeuritis multiplex		Not defined		Due to vasculitis & may not be responsive to antiviral rx. (ArkNeurol 29:139, 1997).

NOTE: All dosage recommendations are for adults (unless otherwise indicated) & assume normal renal function.

TABLE 12 (23)

TYPE OF INFECTION/ORGANISM/ SITE OF INFECTION	SUGGESTED REGIMENS		COMMENTS
	PRIMARY	ALTERNATIVE	
CMV pneumonia—seen predominantly in transplants (esp. bone marrow), **rare in HIV** Rx only when histological evidence present in AIDS pts & other pathogens not identified.	Ganciclovir/valganciclovir: as with retinitis		11/16 pts showed initial improvement with either ganciclovir or foscarnet but disease eventually progressed despite maintenance (CID 23:76, 1996). In BMT recipients, serial measure of pp65 antigen was useful in establishing early dx of CMV interstitial pneumonia with good results if GCV was initiated within 6 days of antigen positivity (Bone Marrow Transplant 26:413, 2000). For preventive therapy, see Table10
Retinitis (most common in AIDS) Still the most common cause of blindness in AIDS patients with <50/mm3 CD4 counts. 19/30 pts (63%) with inactive CMV retinitis who responded to HAART (↑ of ≥60 CD4 cells/ ml) developed immune recovery vitritis (vision ↓ & floaters with posterior segment inflammation—vitreitis, papillitis & macular changes) an average of 43 wks after rx started (JID 179: 697, 1999). Another report 8/21 pts receiving HAART had inflammatory complications (AIDS 14: 1163, 2000). Corticosteroid rx ↓ inflammatory reaction of immune recovery vitritis without reactivation of CMV retinitis, either periocular corticosteroids or short course of systemic steroid.	**For immediate sight-threatening lesions:** Ganciclovir intraocular implant & **valganciclovir** 900mg po q24h. **For peripheral lesions:** **Valganciclovir** 900mg po q12h x14-21d, then 900mg po q24h	Ganciclovir 5mg/kg IV q12h x14-21d, then **valganciclovir** 900mg po q12h **OR** **Foscarnet** 60mg/kg IV q8h or 90mg/kg IV q12h x14-21d, then 90-120mg/kg IV q24h **OR** **Cidofovir** 5mg/kg IV x2wks, then 5mg/kg every other wk, each dose should be administered with IV saline hydration & oral probenecid **OR** Repeated intravitreal injections with fomivirsen (for relapses only, not as initial therapy)	Differential dx: HIV retinopathy, herpes simplex retinitis (Arch Ophthl 114: 834, 1996), varicella-zoster retinitis (rare, hard to diagnose). Valganciclovir po equal to GCV IV in induction of remission: 7/71 progressed on Val & 7/70 on GCV during 1st 4wks & 72% of Val & 77% of GCV-treated pts had satisfactory responses to induction rx. Adverse events were similar (NEJM 346:1119, 2002). Cannot use GCV ocular implant alone as approx. 50% risk of CMV retinitis other eye at 6 mos. & 31% risk visceral disease. Risk ↓ with systemic rx. Non-contralateral retinitis does occur, ganciclovir-resistant mutation often present (JID 189:611, 2004). **Concurrent systemic rx recommended!** Response rates to fomivirsen similar to other therapies (med. time to progression 267–403days). Because of unique mode of action, fomivirsen may have a role if isolates become resistant to other therapies. Retinal detachments 50–60% within 1 yr of dx of retinitis. In 271 AIDS pts with CMV retinitis, both 2nd eye involvement & retinal detachment markedly ↓ with HAART but only if good CD4 cell response: 2nd eye involvement 0.02/person yr with CD4 >200 vs 0.34 with <50/mm3, retinal detachment 0.02/person yr for CD4 >200 vs 0.30 with <50/mm3 (Ophthal 111:2232, 2004). Equal efficacy of IV GCV & FOS. GCV avoids nephrotoxicity of FOS; FOS avoids bone marrow suppression of GCV. Although bone marrow toxicity may be similar to ganciclovir. **Oral valganciclovir should replace both.** Report indicates success of combination rx with GCV at 1/2 dose 5mg/kg q24h & FOS up to 125mg/kg/day for GCV-resistant isolates in solid organ transplants (CID 34:1337, 2002). Hypomagnesemia common complication.

NOTE: All dosage recommendations are for adults (unless otherwise indicated) & assume normal renal function.

TABLE 12 (24)

TYPE OF INFECTION/ORGANISM/ SITE OF INFECTION	SUGGESTED REGIMENS		COMMENTS
	PRIMARY	ALTERNATIVE	
VIRAL INFECTIONS/Retinitis *(continued)*			
Pts who discontinue maintenance rx should undergo regular eye examination for early detection of relapses!	**Suppression, 1°:** Chronic maintenance rx (secondary prophylaxis): **Valganciclovir** 900mg po q24h. Maintenance can be discontinued if CD4 >100/mm³ x6mos.	**Suppression, 2°:** Chronic maintenance therapy: **Cidofovir** 5mg/kg IV every other week with **probenecid** 2gm po 3hrs before the dose followed by 1gm po 2hrs after the dose, & 1 gm by mouth 8hrs after the dose (total of 4 gm); OR **fomivirsen** 1 vial (330 mg) injected into the vitreous, then repeated every 2–4 wks	Potential emergence of resistant CMV. 27.5% pts treated 9mos developed CMV isolates resistant to GCV (*JID 177:770, 1998*), hence may have reason for clinical failure. DC rx a great advantage since IV catheter complications are common: 1.2/person*yr with mortality rate of 5.8% (*AIDS 12:2321, 1999*). Valganciclovir 900mg q24h has similar efficacy (17% progressed over 1 year) & toxicity profile as IV ganciclovir but with fewer IV-related events (*J AIDS 30:392, 2002*). There is also a significant ↓ in cost vs oral vs IV rx (*J AIDS 36:972, 2004*).
Hairy leukoplakia (Epstein Barr virus, EBV)	Usually asymptomatic & no treatment indicated	**Acyclovir** (800mg po 5x/day) or topical podophyllin resin (one application) (not currently FDA-approved for this indication)	Patients usually asymptomatic, lesions respond to rx but recur.
Hepatitis A (*Ln 351:1643, 1998*)	No therapy recommended. If within 2wks of exposure, gamma globulin 0.02ml/kg IM injection x1 is protective.	For vaccine recommendations, *see Table 19 (MMWR 48:RR-12, 1999)*. Based on increased severity of acute hepatitis A superimposed on chronic liver disease, HAV vaccine recommended for all patients with chronic liver disease (*Ann J Med 118:21S, 2005*).	Most common cause of death from acute hepatitis in Italy (*Dig Liver Dis 35:404, 2003*).
Hepatitis B (*see Ln 362:2089, 2003*)			
Acute	No therapy recommended	(See *MMWR 53:100, 2004*)	
Chronic (*ArIM 132:326, 2000*) Prevalence of post-exposure to HBV (presence of anti-HBs is high (90–95%) in HIV+ individuals; active infection only occurs in 10–15%. Prevalence of triple infection with HIV/HCV/ HBV estimated at 1–5%. Incidence of acute HBV was 12.2 cases/1000 person-yrs in HIV-infected CDC cohort (16,248 cases). Risk factors were black race (RR 1.4), alcoholism (RR 1.7), recent injection drug use (1.6%), & history of AIDS (RR 1.5) but risk ↓ with those taking HAART (RR 0.6). Prevalence of chronic HBV was 7.6% (*JID 188:571, 2003*).	For HIV/HBV non-HIV/HBV co-infected pts, see the *Sanford Guide to Antimicrobial Therapy*. Because of lack of controlled studies, it is difficult to make specific recommendations; however, the following seem reasonable: **When ART not indicated** (*see Table 6A*): **Entecavir** (ETV) 0.5mg po fasting q24h. If previous LAM treatment or known YMDD mutation, use 1 mg q24h. Treat 1yr or min. 6mos. after seroconversion. **OR** **Adefovir** (ADV) 10mg po q24h **OR** **PEG INF alfa 2a** 180mcg subcut	**ETV:** Min. toxicity. Active vs YMDD LAM mutants & ADV-resistant strains. Headache & fatigue in 3–4%. More effective with less toxicity than lamivudine in HBeAg-positive & negative HBV. (*NEJM 354:1001,1011, 2006*) **ADV:** Has no activity against HIV at this dose, & unlikely to generate resistant mutations. Active against HBV in HIV co-infected pts: ↓ of 4 log₁₀ HBV DNA & normalization of ALT levels at 48 wks in 11 pts (*Ln 358:718, 2001*). Long-term safety not established in HIV+ pts. **PEG INF alfa 2a** may be superior to standard INF in HIV/HBV co-infection (*J Viral Hepat 10:298, 2003*).

NOTE: All dosage recommendations are for adults (unless otherwise indicated) & assume normal renal function.

TABLE 12 (25)

TYPE OF INFECTION/ORGANISM/ SITE OF INFECTION	SUGGESTED REGIMENS		COMMENTS
	PRIMARY	ALTERNATIVE	
VIRAL INFECTIONS/Hepatitis B (continued)			
HIV infection assoc. with ↑ risk for development of chronic Hep B, ↑ HBV DNA levels, ↑ likelihood of having detectable HBeAg & ↑ risk of liver-related morbidity & mortality. Goal of rx is to reduce HBV-related morbidity & mortality. Surrogate endpoints include sustained suppression of HBV DNA, prevention of liver disease progression & clearance of HBeAg (treated HIV+ pts rarely become HBsAg-). Rx likely ↓ risk of HCC. In general, **consider rx in pts with persistent ↑ of aminotransferase; detectable levels of HBsAg & HBV DNA in serum (levels >10^5 copies/ml) for at least 6mos; active hepatitis on liver bx; & compensated liver disease.**	**Lamivudine-naive pts requiring ART:** (Entecavir (ETV) 0.5mg po fasting q24h **OR** Lamivudine (LAM) 150mg po q24h **+** Tenofovir 300mg po q24h **+** Additional agents to achieve HAART **OR** Tenofovir 300mg + **emtricitabine** 200mg as Truvada™ po q24h looks promising, plus additional agents to achieve HAART **OR** Add adefovir 10mg/day to HAART **OR** Add PEG INF alfa 2a 180mcg subQ/wk to HAART **Lamivudine-experienced pts requiring ART:** lamivudine **OR** Add adefovir 10mg po q24h to HAART regimen		Tenofovir effective in ↓ HBV DNA in retroviral rx-experienced; ↓ 4.9 log$_{10}$ (10 pts) after 10wks vs ↓ 1.2 log$_{10}$ in placebo (2 pts) (p <0.001). Normal rx-naïve: HBV w/tenofovir + lamivudine (5 pts) ↓ by 4 log$_{10}$ with lamivudine alone (1 vts) (p55). (JID 1185, 2004). Other small studies support (Clin Gastro & Hepat 2:87, 2004). Some reports of renal toxicity & hypophosphatemia with tenofovir in HIV co-infected pts. Long term effects on HBV resistance unknown. In non-HIV infected, lamivudine alone effective until YMDD mutations arise; rate of development is approx. 20%/year among HIV/HBV co-infected pts receiving lamivudine alone (Hepatol 30:1320, 1999). Hepatitis flares & occ. hepatic decompensation may occur when "YMDD mutations "break through" (NEJM 351:1521, 2004). Rx with lamivudine for 1 year resulted in seroconversion of HBeAg+ to HBeAb+ in 22% (JID 180:609, 1999). Pts should continue lamivudine for 6-12mos. at least after seroconversion. Optimal duration of rx unknown but flares reported when anti-HBV rx stopped. See above. Duration of INF alfa rx: HBeAg+ rx 16-24wks. HBeAg- min 12mos. See Comments above for lamivudine-naive pts. Addition of lamivudine continued but unlikely to add much when YMDD mutations present (>90% with 4yrs 3TC rx) (Antiviral Therapy 8:257, 2004). HAART should always include HBV therapy to minimize immune reconstitution flares.
Hepatitis C up to 3% of world infected, 4 million in U.S.) See NEJM 345:41, 2001; CID 33:1728, 2001; AnIM 136:747, 2002 **Acute:** Most pts asymptomatic (>75%), occasionally non-specific complaints such as fatigue.	PEG INF + ribavirin, as below, but remains controversial: requires confirmation (NEJM 346:1091, 2002).		Data emerging that early rx of acute hepatitis C with INF alfa 2b may reduce progression to chronic Hep C infection: 43/44 pts in Germany with pos. HCV RNA (mean 54 days to start of rx after exposure/infection) had neg. HCV RNA & normal ALT after 24wks of INF alfa 2b rx (NEJM 345:1452, 2001). A review of published trials (206 pts) concluded that SVR following rx of acute Hep C with INF alfa 2b was 32% vs 4% with placebo (p=0.00007) (Cochrane Database Sys & Rev-CD000369, 2002). No data available in HCV/HIV co-infected pts.

NOTE: All dosage recommendations are for adults (unless otherwise indicated) & assume normal renal function.

TABLE 12 (26)

TYPE OF INFECTION/ORGANISM/ SITE OF INFECTION	SUGGESTED REGIMENS		COMMENTS
	PRIMARY	ALTERNATIVE	
VIRAL INFECTIONS/Hepatitis C *(continued)*	**Ref: www.va.gov/hepatitisc**		Obtain baseline CBC & at wks 2 & 4 of rx *(see Table 13, pg147)*, hemolytic anemia very common with rx.

Chronic: see 2002 NIH consensus statement, http://consensus.nih.gov/cons/116/116cdc_intro.htm.
Genotype 1 is most common in U.S. (>75%), & least responsive to rx in HIV/HCV co-infected pts *(CID 34:831, 2002)*. Once infected only 15% spontaneously clear virus, 85% have chronic infection. 10–15% progress to cirrhosis (med time 28–32 yrs), 4% hepatocellular (HCCA) carcinoma. 5–10,000 deaths in U.S./yr. Hepatitis C & HIV are closely linked conditions & frequently occur in the same pts; >80% of IVDUs & 8–10% of men who have sex with men have HCV compared to 0.4% of routine blood donors in the U.S. 37% of HIV+ persons in the U.S. are also infected with HCV *(CID 34:831, 2002)*. As CD4 cells ↓, HCV titers ↑, resulting in a ↑ in perinatal & sexual transmission of HCV & an acceleration of HCV disease vs 10% of HIV-infected individuals without HCV disease *(Hepatology 34: 1193, 2001)*. The rate of progression to cirrhosis in HCV disease is ↑ by 3.6-fold in HIV-infected individuals *(CID 33:562, 2001; AIDS 17: 1803, 2003)*. endstage liver disease has emerged as a common cause of death in co-infected individuals accounting for 11% of deaths in 1991, 14% in 1994 & 50% in 1998 *(CID 33:492, 2001; AnIM 136:747, 2002 & 138:197, 2003; AIDS 16:813, 2002)*.
The impact of HCV on the progression of HIV disease or response to HAART remains inconclusive *(Ln 362:1687, 2003)*. HCV infection appeared to accelerate HIV progression in 1 study: HR 1.7 for progression to new AIDS-defining event *(CID 36:97, 2003)*. However, in another large (1,955 pts) prospective study, no impact of HCV on progression to AIDS, death, or response to HAART was found *(CID 33:1579, 2002)*.

- Standard HCV antibody testing was falsely negative in 20% of HIV co-infected pts; check HCV RNA by PCR in pts with neg. HCV Ab & ↑ ALT *(Hepatol 36:4, Abst. 746, 53rd AASLD, 2002)*.
- Both HCV & HIV appear to complicate rx of the co-infecting virus. HIV may reduce effectiveness of HCV rx & HCV effectiveness of HAART (↑ X3)
- ↑ risk of HAART hepatotoxicity (↑ X3)

Genotypes 1 & 4 in HIV co-infected patients *(AnIM 140:346, 2004)*

Pegylated INF:	Wt	Ribavirin[+]	
Alfa 2a (Pegasys) 180mcg subQ q wk **OR**		Wt <75kg: nh* (400 mg a.m., 600mg po p.m.)	
Alfa 2b (PEG-Intron) 1.5mcg/kg subQ q wk		>75kg: 600mg po q12h	

Monitor response by quantification: HCV RNA
After 4 wks rx:	<1 log	discontinue Rx
After 12 wks rx:	<2 log	discontinue Rx
	>2 log or undetectable	Rx 48 weeks

Genotype 2 or 3 in HIV co-infected patients
PEG IFN alfa-2a or 2b—dose as for types 1 & 4 above + Ribavirin 400 mg po bid

Monitor response by quantification: HCV RNA
After 4 wks rx:	<1 log	discontinue Rx
After 12 wks rx:	<2 log	discontinue Rx
	>2 log or undetectable	Rx 48 weeks

† Standard ribavirin dose in 3 major clinical trials was 800mg q24h; however, several trials both in HCV & HCV/HIV co-infected pts, doses of ribavirin alone support higher doses recommended here *(ICAAC 2004, Abst. V-1148; AnIM 140: 346, 2004)*.

In nearly 1500 HCV/HIV co-infected pts, 3 prospective randomized trials reported in late 2004 demonstrated superiority of 48 wks of PEG INF (180mcg q wk) + ribavirin (800mg q24hr) over standard INF alfa + ribavirin *(NEJM 351:438 & 451, 2004; JAMA 292:2839, 2004; APRICOT, ACTG, RIBAVIC)*. Sustained viral response (SVR) was lower than previously reported in non-co-infected pts (27%–40% vs 55–60%). **SVR was 14–29% for genotype 1 & 44–73% for genotype 2 or 3.** As in other trials, lack of response at 12wks predicted failure at 48wks: 63 pts (59%) who failed to ↓ HCV 2 logs or to neg, 0 had SVR at 48wks. Of the pts in ACTG study who failed to achieve SVR, 35% had histological response by liver biopsy. 15 pts developed pancreatitis; all were receiving ddI-containing HAART. **Don't give ddI with ribavirin!** 14/133 cirrhotic pts developed hepatic decompensation during rx & 6 died *(APRICOT, AIDS 18:F21, 2004)*. Watch cirrhotic pts carefully during PEG-INF/ribavirin rx.

Higher SVRs may be achieved with ↑ doses of ribavirin. In a preliminary report of 120 HCV/HIV co-infected pts, doses of 1000–1200mg/day achieved 24-week response rate in >70%, with 61% response rate in genotype 1. Although 31% saved dose adjustment & 15% DCd rx, higher doses will likely give better SVR *(ICAAC 44th, Abst V-1148, 2004)*.

- Some would only rx genotypes 2 & 3 for 24wks, but most studies with HCV/HIV co-infected pts have rx for 48wks *(AIDS 19:s3, S166, 2005)*.

NOTE: All dosage recommendations are for adults (unless otherwise indicated) & assume normal renal function.

TABLE 12 (27)

TYPE OF INFECTION/ORGANISM/ SITE OF INFECTION	SUGGESTED REGIMENS		COMMENTS
	PRIMARY	ALTERNATIVE	
VIRAL INFECTIONS/Hepatitis C (continued)			
• Therefore, it seems prudent to rx HCV 1° if HIV is not advanced (CD4 >300 & VL <55,000). Pegylated INF itself may ↓ CD4 counts (↓ 194 cells/mm³) & accelerate HIV (Int AIDS Conf, Barcelona, 2002, Abst. LB Or 16). **If HAART indicated (CD4 200–300/mm3), rx HCV 1°; it is clear now that HAART improves survival in co-infected pts & even ↓ longterm liver-related mortality from HCV** (Ln 362: 1708, 2003). Don't start with both simultaneously—too complicated & ↑ toxicity. • Equally important is treatment of IVDU & alcoholism; both impact negatively on response to rx & will likely reduce compliance to regimens.			Excessive **alcohol consumption** (>5oz/day) **accelerates hepatic fibrosis** from HCV (Ln 349: 825, 1997). Occult HBV or HIV infection might account for lack of response to rx in some pts (NEJM 341:22, 1999; CID 36:1564, 2003). Side effects significant: 10–14% receiving PEG INF-Rib dc rx 2° to side effects (flu-like symptoms, hematological & particularly neuropsychiatric abnormalities. **2002 FDA warning:** Intron can cause or aggravate life-threatening neuropsychiatric, autoimmune, ischemic & infectious disorders—monitor closely). See Table 13, pg147. **Ribavirin is teratogenic & must not be used if pregnancy possible in pt or partner**

NOTE: All dosage recommendations are for adults (unless otherwise indicated) & assume normal renal function.

TABLE 12 (28)

TYPE OF INFECTION/ORGANISM/ SITE OF INFECTION	SUGGESTED REGIMENS		COMMENTS
	PRIMARY	ALTERNATIVE	
VIRAL INFECTIONS/Hepatitis C (continued)			
Prevention **Risk factors:** (1) contaminated blood via transfusion (1/100,000 per unit in U.S.); (2) injection drug use (in IVDU, prevalence of Hep C 79%); (3) occupation exposure—risk of infection from needlestick from HCV+ source is 1.8%, highest from hollow-core needles; (4) sexual activity risk low but male → female > female → male. HCV recovered from 36.4% cervical secretions in 22 HCV+ women (CID 35:966, 2002). Perinatal transmission: infants born to HCV+ mothers have 5-6% risk of infection (when co-infection with HCV + HIV, risk is 14%)		See *MMWR 47(RR-19), Oct. 16, 1998* Although interferon + ribavirin is now approved for rx of chronic hepatitis C (see Table 13, pg147), not recommended for post-exposure prophylaxis. IG not effective. Early treatment of HCV seroconversion in 7 pts (with persistent HCV RNA for 12–20wks following occupational exposure) with INF-alfa alone x1yr achieved sustained response in 7/7 pts (Dig Dis Wk 2000, Abstract 973). Thus, early rx of acute infection may be advisable but data lacking on optimal regimens & duration.	
Herpes simplex virus (HSV) Genital herpes ↑ transmission of HIV			
Treatment Mild	**Acyclovir** 400mg po q8h x7-14d **OR** **Famciclovir** 500mg po q12h x7-14d **OR** **Valacyclovir** 1000mg po q12h x7-14d[(CID 39(Suppl 5):S237, 2004)]	Chronic suppression indicated if frequent recurrences &/or extensive disease. 1% foscarnet cream applied 5x/day in acyclovir-unresponsive ulcers had 65-90% partial to complete response (J AIDS 21:301, 1999).	
Severe—extensive disease, systemic toxicity	**Acyclovir** 5mg/kg IV q8h x10 d [For encephalitis, ↑ to 10mg/kg IV q8h x10 d] After lesions begin to heal, switch to **famciclovir** 500mg po q12h or **valacyclovir** 1000mg po q12h, or **acyclovir** 400mg po q8h. Continue rx until lesions have completely healed.	If acyclovir-resistant: **Foscarnet** 40-60mg/kg q8h IV **OR** **Cidofovir** 5mg/kg IV q w until clinical response	Severe disease not responding to acyclovir may represent resistant virus. Acyclovir-resistant HSV occurs, esp. in large ulcers. Most will respond to IV foscarnet, but recur after drug discontinued [median 6wks (NEJM 325:551, 1991)]. HSV that becomes resistant to both acyclovir & foscarnet will usually remain sensitive to cidofovir (JID 180:487, 1999).
Suppression, post-treatment, only if recurrences are frequent or severe See *CID 39(Suppl.5):S237, 2004*	**Acyclovir** 400mg po q12h or 200mg po q8h indefinitely. 800mg 4x/d more effective in 1 study (5th CRV, Abst. 499) **OR** **Famciclovir** 250-500mg po q12h **OR** **Valacyclovir** 500mg po q12h approved for HIV-infected pts with CD4 count ≥100. If acyclovir-resistant: **Foscarnet** 40mg/kg IV q24h indefinitely		NOTE: For pts taking acyclovir for chronic suppression who then develop CMV retinitis, stop acyclovir when ganciclovir started—GCV active vs H. simplex. Suppressive rx with famciclovir (500mg po q12h) reduced viral shedding & clinical recurrences (total days with lesions 18% vs 5%) in HIV-infected pts (AnIM 128:21, 1998), similar to findings with acyclovir. Valacyclovir (500mg po q12h) rx of HIV-infected pt: at 6mos, 65% were recurrence-free vs 26% receiving placebo (package insert, Valtrex).
Human herpesvirus 8 (Kaposi's sarcoma-associated herpesvirus) See *JCI 113:121, 2004*	See *Table 18, Treatment of HIV-Associated Malignancies.* Effective suppression of HIV-1 replication with ART has best chance of preventing progression of KS or occurrence of new lesions.		Virus appears to be spread by saliva (JID 190:199, 2004). HHV8-associated Castleman disease responds to HAART with immune reconstitution, but relapse of disease still occurred. Survival was 48mos. (CID 35:880, 2002).

NOTE: All dosage recommendations are for adults (unless otherwise indicated) & assume normal renal function.

TABLE 12 (29)

TYPE OF INFECTION/ORGANISM/ SITE OF INFECTION	SUGGESTED REGIMENS		COMMENTS
	PRIMARY	ALTERNATIVE	

VIRAL INFECTIONS (continued)

TYPE OF INFECTION/ORGANISM/ SITE OF INFECTION	PRIMARY	ALTERNATIVE	COMMENTS
Human papillomavirus (HPV): Condyloma acuminatum (CA) (anogenital warts) (MMWR 53:46, 2004.) Progression of disease correlates with ↑ HIV RNA in plasma (JID 179:1405, 1999). Rate of recurrence is high, esp. in HIV+ pts, despite rx. For rx of cervical or anal intraepithelial neoplasia (CIN & AIN), see MMWR 53(RR-15):46 & 91, 2004.	**Patient-applied:** Podofilox 0.5% solution or 0.5% gel. Apply to all lesions q12h x3 consecutive days. Repeat weekly for up to 4wks. OR Imiquimod 5% cream: apply to lesions at bedtime & remove in morning x 3 consecutive nights, weekly for up to 16wks.	**Provider-applied:** Liquid nitrogen cryotherapy—apply until each lesion is thoroughly frozen; repeat every 1–2wks x3–4 times Trichloroacetic acid or bichloroacetic acid cauterization 80–95% aqueous solution—apply to each lesion; repeat weekly for 3–6wks Surgical excision or laser surgery Podophyllin resin 10–25% suspension in tincture of benzoin—apply to area & wash off in a few hrs; repeat weekly for up to 3–6wks	Do not rx cervical warts until results of Pap smear known. Avoid podophyllin & podofilox in pregnant women. Alternatives: cryotherapy with liquid nitrogen, electrocautery. Cidofovir topical gel + surgical excision 100% effective in achieving complete response in 19 pts but 27% relapsed (AIDS 16:447, 2002).
Molluscum contagiosum virus (See Curr Opin Inf Dis 12:185, 1999)	**Treatment:** Usually rx with destructive modalities: cryotherapy with liquid nitrogen, light electrocautery, or curettage. **Suppression:** Retinoic acid (Retin A) applied once nightly to face may ↓ rate of appearance but does not affect established lesions.	3 pts also responded to either IV or topical cidofovir (1% cream) (Ln Abst. 504, Ln 353:2042, 1999).	Interferon alfa is not effective. Spontaneous resolution observed in pts with good response to combination antiretroviral therapy. Retinoic acid cannot be used on eyelids or genitalia. Lesions in disseminated cryptococcosis, histoplasmosis may resemble molluscum.
Parvovirus B-19 "Pure red cell aplasia"	**Immunoglobulin G:** 2gm/kg IVIG given over 2 days. Most pts with <80 CD4/mm³ suffer relapse within 6mos, & require re-rx with IVIG. Maintenance rx effective in 60–70% of relapses (partial) is q2h weekly but necessary if CD4 count >300/mm³ (Am J Hematol 61:16, 1999).		Persistent parvovirus B-19 infection is a cause of anemia in HIV+ pts. Found in 1/3 HIV+ pts (J Invest Med 45:504, 1997). Essentially all pts (27) reported have responded to IVIG (Am J Hematol 61:16, 1999).
Progressive multifocal leukoencephalopathy (PML) (JC virus) Usually in pts with advanced HIV disease (see Table 11, pg61)	HAART ↑ survival (545days vs 60days, p < 0.001) & improved (50%) or stabilized (50%) neurological deficits in 12 pts (AIDS 12:2467, 1999). Pts have experienced ↑ neurological manifestations after initiating HAART—possibly due to IRIS.		Cytarabine of no value in controlled trial (NEJM 338:1345, 1998). Camptothecin, a human topoisomerase I inhibitor, was administered to a single pt with slowing of progression (Ln 349:1366, 1997).
Varicella zoster virus (VZV) ↑ frequency of zoster reported within 2 mos. of starting HAART (7% of 193 pts) (5th CRV, Abst. 501). PCR for VZV DNA in CSF for CNS infection helpful for dx (J Neurovirol 15:172, 1999).	HAART		Treatment must be begun within 72hrs of onset of vesicles. Chronic post-treatment suppression not required. Acyclovir: adjust dose if renal function ↓ . Acyclovir-resistant VZV occurs in HIV pts previously rx with acyclovir & is associated with poor prognosis. However in 11 pts who failed 10 days acyclovir, only 3 had in vitro resistance (mutation of thymidine kinase gene) & no resistance developed on rx. Authors recommend 21 days of rx in such cases (CID 33:2061, 2001). Foscarnet: 4/5 pts rx responded, although 2 relapsed within 14 days (An H 115:19, 1991; J AIDS 7:254, 1994).
Herpes zoster (shingles) Not severe (local dermatomal zoster)	**Acyclovir** 800mg po 5 x/day OR **Famciclovir** 500mg po tid OR **Valacyclovir** 1 gm po tid[NAI] All x7–10 days		
~ Severe (extensive cutaneous, >1 dermatome, trigeminal nerve or visceral involvement)	**Acyclovir** (Zovirax) 10mg/kg IV (infuse over 2hrs) q8h. Continue until cutaneous & visceral disease clearly reacts Comments	**Foscarnet** 40mg/kg IV (infuse over 2hrs) q8h or 60mg IV q12h for 14–26 days. See Comments	

NOTE: All dosage recommendations are for adults (unless otherwise indicated) & assume normal renal function.

TABLE 12 (30)

TYPE OF INFECTION/ORGANISM/ SITE OF INFECTION	SUGGESTED REGIMENS		COMMENTS
	PRIMARY	ALTERNATIVE	
VIRAL INFECTIONS / Varicella zoster virus (VZV) *(continued)*			
Varicella (chickenpox) Mortality high (43%) in AIDS pts *(Int J Infect Dis 6:6, 2002)*	**Acyclovir** 10mg/kg IV (infuse over 1h) q8h x7d	Switch to oral rx (acyclovir 800mg po 5x/day or famciclovir 500mg po q8h or valacyclovir 1gm po q8h) after defervescence if no evidence for visceral involvement *(MMWR 53:99, 2004)*	Adjust dosage if renal function ↓

CAUSATIVE AGENT/DISEASE	MODIFYING CIRCUMSTANCES	SUGGESTED REGIMENS		COMMENTS
		PRIMARY	ALTERNATIVE	
MISCELLANEOUS CONDITIONS				
Aphthous ulcers, recurrent (RAU)		**Thalidomide** 200mg po q24h x14–28d or 400mg po q24h x7d followed by 200mg q24h x7wks.		16/29 pts responded to 200mg q24h vs 2/28 placebo. Side effects: somnolence 7/29 & rash 6/29 *(NEJM 336:1487, 1997).* In another study, 8/11 responded to 200 q24h; 4 had somnolence, 2 rash *(JID 180:61, 1999),* 9/10 responded to high-dose (400 mg q24h) but 8/10 developed rash *(CID 28:892, 1999).* **Teratogenic: do not use in pregnancy!**
Gingivitis (periodontitis/stomatitis) (See Table 11, pg72)		Topical Betadine & chlorhexidine gluconate (Peridex) mouthwash + antibiotics effective vs anaerobes (metronidazole, clindamycin or amoxicillin/clavulanate). [10] Often requires curettage debridement.		
Psoriasis	Mild to moderate	Topical steroids + tar		Methotrexate rx has been associated with rapid immune suppression & death *(AnIM 106:19, 1987).*
	Severe	Skin lesions may improve with ZDV		
Seborrheic dermatitis	Scalp, mild-moderate	Regular use of dandruff shampoo containing selenium sulfide (Selsun), zinc pyrithione (Head & Shoulders, Danex, Zincon) or sulfur/salicylic acid (Vanseb, Sebulex) + medium potency steroid solution (triamcinolone 0.1%), ketoconazole shampoo (2%).		Extremely common in HIV+ patients. Involves hairy areas of scalp, face, chest, back & groin.
	Facial, trunk, &/or groin	Topical imidazole cream (ketoconazole 2%, clotrimazole 1%) + low potency topical steroid (hydrocortisone 1–2.5%, desonide 0.05%) applied 2x q24h		For refractory trunk lesions, ↑ strength of topical steroid. For severe disease, ketoconazole 200–400mg po q24h x2–4wks

Abbreviations: AM/SB = ampicillin/sulbactam; **AUC** = area under the curve (blood concentration vs time); **azithro** = azithromycin; **CIP** = ciprofloxacin; **clarithro** = clarithromycin; **5th CRV** = 5th Conference on Retroviruses & Opportunistic Infections 1998; **ddC** = zalcitabine; **DOT** = directly observed therapy; **DRSP** = drug-resistant S. pneumoniae; **erythro** = erythromycin; **ETB** = ethambutol; **flu** = fluconazole; **FQ** = fluoroquinolones (ciprofloxacin, ofloxacin, levofloxacin, gatifloxacin or moxifloxacin); **IA** = injectable agent, may include aminoglycosides (streptomycin, amikacin, or kanamycin) or the polypeptide capreomycin; **IDSA** = Infectious Diseases Society of America; **IMP** = imipenem cilastatin; **INH** = isoniazid; **itra** = itraconazole; **IVDU** = intravenous drug users; **keto** = ketoconazole; **MRSA** = methicillin-resistant Staph. aureus; **MSSA** = methicillin-sensitive Staph. aureus; **NFDAI** = not FDA-approved for this indication; **NSAID** = non-steroidal anti-inflammatory drug; **NUS** = not available in the U.S.; **oflox** = ofloxacin; **OTC** = over the counter; **PRSP** = penicillinase-resistant synthetic penicillins; **PZA** = pyrazinamide; **RFB** = rifabutin; **RIF** = rifampin; **SM** = streptomycin; **TMP** = trimethoprim; **TMP/SMX** = trimethoprim/ sulfamethoxazole; **VDRL (RPR)** = non-treponemal serologic tests for syphilis (in contrast to FTA/ABS test; **ZDV** = zidovudine

[10]   This is the regimen used by JS Greenspan, *MEDICAL MANAGEMENT OF AIDS,* 6th Ed. Eds.: MA Sande, PA Volberding, W.B. Saunders & Co., 1999

NOTE: All dosage recommendations are for adults (unless otherwise indicated) & assume normal renal function.

TABLE 13: DRUGS USED IN TREATMENT &/OR CHRONIC SUPPRESSION OF AIDS-RELATED INFECTIONS: ADVERSE EFFECTS, COMMENTS, COST

DRUG NAME, GENERIC (TRADE)/ USUAL DOSAGE/COST*	ADVERSE EFFECTS/COMMENTS
ANTIFUNGAL DRUGS	
Non-lipid amphotericin B deoxycholate (Fungizone): 0.3–1mg/kg/day as single infusion 50mg $36.55 Mixing ampho B with lipid emulsion results in precipitation & is discouraged *(Am J Hlth Pharm 52:1463, 1995)*	**Admin:** Ampho B is a colloidal suspension that must be prepared in electrolyte-free D5W at 0.1 mg/ml to avoid precipitation. No need to protect drug suspensions from light. Ampho B infusions cause chills/fever, myalgia, anorexia, nausea, rarely hemodynamic collapse/hypotension. Postulated due to proinflammatory cytokines but does not appear to be histamine release *(Pharmacol 23:966, 2003)*. Manufacturer recommends a test dose of 1 mg, but often not done (1st few ml of 1st dose is a test dose). Duration of infusion usually 4 or more hrs. No difference found in 1- vs 4-hr infusions *(AAC 34:1402, 1992)* except chills/fever occurred sooner with 1-hr. infusion. Febrile reactions decrease with repeated doses. Rare pulmonary reactions (severe dyspnea & focal infiltrates suggesting pulmonary edema) associated with rapid infusion *(CID 33:75, 2001)*. Severe rigors respond to meperidine (25–50mg IV). Premedication with acetaminophen, diphenhydramine, hydrocortisone (25–50mg) & heparin (1000 units) had no influence on rigors/fever *(CID 70:755, 1995)*. If cytokine postulate correct, NSAIDs or high-dose steroids may prove efficacious but their use may risk worsening infection under rx or increased risk of nephrotoxicity (i.e., NSAIDs). Clinical side effects ↓ with ↑ age *(CID 26:334, 1998)*. **Toxicity:** Major concern is nephrotoxicity (15% of 102 pts surveyed, *CID 26:334, 1998*). Manifest initially by kaliuresis & hypokalemia, then fall in serum Can reduce risk of renal injury by **(a) pre- & post-infusion hydration with 500ml saline (if clinical status will allow salt load)**, (b) avoidance of other nephrotoxins, e.g., radiocontrast, aminoglycosides, cis-platinum, (c) use of lipid prep of ampho B. Use of low-dose dopamine did not significantly reduce renal toxicity *(AAC 42:3103, 1998)*. In a single randomized controlled trial of 80 neutropenic pts with refractory fever & suspected or proven invasive fungal infection, 0.97mg/kg/day amphotericin **continuously infused over a 24-hr period** was compared to the classical **rapid infusion** of 0.95mg/kg/day **infused over 4hrs**. Continuous infusion produced less nephrotoxicity [26% ↓ in max. serum Cr (p=0.005)], a reduction in fever, chills & vomiting (p <0.02–0.0003) & appeared as effective as rapid infusion but in very few proven fungal infections (7 & 3, respectively) *(BMJ 322:1, 2001)*. Continuous infusion also allows a dramatic ↑ in administered dosage without sig. toxicity *(CID 36:943, 2003)*. It is disturbing that these exciting observations have not led to controlled trials examining efficacy in rx of life-threatening fungal infections *(CID 36:952, 2003)*. Await trials of efficacy in larger number of proven fungal infections! *(IDCP 12:321, 2004)*
Lipid-based ampho B products:[1,2] Amphotericin B lipid complex (ABLC) (Abelcet): 5mg/kg/day as single infusion 100mg IV $255 ($890/350 mg)	**Admin:** Consists of ampho B complexed with 2 lipid bilayer ribbons. Compared to standard ampho B, larger volume of distribution, rapid blood clearance & high tissue concentrations (liver, spleen, lung). Dosage: **5mg/kg q24h**; infuse at 2.5mg/kg/hr; adult & ped. dose the same. Do NOT use an in-line filter. Do not dilute with saline or mix with other drugs or electrolytes.[3] **Toxicity:** Fever & chills in 14–18%; nausea 9%, vomiting 8%; serum creatinine ↑ in 11%; renal failure 5%; anemia 4%; ↓ K 5%; rash 4%.
Liposomal amphotericin B (L-AmB, AmBisome): 1–5mg/kg/day as single infusion. 50mg $196 ($1372/350mg)	**Admin:** Consists of vesicular bilayer liposome with ampho B intercalated within the membrane. Dosage: **3–5mg/kg/day** IV as single dose infused over a period of approx. 120min. If infusion is well tolerated, infusion time can be reduced to 60min.[2] 1mg/kg/day was as effective as 4mg/kg/day (6mos. survival rates 43% vs 37%, respectively) in pts with invasive aspergillosis complicating bone marrow transplant &/or neutropenia from malignancy *(CID 27:1406, 1998)*. **Major toxicity:** Generally less than ampho B. Nephrotoxicity 18.7% vs 33.7% for ampho B, chills 47% vs 75%, nausea 39.7% vs 38.7%, vomiting 31.8% vs 43.9%, rash 24% for both, ↓ Ca 18.4% vs 20.9%, ↓ K 20.4% vs 25.6%, ↓ Mg 20.4% vs 25.6%. Acute infusion-related reactions are common with liposomal ampho B, 20–40%. 86% occurred within 5 min. of infusion, including chest pain, dyspnea & hypoxia or severe abdominal, flank or leg pain; 14% developed flushing & urticaria near the end of 4-hr infusion. All responded to diphenhydramine (1mg/kg) & interruption of L-AmB infusion. These reactions may be due to complement activation by the liposome *(CID 36:1213, 2003)*.

1 Published data from patients intolerant of or refractory to conventional ampho B deoxycholate (Amp B). **None of the lipid ampho B preps has shown superior efficacy compared to ampho B in prospective trials (except liposomal ampho B was more effective vs ampho B in rx of disseminated histoplasmosis at 2wks** *(AnIM 137:105, 2002; CID 37:415, 2003)*. **Dosage equivalency has not been established** *(CID 36:1500, 2003)*. Nephrotoxicity ↓ with all lipid ampho B preps *(IDCP 7:516, 1998; CID 27:603, 1998; NEJM 340:764, 1999)*.

2 Comparisons between Abelcet & AmBisome suggest higher infusion-assoc. toxicity (rigors) & febrile episodes with Abelcet (70% vs 36%) but a higher frequency of mild hepatic toxicity with AmBisome (59% vs 38%, p=0.05). Mild elevations in serum creatinine were observed in 1/3 of both *(BJ Hemat 103:198, 1998; Focus on Fungal Inf #9, 1999; Bone Marrow Tx 20:39, 1997; CID 26:1383, 1998)*.

TABLE 13 (2)

DRUG NAME, GENERIC (TRADE)/ USUAL DOSAGE/COST*	ADVERSE EFFECTS/COMMENTS
ANTIFUNGAL DRUGS (continued)	
Amphotericin B cholesteryl complex, (amphotericin B colloidal dispersion, ABCD, Amphotec): 3–4mg/kg/day as single infusion. 100mg/day $160	**Admin.:** Consists of ampho B deoxycholate stabilized with cholesteryl sulfate resulting in a disc-shaped colloidal complex. Compared to standard ampho B, larger volume of distribution, rapid blood clearance, high tissue concentrations. Dosage: Initial dose for adults & children: **3–4mg/kg/day.** If necessary, can ↑ to 6mg/kg/day. Dilute in D5W & infuse at 1 mg/kg/hr. Do NOT use in-line filter. **Toxicity:** Chills 50%, fever 33%, ↑ serum creatinine 12–20%, ↓ Ca 6%, ↓ K 17%.
Caspofungin (Cancidas) 70mg IV on day 1 followed by 50mg IV q24h (reduce to 35 mg IV q24h with moderate hepatic insufficiency) 70 mg $424; 50 mg $329 Ref.: *Ln* 362:1142, 2003	An echinocandin which inhibits synthesis of β-(1,3)-D-glucan, a critical component of fungal cell walls. Fungicidal against candida (MIC <2 mcg/ml) including those resistant to other antifungals & active against aspergillus (MIC 0.4–2.7 mcg/ml). Serum levels on rec: dosages = peak 12, trough 1.3 (24hrs) mcg/ml. Approved for rx of candidemia & other candida infections (intra-abdominal abscess, esophageal peritonitis, pleural space infection) & refractory aspergillus infections & was 48.9% successful in 57 pts with invasive aspergillus infections in severely impaired hosts who had failed other antifungals. **Toxicity:** remarkably non-toxic with no nephrotoxicity reported. Only 2% of 263 pts in double-blind trial dc drug due to drug-related adverse event (*Transpl Inf Dis* 1:25, 2002). 14% had ↑ transaminases (similar to triazoles). Most common adverse effect: pruritus at infusion site & headache, fever, chills, vomiting, & diarrhea associated with infusion. Drug metabolized in liver & dosage ↓ to 35mg in moderate to severe hepatic failure. Class C for pregnancy (embryotoxic in rats & rabbits), so only use if potential benefits outweigh risks. *See Table 16 for drug-drug interactions, esp. cyclosporine (hepatic toxicity) & tacrolimus (drug level monitoring recommended)* (*Curr Med Res Opin* 19:263, 2003; *JAC* 49:889, 2002).
Micafungin (Mycamine) 50mg per day for prophylaxis post-bone marrow stem cell transplant: $95/day 150mg/day per day for rx: $280.50/day (50mg vials): $5890.30 for 150mg IV q24h for 21 days (*Med Lett* 47:52, 2005)	The 2nd echinocandin approved by the FDA (March 2005) for rx of esophageal candidiasis & for prophylaxis against candida infections in HSCT recipients. Fungicidal against most strains of candida sp. & aspergillus sp. including those resistant to fluconazole such as C. glabrata & C. krusei. No antagonism seen when combined with other antifungal drugs & occ. synergism with ampho B (*JAC* 49:2294, 2005). No dosage adjustment for severe renal failure or moderate hepatic impairment. Watch for drug-drug interactions with sirolimus or nifedipine. Micafungin is well tolerated & common adverse events include nausea 7.8%, vomiting 7.3%, & headache 2.4%. Transient ↑ LFTs, BUN, creatinine reported; rare cases of significant hepatitis & renal insufficiency *(package insert for micafungin).*
Anidulafungin (Eraxis) 200mg IV on day 1 followed by 100mg/day IV for esophageal can-didiasis 100mg IV times 1, then 50mg IV q24h (no cost data available) Cost per day $90	An echinocandin with antifungal activity (cidal) against candida sp. & aspergillus sp. including ampho B- & triazole-resistant strains. Effective in clinical trials of esophageal candidiasis & in 1 trial was superior to fluconazole in rx of invasive candidiasis/candidemia in 245 pts (75.6% vs 60.2%) (*ICAAC* Abst 49:2984, 2005). Like other echinocandins, remarkably non-toxic; most common side effects: nausea, vomiting, ↓ Mg, ↓ K & headache in 11–13% of pts. No dose adjustments for renal or hepatic insufficiency. Few drug-drug interactions.
Fluconazole (Diflucan) (available generically) 100mg tabs NB.80, G 1.73 150mg tabs NB16, G $7 200mg tabs N$B$16, G $1 400mg IV N$B$170,G$152 Oral suspension: 50mg/5ml, $40/35ml NB	IV=oral dose because of excellent bioavailability. **Pharmacology:** absorbed po, water solubility enables IV. Peak serum levels *(see Table 14.)* T ½ 30 hrs (range 20–50hrs); 12% protein bound. **CSF levels 50–90% of serum in normals.** No effect on mammalian steroid metabolism. **Drug-drug interactions common, see Table 16.** Side effects overall 16% [more common in HIV+ pts (21%)]. Nausea 3.7%, headache 1.9%, skin rash 1.8%, abdominal pain 1.7%, vomiting 1.7%, diarrhea 1.5%. ↑ SGOT 20%. Alopecia (scalp, pubic crest) in 12–20% pts of women receiving a median of 3mos (reversible in approx 6mos) (*AnIM* 123:354, 1995). Rare: severe hepatotoxicity, exfoliative dermatitis. Anaphylaxis (*CID* 13:81, 1993), thrombocytopenia, leukopenia. Good reference: *NEJM* 330:263, 1994
Flucytosine (Ancobon) 500mg cap $9	**AEs:** Overall 30%. GI 6% (diarrhea, anorexia, nausea, vomiting); hematologic 22% (leukopenia, thrombocytopenia, when serum level > 100mcg/ml (esp. in azotemic pts)]; hepatotoxicity (asymptomatic ↑ SGOT, reversible); skin rash 7%, aplastic anemia (rare—2 or 3 cases). False ↑ in serum creatinine on EKTACHEM analyzer. *(JAC* 26:171, 2000)

TABLE 13 (3)

DRUG NAME, GENERIC (TRADE)/ USUAL DOSAGE/COST*	ADVERSE EFFECTS/COMMENTS
ANTIFUNGAL DRUGS *(continued)*	
Griseofulvin (Fulvicin, Grifulvin, Grisactin) 500mg G $3.45, susp 125mg/ml: 120ml $452	Photosensitivity, urticaria, GI upset, fatigue, leukopenia (rare). Interferes with warfarin drugs. Increases blood & urine porphyrins, should not be used in patients with porphyria. Minor disulfiram-like reactions. Exacerbation of systemic lupus erythematosus.
Imidazoles, topical For vaginal &/or skin use	Not recommended in 1st trimester of pregnancy. Local reactions: 0.5-1.5%: dyspareunia, mild vaginal or vulvar erythema, burning, pruritus, urticaria, rash. Rarely similar symptoms in sexual partner.
Itraconazole (Sporanox) 100mg cap $10 _____ 10mg/ml oral solution (fasting state) (150 ml: $141) (AAC 42:1862, 1998) _____ IV usual dose 200mg q12h x 4 doses followed by 200mg q24h for a maximum of 14 days ($213/250mg)	**Itraconazole tablet & solution forms are not interchangeable, solution preferred.** Many authorities recommend measuring drug serum concentration after 2 wks on prolonged rx to ensured satisfactory absorption. To obtain the highest plasma concentration, the tablet is given with food & acidic drinks (e.g. cola) while the solution is taken in the fasted state; under these conditions, the peak conc. of the capsule is approx. 3 mcg/ml & of the solution 5.4mcg/ml. Peak levels are reached faster (2.2 vs 5hrs) with the solution. **Peak plasma concentrations after IV injection (200mg) compared to oral capsule (200mg): 2.8mcg/ml (on day 7 of rx) vs 2mcg/ml (on day 36 of rx).** Protein-binding for both preparations is over 99%, which explains the virtual absence of penetration into the CSF (**do not use to treat meningitis**). Most common adverse effects are dose-related nausea 10%, diarrhea 8%, vomiting 6%, & abdominal discomfort 5.7%. Allergic rash 8.6%, ↑ bilirubin 6%, edema 3.5%, & hepatitis 2.7% reported. ↑ doses may produce hypokalemia 8% & ↑ blood pressure 3.2%. Thrombocytopenia & leukopenia reported (AnIM 125:157, 1996). Delirium reported (Psychosomatics 44:260, 2003). Hypokalemia & rhabdomyolysis reported (PID 22:1024, 2003; Respiration 71:289, 2004). **Reported to produce Impairment in cardiac function** (See Ln 357:1766, 2001). Other concern, as with fluconazole & ketoconazole, is **drug-drug interactions; see Table 16**. Some interactions can be life-threatening (CID 38:e73, 2004; Ann Pharmacother 38:46, 2004).
Ketoconazole (Nizoral) 200 mg tab $2.25	Gastric acid required for absorption—cimetidine, omeprazole, antacids block absorption. In achlorhydria, dissolve tablet in 4ml 0.2N HCl, drink with a straw. Coca-Cola ↑ absorption by 65% (AAC 39:1671, 1995). CSF levels "none". **Drug-drug interactions important, see Table 16. Some interactions can be life-threatening, Dose-dependent nausea & vomiting.** Liver toxicity of hepatocellular type reported in about 1:10,000 exposed pts—usually after several days to weeks of exposure. At doses of ≥800mg/day serum testosterone & plasma cortisol levels fall. With high doses, adrenal (Addisonian) crisis reported.
Miconazole (Monistat IV) 200 mg —not available in U.S.	IV miconazole indicated in patient critically ill with Pseudallescheria boydii. Very toxic due to vehicle needed to get drug into solution.
Nystatin (Mycostatin) 30 gm cream NB $28, G $2.30 500,000 units oral tab $0.36	Topical: virtually no adverse effects. Less effective than imidazoles & triazoles. PO: large doses give occasional GI distress & diarrhea.
Terbinafine (Lamisil) 250 mg tab $10.50	Rare cases (8) of idiosyncratic & symptomatic hepatic injury & more rarely liver failure leading to death or liver transplantation reported in pts receiving terbinafine for onychomycosis. Therefore, the drug is **not recommended** for pts with **chronic or active liver disease** although hepatotoxicity may occur in pts with or without pre-existing disease (An Hepatol 2:47, 2003). Pretreatment screening of serum transaminases (ALT & AST) is advised & alternate rx used for those with abnormal levels. Pts started on terbinafine should be warned about symptoms suggesting liver dysfunction (persistent nausea, anorexia, fatigue, vomiting, RUQ pain, jaundice, dark urine or pale stools). If symptoms develop, drug should be discontinued & liver function immediately evaluated. In controlled trials, changes in ocular lens & retina reported—clinical significance unknown. Major drug-drug interaction is 100% ↑ in rate of clearance by rifampin. Less frequent, transient & rarely caused discontinuation of rx. % with AE: terbinafine vs placebo: nausea/diarrhea 2.6–5.6 vs 2.9; rash 5.6 vs 2.2; taste abnormality 2.8 vs 0.7. Inhibits CYP2D6 enzymes.

TABLE 13 (4)

DRUG NAME, GENERIC (TRADE)/ USUAL DOSAGE/COST*	ADVERSE EFFECTS/COMMENTS
ANTIFUNGAL DRUGS (continued)	
Voriconazole (Vfend) IV: Loading dose 6mg/kg q12h x1 day, then 4mg/kg q12h IV for invasive aspergillus & serious mold infections; 3mg/kg q12h IV for serious candida infections **Oral:>40kg body weight:** 400mg po q12h x1 day, then 200mg po q12h; **<40kg body weight:** 200mg po q12h x1 day, then 100mg po q12h Take oral dose 1hr before or 1hr after eating. Oral suspension (40mg/ml) $36.49/200mg dose. Oral suspension dosing: Same as for oral tabs. Reduce to 1/2 maintenance dose for moderate hepatic insufficiency.	A triazole with activity against Aspergillus sp. including Ampho resistant strains of A. terreus (*JCM 37:2343, 1999*). Active vs Candida sp. (including krusei), Fusarium sp., & various molds. Steady state serum levels reach 2.5–4 g/ml. Toxicity similar to other azoles/triazoles (*CID 39:1241, 2004*) including uncommon serious hepatic toxicity (hepatitis, cholestasis & fulminant hepatic failure. Liver function tests should be monitored during rx & drug dc" if abnormalities develop. Rash reported in up to 20%, occ. photosensitivity & rare Stevens-Johnson, & anaphylactoid infusion reactions with fever & hypertension (*Clin Exp Dermatol 26:648, 2001*). 1 case of QT prolongation with ventricular tachycardia in a 15 y/o pt with ALL reported (*CID 39:984, 2004*). **Approx. 30% experience a transient visual disturbance** following IV or po. ("altered/enhanced visual perception", blurred or colored visual change or photophobia) within 30–60min. Visual changes resolve within 30–60min. after administration & are attenuated with repeated doses **(do not drive at night for outpatient rx)**. No persistence of effect reported. Cause unknown. Accumulate. Potential for drug-drug interactions high—see *Table 16 (CID 36:630, 1087, 1122, 2003)*. **NOTE:** Not in urine in active form. **Cost:** 50mg tab $9; 200 mg tab $35; 200mg IV $109
ANTIMYCOBACTERIAL DRUGS	
First Line Drugs	
Isoniazid (INH) (Nydrazid, Laniazid, Teebaconin) 300mg/day po 300mg tab $0.02 100mg/ml in 10 ml vials (IM) (Nydrazid, Apothecon) $16.64	**Adverse effects:** Overall <1%. **Peripheral neuropathy** (<1%); pyridoxine 25mg q24h will ↓ incidence; other neurologic sequelae, convulsions, optic neuritis, toxic encephalopathy, psychosis, muscle twitching, dizziness & alterations of sensorium, coma (all rare); allergic skin rashes, lymphadenopathy & vasculitis (SLE-like syndrome), fever, minor disulfiram-like reaction, flushing after Swiss cheese, constipation, **hepatitis** (children 10% mild ↑ SGOT, normalizes with continued rx, age <20yrs rare, 20–34yrs 0.3%, 35–49yrs 1.2%, ≥50yrs 2.3%) (also ↑ with daily alcohol); acute liver failure (fatal if requiring transplantation (*Lancet 345:555, 1995*); blood dyscrasias (rare); + antinuclear antibody 20%.
Rifampin (Rifadin, Rimactane, Rifocin) 600mg/day po 300mg cap $1.90 (IV available, Aventis. 600mg $90.28)	**Adverse effects:** Produces an orange-brown discoloration of urine, tears (can stain contact lens), semen, & sweat. Can falsely elevate lab measurements of bilirubin. **Drug-drug interactions:** Many (*see Table 16*): induces liver cytochrome P450 system (CYP3A) to ↑ drug metabolism, e.g., ↑ Coumadin requirement, ↑ steroid dosage in pts with Addison's disease or asthmatics,; ↓ effectiveness of oral contraceptives (uterine bleeding, pregnancies), methadone less effective, reduced levels of azole antifungals, e.g., fluconazole. 16 deaths reported in 500,000 recipients. Minor enzyme changes common & resolve while continuing rx. **Flu syndrome** Manifest as fever/chills, headache, bone pain, dyspnea if rifampin ingestion irregular. Hepatotoxicity: Hepatotoxicity (~1% of rx). Interstitial nephritis reported.
Ethambutol (Myambutol) 15–25mg/kg/day po 400mg tab $1.78	**Adverse effects: Optic neuritis** with decreased visual acuity, central scotomata, & loss of green & red perception at 25mg/kg/day (not at 15mg/kg/day; peripheral neuropathy & headache (~1%), rashes (rare), arthralgia (rare), hyperuricemia (rare). Monthly evaluation of visual acuity (>10% loss considered significant), red/green color discrimination; usually reversible if drug discontinued. Anaphylactoid reaction. **Comment** Disrupts outer cell membrane in M. avium with ↑ activity with ↑ of other drugs.

TABLE 13 (5)

DRUG NAME, GENERIC (TRADE)/ USUAL DOSAGE/COST*	ADVERSE EFFECTS/COMMENTS
ANTIMYCOBACTERIAL DRUGS/First Line Drugs *(continued)*	
Pyrazinamide (PZA) 25mg/kg/day po 500 mg tab $1.09	**Adverse effects: Arthralgia; hyperuricemia** (with or without symptoms); hepatitis (not over 2% if recommended dose not exceeded); gastric irritation; photosensitivity (rare). Serum uric acid if symptomatic gouty attack occurs. **Comment:** Maximum dose 2gm/day.
Streptomycin 0.75–1gm/day IM (or IV) 1gm $9.10	**Adverse effects:** Overall 8%. **Ototoxicity,** vestibular dysfunction (vertigo): paresthesias, dizziness & nausea (all less in pts receiving 2–3 doses/wk); tinnitus & high frequency loss 1%; nephrotoxicity (rare); peripheral neuropathy (rare); allergic skin rashes 4–5%; drug fever. Available from Pfizer/Roerig 1-800-254-4445, Reference for IV use. *CID 19:1150, 1994.*
Rifabutin* (see Comment for content) 2 tablets single dose po q24h (1hr before meal). 1 tab $2.65	**Adverse effects:** Same as individual components. **Comments** : 1 tablet contains 150mg INH, 300mg Rif.
Rifater* (See Comment for content) If pt not >55kg: 6 tablets single dose po q24h (1hr before meal). 1 tab $1.96	**Adverse effects:** Same as individual components. **Comments** : 1 tablet contains 50mg INH, 120mg RIF. 300mg PZA. Used in 1st 2mos of rx. (PZA 25mg/kg). Purpose is convenience in dosing. ↑ compliance (*AnIM 122:951, 1995*) but costs 1.5x more.
SECOND LINE DRUGS	
Para-aminosalicylic acid (PAS) (Na⁺ or K⁺ salt) (Paser) 4–6gm po q12h (200mg/kg/day) 450mg tab $0.08	**Adverse effects: Gastrointestinal irritation** 10–15%; goitrogenic action (rare); depressed prothrombin activity (rare); G6PD-mediated hemolytic anemia (rare), drug fever, rashes, hepatitis, myalgia, arthralgia. Retards hepatic enzyme induction, may ↓ INH hepatotoxicity. Available from Jacobus Pharm. Co. (609) 921-7447, CDC (404) 639-3670.
Ethionamide (Trecator-SC) 500–1000mg/day (15–20mg/kg/day) po as 1–3 doses 250 mg tab $3.09	**Adverse effects: Gastrointestinal irritation** (up to 50% on large dose); goiter, peripheral neuropathy (rare); convulsions (rare); changes in affect (rare); difficulty in diabetes control; rashes; hepatitis; purpura, stomatitis, gynecomastia, menstrual irregularity. Give drug with meals or antacids; 50–100mg pyridoxine per day concomitantly; SGOT monthly. Possibly teratogenic.
Cycloserine (Seromycin) 750–1000mg/day (15mg/kg/day) po as 2–4 doses. 250mg cap $3.50	**Adverse effects:** Convulsions, **psychoses** (5–10% of those receiving 1gm/day); headache, somnolence, hyperreflexia, increased CSF protein & pressure, peripheral neuropathy, contraindicated in epileptics & active alcoholics; 50mg pyridoxine for every 250mg cycloserine should be given concomitantly.
Amikacin (Amikin) 7.5–10mg/kg/day IV or IM 500mg vial $7.80	**Adverse effects:** Nephrotoxicity, **ototoxicity** [usually high frequency loss—especially with larger total dose (>10gm), longer duration (>10 days), prior aminoglycosides, pos. family history, assoc. renal impairment & rising trough level (>10μg/ml). All aminoglycosides may cause or ↑ neuromuscular blockade. Use with caution in pts with myasthenia gravis, Parkinsonism, botulism, with neuromuscular blocking agents (*Table 16*), or with massive transfusion of citrated blood. Avoid concurrent use with ethacrynic acid, furosemide or methoxyflurane. ↑ risk of nephrotoxicity with cis platinum, vancomycin, radiocontrast agents. **Comments:** With edema, ascites, &/or obesity, base calculation of est. creatinine clearance on lean body mass & ideal body weight. For dosing with renal impairment, see *Table 16*.
Capreomycin sulfate (Capastat sulfate) 1gm/day (15mg/kg/day) as 1 dose IM 1gm $25.54	**Adverse effects: Nephrotoxicity** 36%, **ototoxicity** (auditory 11%), eosinophilia, leucopenia, skin rash, fever, hypokalemia, neuromuscular blockade. Abnormal liver function tests, ? related. Capreomycin is an aminoglycoside & shares group side-effects of nephrotoxicity, ototoxicity, & potential neuro-muscular blockade.

TABLE 13 (6)

DRUG NAME, GENERIC (TRADE)/USUAL DOSAGE/COST*	ADVERSE EFFECTS/COMMENTS
Antimycobacterial Drugs/Second Line Drugs (continued)	
Amithiozone (Thiacetazone, Tibione, Thioparamizone) (NOT MARKETED IN U.S.) 150mg/day po	**Adverse effects:** Common: nausea, vomiting, skin rash, dizziness. Uncommon: bone marrow depression, jaundice 0.2%, & renal toxicity. Marked differences in frequency of side effects between racial groups noted. Asia > Africa. Total incidence 21–38%, 1/2 lasted 6 days or less, 1/2 mild. **Comments: Skin reactions** reported in 20% of HIV+ pts. Felt to be responsible for a 3% **mortality** (Lancet 1.627, 1991). In trial comparing RIF/INH/PZA (RHZ) with SM/thiacetazone/INH (STH), relative risk of death with STH 1.6, drug reactions 11.7 & sputum negative at 2mos RHZ 74% vs 37% in STH (Lancet 344.323, 1994; ibid, 345.62, 1995).
Clofazimine (Lamprene) 50mg/day po (with meals) 50mg $0.20	**Adverse effects: Skin pigmentation (reddish brown to brownish black)** 75–100%, dryness 20%, pruritus 5%. GI abdominal pain 50% (rarely severe leading to exploratory laparoscopy), splenic infarction (very rare), bowel obstruction (very rare), GI bleeding (very rare). Eye: conjunctival irritation, retinal crystal deposition.
Rifabutin (Mycobutin) 300mg/day po (prophylaxis or treatment) 150mg $7.19	**Adverse effects:** Similar to rifampin: rifabutin-related adverse effects occurred in 77% of pts receiving 600mg (high dose) rifabutin with either clarithro or azithro. Most common was a fall in WBC, then nausea/vomiting/diarrhea in 42%, diffuse polyarthralgia in 19%, & anterior uveitis in 8% (CID 21.594, 1995). Uveitis responds to topical steroids & cycloplegics (CID 22(Suppl. 1).S43, 1996). Subsequently, max. dose of rifabutin reduced to 300mg. Other adverse effects similar to rifampin: skin rash 11%, orange-tan to brown skin pigmentation (CID 21.1515, 1995). Discolored (reddish) urine 30%. Lab: ↑ SGOT/SGPT 8%.
Rifapentine (Priftin) 600mg po twice weekly for first 2mos. then 600mg po q week 150mg tabs $3.00	**Adverse effects:** Similar to other rifamycins (see RIF; RFB). Hyperuricemia seen in 21%. Causes red-orange discoloration of body fluids. Note ↑ prevalence of RIF resistance in pts on weekly rx (Ln 353.1843, 1999).
Fluoroquinolones	**Review drug-drug interactions.** **Children:** No FQ approved for use under age 16 based on joint cartilage injury in immature animals. Articular SEs in children est. at 2–3% (Ln ID 3.537, 2003). **CNS toxicity:** Poorly understood. Varies from mild (lightheadedness) to moderate (confusion) to severe (seizures). May be aggravated by NSAIDs. **Gatifloxacin** contraindicated in patients with diabetes mellitus due to reports of hypo- & hyperglycemia. Risk factors: older age, use of oral hypoglycemic drugs & renal insufficiency. **Opiate screen false-positives:** FQs can cause **false-positive urine assay for opiates** (JAMA 286.3115, 2001). **Photosensitivity** **QT$_c$ (corrected QT) interval prolongation:** ↑ QT$_c$ (>500 msec or >60 msec from baseline) with any FQ, can lead to torsades de pointes & ventricular fibrillation. Risk low with current marketed drugs. Risk ↑: women, ↓ K$^+$, ↓ Mg^{++}, bradycardia. (Refs: NEJM 35.11053 & 1089, 2004). Major problem is ↑ risk with concomitant drugs. For list, see SANFORD GUIDE TO ANTIMICROBIAL THERAPY, Table 10B or www.qtdrugs.org. **Avoid concomitant drugs with potential to prolong QT$_c$.** **Skin rash with gemifloxacin:** Maculopap rash after 8–10 d of Rx. Highest frequency in females <age 40 treated for 14 d (22.6%). Mechanism unclear. Self-limited. No known cross-reactivity with other FQs. **Tendinopathy:** Over age 60, approx. 2–6% of all Achilles tendon ruptures attributable to use of FQ (AnIM 163.1801, 2003). ↑ risk with concomitant steroid or renal disease (CID 36.1404, 2003).
Ciprofloxacin (Cipro) & **Ciprofloxacin-extended release** (Cipro XR) **500–750mg po q12h.** **Urinary tract infection: 250mg po q12h or Cipro XR 500mg q24h.** Parenteral rx 200–400mg IV q12h. 500mg po $5.80, Cipro XR 500mg $8.66, 400 mg IV $30.00	
Gatifloxacin (Tequin) (see comment) 200–400mg IV/po q24h. 400 mg po $9.99, 400mg IV $38.20	
Gemifloxacin (Factive) 320 mg po q24h 320 mg $18.78	
Levofloxacin (Levaquin) 250–750mg po q24h 750mg po $12.11, 750mg IV $58 400 mg po/IV q24h	
Moxifloxacin (Avelox) 400 mg po/IV q24h 400 mg po $10/IV $44	
Ofloxacin (Floxin) 200–400mg po q12h, 400mg po q24h $6.80	

TABLE 13 (7)

DRUG NAME, GENERIC (TRADE)/USUAL DOSAGE/COST*	ADVERSE EFFECTS/COMMENTS
Antimicrobacterial Drugs/Second Line Drugs *(continued)*	
Clarithromycin (Biaxin) 500mg po q12h or extended release (Biaxin XL) 2 tabs po q24h with food 500mg $5.00; 500mg ER $4.93 *investigational for other atypical/myco-bacteria, not effective vs MAC.* (FDA approved for MAC; *investigational vs M. tuberculosis*)	**Adverse effects:** Overall −13%, −3% discontinued drug secondary to side effects. GI −13%: diarrhea 3%, nausea 3%, abnormal taste 3%, abdominal pain 2%, dyspepsia 2%. 1 case report of corneal opacities *(JAC 34:605, 1994)*. CNS: headache 2%. Lab (each <1%): ↑ SGOT, alk p'tase, ↓ WBC, ↑ prothrombin time 1%, ↑ BUN 4%, ↑ creatinine <1%. Should not be used in pregnant women, has demonstrated adverse effects in animals at blood levels 2–17x higher than achieved in humans. **Remember** potential prolongation of QTc interval by clarithro, erythro & other macrolides, esp. in combination with other drugs capable of prolonged QTc *(NEJM 312:301, 2005).* **Check drug-drug interactions, Table 16.**
Azithromycin (Zithromax) 250–500mg po q24h, 1200mg po once weekly 250mg $8.30; 600mg $20.00 *(Investigational in T. gondii, not effective vs M. tuberculosis)*	**Adverse effects:** Overall 12%, 0.7% discontinued drug secondary to side effects. GI 12.8%: diarrhea 4%, nausea 3%, abdominal pain 2%, vomiting 1%. CNS 1%, ototoxicity (3/21 pts 3-30-90 days after 500 mg/day, *Lancet 343:241, 1994*). Lab: ↑ SGOT 1.5%, WBC ↓ or ↑ 1%, others <1%. Has not been studied in pregnant women. In rats at dose of 60x human total dose.
Imipenem-cilastatin (Primaxin) 500mg q6h IV 500mg $33.10	Active in vitro vs M. tuberculosis. Being used in some trials. **Adverse effects:** Local: phlebitis 3%. Hypersensitivity 2.5%: rash, pruritus, eosinophilia <1%. Blood: ↑ Coombs 1%, neutropenia <1%. Renal: oliguria <0.2%. Hepatic: ↑ SGOT, SGPT, alk p'tase <1%. CNS (0.2%): confusion, seizures (with 0.5 gm q6h 0.5–1.0% but with 1 gm q6h ~10%). GI: nausea 2%, vomiting 2%, diarrhea 3%. **Comment** Tbc treatment is not an FDA-approved indication., i.e., use is investigational
ANTIPARASITIC DRUGS	
Albendazole (Albenza) Doses vary with indication. 200–400mg po q12h ─200mg tab $1.58	**Adverse effects: Teratogenic, Pregnancy Cat. C.** Give after negative pregnancy test. Abdominal pain, nausea/vomiting, alopecia, ↑ serum transaminase. Rare reports of bone marrow suppression.
Atovaquone (Mepron) 750mg po q12h x21 days for PCP rx, 1500mg po q24h for PCP prophylaxis 750mg/5ml suspension, cost 210ml $744 Ref.: *AAC 46:1163, 2002*	**Adverse effects:** Discontinuation rate 9%. Skin rash 23%, only 4% required discontinuation of rx, pruritus 5%. GI: nausea 21%, diarrhea 19%, vomiting 14% abdominal pain 4%. CNS: headache 16%, insomnia 19%, dizziness 3%. General: fever 14%. Lab: anemia (Hgb <8.0gm/day), 6%), neutropenia (<750/mm³, 3%), ↑ AST 4%, ↑ amylase 7%. **Comments:** Has not been evaluated in severe PCP. Better absorbed with meals. Plasma concentration 3x higher when taken with fatty (>23 gm) meal.
Clindamycin (Cleocin) 600mg po or IV q6h 300mg cap $3.76 (generic) 600mg IV NB $7.29 Q $4.31	**Adverse effects:** Diarrhea ± *C. difficile* toxin, nausea, rash, neutropenia, eosinophilia
Dapsone (Dapsone USP) 100mg po q24h or 2x weekly 100mg $0.20 Ref.: *CID 27:191, 1998*	**Adverse effects:** Nausea, vomiting, rash & oral lesions *(CID 18:630, 1994)*. Hemolytic anemia (if G6PD deficient, methemoglobinemia (usually asymptomatic but if pts has dyspnea, O₂ saturation disproportionately low to pO₂, check for methemoglobinemia—if >10–15%, discontinue dapsone). Peripheral neuropathy (rare). **Comment:** Usually tolerated even if rash after TMP/SMX.
Iodoquinol (Yodoxin) ─650mg $0.47	**Adverse effects:** Nausea, abdominal cramps, rash, acne, increase in thyroid size & PBI. Optic atrophy risk if daily dose over 2 gm. Contraindicated if iodine intolerant.

TABLE 13 (8)

DRUG NAME, GENERIC (TRADE)/USUAL DOSAGE/COST*	ADVERSE EFFECTS/COMMENTS
ANTIPARASITIC DRUGS *(continued)*	
Ivermectin (Stromectol) Strongyloidiasis: 200mcg/kg x1 dose po Onchocerciasis: 150mcg/kg x1 po Scabies: 200mcg/kg x1 po 3mg tabs $4.35	**Adverse effects:** Mild side-effects—fever, pruritus, rash. Host may experience inflammatory reaction due to death of adult worms (Mazzotti reaction): fever, urticaria, asthma, GI upset.
Metronidazole (Flagyl) 500-750mg po q12h-q8h 500mg G $0.21	**Adverse effects:** GI: nausea, vomiting, metallic taste. Neuro: headache, paresthesias, avoid alcohol during & 48 hours post-rx (disulfiram-like reaction). Peripheral neuropathy possible.
Nitazoxanide (Alinia) Ages 1-4: 100mg po q12h x3 days Ages 4-11: 200mg po q12h x3 days Adults: 500mg po q12h 500mg $13.02	**Adverse effects:** Only approved for otherwise healthy children with infection due to Giardia lamblia or Cryptosporidium parvum. Caution in diabetics: 5 ml suspension contains 1.5gm sucrose. AEs in <1%. Discolored eyes & urine.
Paromomycin (Humatin) 500mg q8h or q6h po 250mg $3.37	**Adverse effects:** GI: doses of >3gm, nausea, abdominal cramps, diarrhea. CNS: vertigo, headache. Skin: rash. **Comment:** This is an aminoglycoside similar to neomycin ("non-absorbed", ~3% of dose is absorbed). Discontinue promptly if patient complains of tinnitus, ↓ in hearing, or vertigo.
Pentamidine isethionate (IV) (Pentam 300) 4mg/kg/day IV 300mg $98.75	**Adverse effects:** Hypotension with rapid IV administration, rash, nausea, vomiting, nephrotoxicity, cardiac arrhythmia (ventricular tachycardias including torsade de pointes), neutropenia (15%), thrombocytopenia, pancreatitis, hypocalcemia, hypoglycemia followed by hyperglycemia. Sterile abscesses after IM administration. **Comments:** Pentamidine inhibits distal nephron absorption of Na+ with resultant hyperkalemia similar to K-sparing diuretics (AnIM 122;193, 1995).
Pentamidine (aerosol) (NebuPent) 300mg/month (prophylaxis) 300mg $98.75	**Adverse effects:** Cough may respond to bronchodilator, upper lobe pneumocystis may occur if given with patient sitting. **Comment:** Risk of extrapulmonary pneumocystis & pneumothorax greater than with systemic prophylaxis. Use aerosol only in patients intolerant of oral drugs.
Primaquine: Primaquine phosphate 26.3mg = 15mg of base 15mg (base) po q24h 26.3mg $0.77	**Adverse effects:** Hemolytic anemia if G6PD deficient; may cause clinically significant methemoglobinemia; nausea/abdominal pain if taken on empty stomach.
Pyrimethamine (Daraprim, Malocide) 50-75mg po q24h; 25mg $0.43 (Leucovorin tablet 5mg $2.36 —see Comments)	**Adverse effects:** Major problem hematologic: megaloblastic anemia, ↓ WBC, ↓ platelets. PO folinic acid 5mg/day will ↓ heme adverse effects & not interfere with efficacy of rx. If high-dose pyrimethamine, ↑ folinic acid to 10-50 mg/day. Pyri + sulfadiazine can cause mental changes due to carnitine deficiency (AJM 95:112, 1993). Other: rash, vomiting, diarrhea, xerostomia
Sulfadiazine 1-1.5gm po q6h 500mg tablet $0.34	**Adverse effects:** Compared to non-HIV pts, dramatic ↑ in incidence of pruritus, rash, Stevens-Johnson syndrome, myalgia/arthralgia. Traditionally thought on hypersensitivity basis. New data support postulate of dose-dependent accumulation of toxic sulfonamide metabolites that fail to clear due to concomitant glutathione deficiency in the AIDS pt (Brit J Pharm 39:621, 1995; JAC 34;1, 1994). In addition, can cause hemolytic anemia in G6PD-def. pts. All sulfonamides can cause crystalluria. Do not use in newborns or late stages of pregnancy.

TABLE 13 (9)

ANTIPARASITIC DRUGS (continued)

DRUG NAME, GENERIC (TRADE)/USUAL DOSAGE/COST*	ADVERSE EFFECTS/COMMENTS
Trimethoprim (Proloprim) 5mg/kg po q8h ___100mg $0.15 (generic)	**Adverse effects:** Rash, pruritus, marrow suppression rare. Rare cases of aseptic meningitis [fever, headache, CSF ↑ cells (monos), ↑ protein] reported (CID 19:431, 1994). **Comment:** Fewer reactions than TMP/SMX.
Trimethoprim (TMP)- sulfamethoxa- zole (SMX) (Cotrim, Bactrim, Septra) (Dosage depends on indication) 1 double-strength tab (160 TMP/ 800mg SMX) $0.15; 160/800mg IV $11.21	**Adverse effects:** Compared to non-AIDS pts, dramatic dose-dependent ↑ in pruritus, skin rash, Stevens-Johnson syndrome. In pts given TMP/SMX + steroids for PCP, % skin reactions ↓ from 47 to 13 (CID 18:319, 1994). Initially describe hypersensitivity was reason; accumulating data support hypothesis of dose-dependent accumulation of toxic sulfonamide metabolites (hydroxylamine). Clearance of metabolites requires glutathione & AIDS pts are deficient (Brit J Pharm 39:621, 1995; JAC 34:1, 1994). May explain ability 2/3 of time to rx continuing rash (Arch Derm 130:1383, 1994). Beware progressive exanthem—some pts progress to exfoliation &/or Stevens-Johnson syndrome. Tremors associated with high dose (CID 22:598, 1996). TMP competes with creatinine for tubular secretion & can ↑ serum creatinine (reversible); TMP also blocks distal tubular reabsorption of Na & secretion of K⁺. ↑ serum K⁺ in 21% of pts (AnIM 124:316, 1996).

ANTIVIRAL DRUGS (other than retroviral)

DRUG NAME(S) GENERIC (TRADE)	DOSAGE/ROUTE/COST*	COMMENTS/ADVERSE EFFECTS
CMV		
Cidofovir (Vistide)	5mg/kg IV q week x2, then q2wks. (375mg $888) Properly timed IV prehydration with normal saline & oral probenecid **must be used with each cidofovir infusion** (see pkg insert for details). Renal function (serum creatinine & urine protein) must be monitored prior to each dose (see pkg insert for details).	**Adverse effects: Nephrotoxicity:** dose-dependent proximal tubular injury (Fanconi-like syndrome): proteinuria, glycosuria, bicarbonaturia, phosphaturia, polyuria (nephrogenic diabetic insipidus now reported, Ln 350:413, 1997), ↑ creatinine. Concomitant saline prehydration, probenecid, extended dosing intervals allowed use. 25% of pts do IV cidofovir due to nephrotoxicity. Other toxicities: nausea 48%, fever 31%, alopecia 16%, myalgia 16%, probenecid hypersensitivity 16%, neutropenia 29%. No effect on hematocrit, platelets, LFTs. **Comment:** Recommended dosage, frequency or infusion rate of cidofovir must not be exceeded. Dose must be reduced or discontinued if changes in renal function occur during rx. For ↑ of 0.3–0.4mg/dl in serum creatinine, cidofovir dose must be ↓ from 5 to 3 mg/kg; discontinue cidofovir if ↑ of ↑ 0.5mg/dl above baseline or 3+ proteinuria develops (for 2+ proteinuria, observe pts carefully & consider discontinuation).
Foscarnet (Foscavir)	90mg/kg q12h IV (induction) 90mg/kg q24h (maintenance) Dosage adjustment with renal dysfunction (see Table 15) (6gm $83)	**Adverse effects: Major clinical toxicity is renal impairment (1/3 of patients):** —↑ creatinine, proteinuria, nephrogenic diabetes insipidus, ↓ K⁺, ↓ Ca⁺⁺, ↓ Mg⁺⁺. Toxicity ↑ with other nephrotoxic drugs (amphotericin B, aminoglycosides or pentamidine (especially severe ↓ Ca⁺⁺)). Adequate hydration may ↓ toxicity. Other: headache, mild (100%), fatigue (100%), nausea (80%), fever (25%). CNS: seizures. Hematol: ↓ WBC, ↓ Hgb. Hepatic: liver function tests ↑. Genital ulcers.
Ganciclovir (Cytovene)	IV: 5mg/kg q12h x14 days (induction) 5mg/kg IV q24h or 6mg/kg 5x/wk (maintenance) Dosage adjustment with renal dysfunction (see Table 15) (500mg IV $45) Oral: 1gm q8h with food (fatty meal) (500mg cap $9.60)	**Adverse effects:** Absolute neutrophil count dropped below 500/mm³ in 15%, thrombocytopenia 21%, anemia 6%. Fever 48%. GI 50%: nausea, vomiting, diarrhea, abdominal pain 19%, rash 10%. Retinal detachment 11% (relationship to ganciclovir?). Confusion, headache, psychiatric disturbances, & seizures. Neutropenia may respond to granulocyte colony stimulating factor (G-CSF or GM-CSF). Severe myelosuppression may be ↑ with coadministration of zidovudine or azathioprine. 32% dc/interrupted rx, principally for neutropenia. Hematologic less frequent than with IV. Granulocytopenia 18%, anemia 12%, thrombocytopenia 6%, GI, skin same as with IV. Retinal detachment 8%.

TABLE 13 (10)

DRUG NAME(S) GENERIC (TRADE)	DOSAGE/ROUTE/COST*	COMMENTS/ADVERSE EFFECTS
ANTIVIRAL DRUGS (other than retroviral)/CMV (continued)		
Valganciclovir (Valcyte)	900mg (two 450mg tabs) po q12h x21 for induction, followed by 900mg po q24h. Take with food. (450mg cap $31.50; ~$1,890 for 60 caps)	A prodrug of ganciclovir with better bioavailability: 60% with food. **Adverse effects:** Similar to ganciclovir.
Herpesvirus (Non-CMV)		
Acyclovir (Zovirax or generic)	Doses: see Table 12 400mg tab NB $2; GA $0.44 IV 500mg NB $2.59-60 Suspension 200mg/5ml: $90 Ointment 5% 15gm $90	**po:** Generally well-tolerated with occ. diarrhea, vertigo, arthralgia. Less frequent rash, fatigue, insomnia, fever, menstrual abnormalities, acne, sore throat, muscle cramps, lymphadenopathy. **IV:** Phlebitis, caustic with vesicular lesions with IV infiltration. CNS (1%): lethargy, tremors, confusion, hallucinations, delirium, seizures, coma (CID 21:435, 1995). Improve 1-2wks after rx stopped. Renal (5%): ↑ creatinine, hematuria. With high doses may crystallize in renal tubules → obstructive uropathy (rapid infusion, dehydration, renal insufficiency & ↑ dose ↑ risk). Adequate pre-hydration may prevent such nephrotoxicity. Hepatic: ↑ ALT, AST. Uncommon: neutropenia (CID 20:1557, 1995), rash, diaphoresis, hypotension, headache, nausea
Famciclovir (Famvir)	250mg cap $4.70 500mg cap $9.33	Metabolized to penciclovir. **Adverse effects:** similar to acyclovir, included headache, nausea, diarrhea, & dizziness but incidence did not differ from placebo (JAMA 276:47, 1996). May be taken without regard to meals. Dose should be reduced if CrCl <60 ml/min (see package insert & Table 12, pg234 & Table 15, pg154).
Penciclovir (Denavir) Trifluridine (Viroptic)	Topical 1% cream 1.5gm $26 1 drop 1% solution q2h (max. 9 drops/.) for max. of 21. (7.5ml 1% solution $105).	Apply to area of recurrence of herpes labialis with start of sx, then q2h while awake x4. Well tolerated. Mild burning (5%), palpebral edema (3%), punctate keratopathy, stromal edema
Valacyclovir (Valtrex)	500mg cap $5.00	An ester pro-drug of acyclovir that is well-absorbed; bioavailability 3-5x greater than acyclovir. **Adverse effects** similar to acyclovir (see JID 186:540, 2002). thrombotic thrombocytopenic purpura/hemolytic uremic syndrome reported in pts with advanced HIV disease & transplant recipients participating in clinical trials at doses of 8gm/day.
Hepatitis		
Adefovir dipivoxil (Hepsera)	10mg po q24h (with normal CrCl) 20-50 CrCl: 10mg q48h 10-19 CrCl: 10mg q72h Hemodialysis: 10mg q7 days following dialysis. Each tab contains 10mg ($18)	Adefovir dipivoxil is a diester prodrug of the active moiety adefovir. It is an acyclic nucleotide analog with activity against hepatitis B (HBV) at 0.2-2.5mM (IC₅₀). Peak plasma concentration after 10mg po was 18.4 ± 6.26ng/ml. 1-4hrs after dose. Terminal elimination $t_{1/2}$ was 7.48 ± 1.65hrs. Primarily renal excretion—adjust dose. No food interactions. Remarkably few side effects. Nephrotoxicity at 30 mg/d.; not yet reported at 10 mg/d. Monitor renal function, esp. with pts with pre-existing or other risks for renal impairment. Lactic acidosis reported with nucleoside analogs, esp. in women. Pregnancy Category C. Hepatitis may exacerbate when rx dc. 6-25% of pts developed ALT ↑ 10x normal within 12 wks, usually responds to re-treatment or self-limited, but hepatic decompensation has occurred.
Entecavir (Baraclude)	0.5mg q24h. If refractory to lamivudine: 1mg per day ($714.60 per month)	A nucleoside analog active against HBV including lamivudine-resistant mutants. Minimal adverse effects reported: headache, fatigue, dizziness, & nausea reported in 22% of pts. Potential for lactic acidosis but not reported to date. Adjust dosage in renal impairment.

TABLE 13 (11)

DRUG NAME(S) GENERIC (TRADE)	DOSAGE/ROUTE/COST*	COMMENTS/ADVERSE EFFECTS
ANTIVIRAL DRUGS (other than retroviral) *(continued)*		
Interferon alfa is available as alfa-2a (Roferon-A), Intron A), (Intron-A) PEG interferon alfa-2b (PEG-Intron)	3 million units: (Roferon $40, Intron $39; Infergen 9mcg $52) 0.5–1.5mcg/kg subQ q wk (120mcg $391)	**Adverse effects:** Flu-like syndrome is common, esp. during 1st wk of rx: fever 98%, fatigue 89%, myalgia 73%, headache 71%. GI: anorexia 46%, diarrhea 21%. Rash 18%; later profound fatigue & psychiatric symptoms in up to 1/2 of pts (*J Clin Psych 64:708, 2003*) (depression, anxiety, emotional lability & agitation), alopecia, ↑ TSH, autoimmune thyroid disorders with hypo– or hyperthyroidism. Hematol.: ↓ WBC 49%, ↓ Hgb 27%, ↓ platelets 35%. Consider prophylactic antidepressant in pts with history. Acute reversible hearing loss &/or tinnitus in up to 1/3 (*Ln 343:1134, 1994*). Optic neuropathy (retinal hemorrhage, cotton wool spots, ↓ in color vision) reported (*AIDS 18:1805, 2004*). Side-effects ↑ with ↑ doses & dose reduction necessary in up to 46% receiving chronic rx for HBV.
Pegylated-40k interferon alfa-2a (Pegasys)	180mcg subQ q wk x48wks (180mcg $404)	Attachment of INF to polyethylene glycol (PEG) prolongs half-life & allows weekly dosing. Better efficacy data with similar adverse effects profile compared to regular formulation.
Lamivudine (3TC) (Epivir-HBV)	**Adverse effects:** *See Table 6B.* NOTE: 100mg po q24h x1 yr for hepatitis B. (100mg tab $7)	

Ribavirin–interferon alfa-2b combination pack (Rebetron)	Combination kit contains 2wk supply of INF & 42, 70, or 84 caps of 200mg ribavirin.
	Dose: INF 3 million units subQ 3x/wk & ribavirin 400mg po a.m. & 600mg po p.m. (<75kg) or 600mg po q12h (≥75kg). Rebetron (1000mg/ribavirin dose pack) ($3652/24wk course)
		Side-effects common with flu-like symptoms (>50%), *see interferon alfa above*. Hemolytic anemia common (mean reduction in Hgb 3 gm/dl) but usually responds to ↓ ribavirin dosage *(see package insert)*. **Severe psychiatric effects, esp. depression, most common (23–36%) reason for discontinuation of rx. Suicidal behavior reported.** Hyper– & hypothyroidism, alopecia (30%) & pulmonary disease reported (*Mayo Clin Proc 74:367, 1999*). **Since ribavirin is teratogenic, drug should not be used during pregnancy or within 6 mos of pregnancy. Also should not be used in pts with endstage renal failure, severe heart disease, or hemoglobinopathies.** ARDS reported (*Chest 124:406, 2003*).
		
		Dose changes:
		Ribavirin
		Hgb: <10 → ↓ to 200 mg q a.m., 400 mg q p.m.
		               <8.5 → DC
		WBC: <1000 → No change
		           <750 → DC
		Abs. PMNs <750 → No change
		          <500 → DC
		Platelets: <50,000 → No change
		          <25,000 → DC
		
		Interferon
		Hgb: No change
		     DC
		WBC: → to 1.5mU subQ 3x/wk
		     DC
		Abs. PMNs → to 1.5mU subQ 3x/wk
		Platelets: No change
		     → to 1.5mU subQ 3x/wk

Ribavirin (Rebetol)	For use with an interferon for hepatitis C & was unbundled from the combination Rebetron *(see above)* mostly for use with the pegylated interferons (alfa-2a & 2b). Available as 200mg capsules. Dose: <75kg BW 2 caps in a.m. & 3 caps in p.m. >75kg BW 3 caps in a.m. & 3 caps in p.m. Cost: 200mg $10.60	Response of immune complex renal disease. *AJM 106:347, 1999.* Side-effects as above, esp. hemolytic anemia (during 1st 1–2 wks of rx) with hemoglobin ↓ of 3–4 gm. Should not be used with CrCl <50 ml/min & cautiously with cardiac disease.
Warts *(See CID 28:S37, 1999)*		
Interferon alfa-2b, or alfa-n3 (Alferon-N)	Apply 1 million units, into lesion 3.5ml for topical application, $130	Interferon alfa-2b 3 million units/0.5 ml, interferon alfa-n3 5 mU/1 ml. Cost: $10 **Side-effects:** Local reactions—pain, burning, inflammation in 50%. No systemic effects
Podofilox (Condylox)	Cream applied 3x/week to maximum of 16wks. 250mg packets $15	Mild erythema, erosions, itching & burning
Imiquimod (Aldara)		

TABLE 14: SELECTED PHARMACOLOGIC FEATURES OF ANTIMICROBIAL AGENTS USED IN HIV-ASSOCIATED INFECTIONS IN ADULTS *

Drug	Dose, Route of Administration	Take Drug (PO Dosing)	% AB	Peak Serum Level mcg/ml	Protein Binding, %	Serum T½ Hours	Biliary Excretion, %	CSF/Blood, %	CSF Level Potentially Therapeutic
ANTIFUNGALS									
Amphotericin B									
Standard: 0.4–0.7mg/kg IV				0.5–3.5		24		0	
Ampho B lipid complex (ABLC): 5mg/kg IV				1–2.5		24			
Ampho B cholesteryl complex: 4mg/kg IV				2.9		39			
Liposomal ampho B: 5mg/kg IV				58 ± 21		7–10/100			
Caspofungin	70mg IV x1, then 50mg IV q24h				97	9–11			
Flucytosine	2.5 gm po	With/Without	78–90	30–40		3–6		60–100	Yes
Azoles									
Fluconazole	400mg po/IV	With/Without	90	6.7		20–50		50–94	Yes
	800mg po/IV	With/Without	90	Approx. 14		20–50			
Itraconazole	100mg po/IV	With food	Low			35		0	No
	Oral soln 200 mg po	Without food	90	0.3–0.7	99.8				
Voriconazole	200 mg po	Without food	96		58	6		22–100	Yes (CID 37:728, 2003)
ANTIMYCOBACTERIALS									
Ethambutol	25mg/kg po	With food	80	2–6	10–30	4		25–50	No
Isoniazid	300mg po	Without food	100	3–5	5–10	0.7–4		20–90	Yes
Pyrazinamide	20–25mg/kg po		95	30–50	5–10	10–16		100	Yes
Rifampin	600mg po	Without food	70–90	4–32	80	1.5–5	10,000	7–56	Yes
Streptomycin	1gm IV (see table 13, pg141)			25–50	0–10	2.5	10–60	0–30	No. Intrathecal: 5–10 mg
ANTIPARASITICS									
Albendazole	400mg po	With food		0.5–1.6	70	8–9			No
Atovaquone suspension:	750mg po	With food	47	15	99.9	67		<1	
Dapsone	100mg po		100			10–50			
Ivermectin	12mg po	Without food		0.05–0.08	98				
Mefloquine	1.25gm po	With food		3	99	13–24 days			
Nitazoxanide	200mg po				99				
Proguanil	200mg po			0.1–2.0	75				
Pyrimethamine	25mg po	With/Without	"High"	0.2–0.3	87	96			
Praziquantel	20mg/kg po	With food	80			0.8–1.5			
Tinidazole	2gm po	With food	48		12	13	Chemically similar to metronidazole		
ANTIVIRAL DRUGS — NOT HIV									
Acyclovir	400 mg po	With food	10–20	1.21	9–33	2.5–3.5		50	No
Adefovir	10 mg po	With/Without	59	0.02	4	7.5			
Entecavir	0.5 mg po	With/Without	100	4.2 ng/ml	13	128–149			
Famciclovir	500 mg po	With food	77	3–4	<20	2–3			
Foscarnet	60 mg/kg IV			155		4		<1	
Ganciclovir	5 mg/kg IV	With/Without		8.3	1–2	3.5			No
Oseltamivir	75 mg po	With/Without	75	0.65/3.5	3	1–3			
Ribavirin	600 mg po	With/Without	64	0.8		44			
Rimantadine	100 mg po	With/Without		0.1–0.4		25			

See next page for footnotes

TABLE 14 (2)

ANTIVIRAL DRUGS—NOT HIV

Drug	Dose, Route of Administration[1]	With Food	Without Food[2]	With/ W/O Food	% AB[3]	Peak Serum Level mcg/ml[4]	Protein Binding, %	Serum T½ Hours[5]	Biliary Excretion, %[6]	CSF/Blood, %[7]	CSF Level Potentially Therapeutic[8]
Valacyclovir	1000 mg po			X	55	5.6	13-18	3			
Valganciclovir	900 mg po	X			59	5.6	1-2	4			

ANTIRETROVIRAL DRUGS

Drug	Dose, Route of Administration[1]	With Food	Without Food[2]	With/ W/O Food	% AB[3]	Peak Serum Level mcg/ml[4]	Protein Binding %	Intracellular T½ Hours (See footnote[11])	Serum T½ Hours[5]	Cytochrome P450	CSF/Blood, %[7]
Abacavir	300 mg po			X	83	3.0	50	20.6	1.5		3.9
Amprenavir	1200 mg po			X	No data	6-9	90		7-11	Inhibitor	
Atazanavir	400 mg po	X			"Good"	2.5	86		7	Inhibitor	
Delavirdine	400 mg po			X	85	19 ± 11	98		5.8	Inhibitor	0
Didanosine	400 mg EC**[12] po		X		30-40		<5	25-40	1.4		0
Efavirenz	600 mg po		X		42	13 µM	99		52-76	Inducer/inhibitor	
Emtricitabine	200 mg po			X	93	1.8	<4	3.8	10		
Enfuvirtide	90 mg subQ				84	5	92	No data	4		
Fosamprenavir	700 mg po w/100 mg ritonavir po			X	No data	6	90		7.7	Inhibitor	
Indinavir	800 mg po		X		65	12.6 µM	60		1.2-2	Inhibitor	11
Lamivudine	300 mg po			X	86	2.6	<36	16	5-7		23
Lopinavir	400 mg po	X			No data	9.6	98-99		5-6	Inhibitor	0
Nelfinavir	750 mg po	X			20-80	3-4	98		3.5-5	Inducer	
Nevirapine	625 mg po			X	>90	2	60		25-30		63
Ritonavir	300 mg po	X			65	7.8	98-99		3-5	Potent inhibitor	0
Saquinavir (gel)	100 mg po (with ritonavir 100 mg)			X	4	3.1	97		1-2	Inhibitor	
Stavudine	100 mg XR**[13] po			X	86	1.4	<5	3.5	1		
Tenofovir	300 mg po			X	39	0.12	<7	10->60	17		20
Tipranavir	500 mg po + 200 mg ritonavir	X				95 µM	99.9		5.5-6		
Zalcitabine	0.75 mg po			X	85	0.03		3	1.2		
Zidovudine	300 mg po			X	60	1-2	<38	3	1.1		2

FOOTNOTES:

1 For adult oral preps; not applicable for peds suspension
2 Food decreases rate &/or extent of absorption
3 % absorbed under optimal conditions
4 Total drug; adjust for protein binding to determine free drug concentration
5 Assumes CrCl >80 mg/min
6 Peak concentration in bile/peak concentration in serum x 100. If blank, no data.
7 CSF levels with inflammation
8 Judgment based on drug dose & organ susceptibility. CSF concentration ideally ≥10 above MIC.
9 Given with atovaquone as Malarone for malaria prophylaxis

10 Oseltamivir/oseltamivir carboxylate
11 Methods for calculating intracellular concentration not standardized. Based on in vitro & in vivo studies, hierarchy of ratio of intracellular/extracellular concentrations of protease inhibitors is: nelfinavir > saquinavir > fosamprenavir > lopinavir ≥ ritonavir > indinavir (JAC 54:982, 2004)
12 EC = enteric-coated
13 XR = extended release
14 CID = 41:1787,2005

TABLE 15A: DOSAGE OF ANTIMICROBIAL DRUGS IN ADULT PATIENTS WITH RENAL IMPAIRMENT

Adapted from *Drug Prescribing in Renal Failure*, 4th Ed., Aronoff et al (Eds.), American College of Physicians, 1999, & Berns et al. "Renal Aspects of Antimicrobial Therapy for HIV Infection" in: P. Kenimel & J. Berns, Eds., *HIV Infection & the Kidney*, Churchill-Livingstone, 1995, pp. 195–236. **UNLESS STATED, ADJUSTED DOSES ARE AS % OF DOSE FOR NORMAL RENAL FUNCTION.**

Drug adjustments are based on the patient's estimated endogenous creatinine clearance, which can be calculated as:

$\dfrac{(140-age)(ideal\ body\ weight\ in\ kg)}{(72)(serum\ creatinine,\ mg/dl)}$ for men (x 0.85 for women)	Ideal body weight for men: 50.0kg + 2.3kg per inch over 5ft
	Ideal body weight for women: 45.5kg + 2.3kg per inch over 5ft

For alternative method to estimate C/rCl, see AnIM 130:461, 1999

NOTE: For summary of drugs that do not require dosage adjustment with renal failure, see Table 15B

The following is a selected list of drugs commonly used in the care of HIV-infected patients. For data on additional antimicrobials, see Table 17 of the *Sanford Guide to Antimicrobial Therapy 2006*.

ANTIMICROBIAL	HALF-LIFE (NORMAL/ESRD) hr	DOSE FOR NORMAL RENAL FUNCTION[1]	METHOD* (see footnote)	ADJUSTMENT FOR RENAL FAILURE Estimated creatinine clearance (CrCl), ml/min			SUPPLEMENT FOR HEMODIALYSIS, CAPD* (see footnote)		COMMENTS ± DOSAGE FOR CAVH/CVVH[1]
				>50-90	10-50	<10			
ANTIBACTERIAL ANTIBIOTICS									
Aminoglycoside Antibiotics: Traditional multiple daily doses—adjustment for renal disease									
Amikacin	1.4-2.3/17-150	7.5mg/kg q12h	D&I	60-90% q12h	30-70% q12-18h **Same dose for CAVH[1]**	20-30% q24-48h	HEMO:	Extra 3.8mg/kg after dialysis	High flux hemodialysis membranes lead to unpredictable aminoglycoside clearance, measure post-dialysis drug levels for efficacy & toxicity. With CAPD, pharmacokinetics highly variable—**check serum levels.**
							CAPD:	15-20mg/L dialysate/day¶ (see Comment)	[1]Usual method for CAPD: 2 liters of dialysis fluid placed q6h
Gentamicin, Tobramycin	2-3/20-60	1.7mg/kg q8h	D&I	60-90% q8-12h	30-70% q12h **Same dose for CAVH[1]**	20-30% q24-48h	HEMO:	Extra 0.9mg/kg after dialysis	Biters/day (give 8L20mg lost/L = 160mg of amikacin supplement IV per day)
							CAPD:	3-4mg lost/L dialysate/day	Adjust dosing weight for obesity: [ideal body weight + 0.4(actual body weight − ideal body weight)] [CID 25:112, 1997]
Netilmicin[NUS]	2-3/35-72	2mg/kg q8h	D&I	50-90% q8-12h	20-60% q12h **Same dose for CAVH[1]**	10-20% q24-48h	HEMO:	Extra 1mg/kg after dialysis	
							CAPD:	3-4mg lost/L dialysate/day	
Streptomycin	2-3/30-80	15mg/kg (max. of 1gm) q24h	I	50% q24h	q24-72h **Same dose for CAVH[1]**	q72-96h	HEMO:	Extra 7.5mg/kg after dialysis	
							CAPD:	20-40mg/L dialysate/day	

[1] **CAVH** = continuous arteriovenous hemofiltration (*NEJM* 336:1303, *1997*) usually results in CrCl of approx. 30 ml/min.; **CVVH** = Continuous Venovenous Hemofiltration (*CID* 41:1159, 2005; & 42:435, 2006). Clearance dependent on ultrafiltration rate (L/h).* **AD** = after dialysis. **'Dose AD' refers only to timing of dose. Supplement is to replace drug lost via dialysis; "extra drug" in addition to regimen used for CrCl <10 ml/min.**

TABLE 15A (2)

ANTIMICROBIAL	HALF-LIFE (NORMAL/ESRD) hr	DOSE FOR NORMAL RENAL FUNCTION*	METHOD* (see footnote)	ADJUSTMENT FOR RENAL FAILURE Estimated creatinine clearance (CrCl), ml/min >50-90	10-50	<10	SUPPLEMENT FOR HEMODIALYSIS, CAPD* (see footnote)	COMMENTS = DOSAGE FOR CAVH/CVVH*
ANTIBACTERIAL ANTIBIOTICS								
ONCE-DAILY AMINOGLYCOSIDE THERAPY: ADJUSTMENT IN RENAL INSUFFICIENCY								

Once-Daily Aminoglycoside dosing by Creatinine Clearance (ml/min)

Drug	>80	60-80	40-60	30-40	20-30	10-20	<10
		Dose q24h (mg/kg)				Dose q48h (mg/kg)	
Gentamicin/Tobramycin	5.1	4	3.5	2.5	4	3	2
Amikacin/kanamycin/streptomycin	15	12	7.5	4	7.5	4	3
Isepamicin[NUS]	8	8	8	8	8 q48h	8 q72h	8 q96h
Netilmicin	6.5	4	4	2	2.5	2.5	2

Cephalosporins; Penicillins; Beta-lactam/beta-lactamase inhibitors; Carbapenems—see Table 17, Sanford Guide to Antimicrobial Therapy 2006

Fluoroquinolone Antibiotics: adjust dosage of trovafloxacin in patients with hepatic insufficiency (see package inserts)

ANTIMICROBIAL	HALF-LIFE (NORMAL/ESRD) hr	DOSE FOR NORMAL RENAL FUNCTION*	METHOD*	>50-90	10-50	<10	SUPPLEMENT FOR HEMODIALYSIS, CAPD*	COMMENTS = DOSAGE FOR CAVH/CVVH*
Ciprofloxacin	4/6-9	500-750mg po (or 400 mg IV) q12h	D	100%	50-75%	50%	HEMO: 250-500mg po or 200mg IV q12h; CAPD: 250mg po or 200mg IV q8h	CAVH*: 200mg IV q12h
Gatifloxacin	7-14/36	400mg po/IV q24h	D	400 mg q24h	200 mg q24h Same dose for CAVH	200mg q24h	HEMO: 200mg q24h AD*; CAPD: 200mg q24h	CAVH*: As for CrCl 10-50
Gemifloxacin	7/>7	320mg po q24h	D	320mg q24h	160mg q24h	160mg q24h	HEMO: 160mg q24h AD*; CAPD: 160mg q24h	
Levofloxacin	4-8/76	750mg IV, PO q24h	D&I	750 mg q24h	750mg x1, then 500mg q24-48h	750mg x1, then 500mg q48h	HEMO/CAPD: Dose for CrCl <10	CAVH*: As for CrCl 10-50

Macrolide Antibiotics: adjust dose of azithromycin in patients with hepatic insufficiency (see package insert)

ANTIMICROBIAL	HALF-LIFE (NORMAL/ESRD) hr	DOSE FOR NORMAL RENAL FUNCTION*	METHOD*	>50-90	10-50	<10	SUPPLEMENT FOR HEMODIALYSIS, CAPD*	COMMENTS = DOSAGE FOR CAVH/CVVH*
Clarithromycin	5-7/22	0.5-1gm q12h	D	100%	75%	50-75%	HEMO: Dose AD*; CAPD: None	ESRD dosing recommendations based on extrapolation
Erythromycin	1.4/5-6	250-500mg q6h	I	100%	100%	50-75%	HEMO/CAPD/CAVH*: None	Ototoxicity with high doses in ESRD. Vol. of distribution increases in ESRD

Tetracycline Antibiotics

ANTIMICROBIAL	HALF-LIFE (NORMAL/ESRD) hr	DOSE FOR NORMAL RENAL FUNCTION*	METHOD*	>50-90	10-50	<10	SUPPLEMENT FOR HEMODIALYSIS, CAPD*	COMMENTS = DOSAGE FOR CAVH/CVVH*
Tetracycline	6-10/57-108	250-500mg qid	I	q8-12h	q12-24h Same dose for CAVH*	q24h	HEMO/CAPD: None	Avoid in ESRD

* Regardless of CrCl, 1st dose is 500mg, then adjust dose & interval

* CAVH = continuous arteriovenous hemofiltration (NEJM 336:1303, 1997) usually results in CrCl of approx. 30 ml/min.; CVVH = Continuous Venovenous Hemofiltration (CID 41:1159, 2005, & 42:435, 2006). Clearance dependent on ultrafiltration rate (L/hr).* AD = after dialysis. "Dose AD" refers only to timing of dose. Supplement is to replace drug lost via dialysis; "extra drug" in addition to regimen used for CrCl <10 ml/min.

TABLE 15A (3)

ANTIMICROBIAL	HALF-LIFE (NORMAL/ ESRD) hr	DOSE FOR NORMAL RENAL FUNCTION	METHOD* (see footnote)	ADJUSTMENT FOR RENAL FAILURE Estimated creatinine clearance (CrCl), ml/min >50-90	10-50	<10	SUPPLEMENT FOR HEMODIALYSIS, CAPD† (see footnote)	COMMENTS ± DOSAGE FOR CAVH/CVVH‡
ANTIBACTERIAL ANTIBIOTICS *(continued)*								
Miscellaneous Antibacterial Antibiotics								
Linezolid	6.4/7.1	600mg po/IV q12h	None	600mg q12h	600mg q12h Same dose for CAVH‡	600mg q12h, AD†	HEMO: As for CrCl <10 CAPD: No data	If high ultrafiltration rate might need 600 mg q8h (*CID* 42:435,2006) Accumulation of 2 metabolites—risk unknown.
Metronidazole	6–14/7–21	7.5mg/kg q6h	D	100%	100% Same dose for CAVH‡	50%	HEMO: Dose AD† CAPD: Dose for CrCl <10	Hemo clears metronidazole & its metabolites (*AAC* 29:235, 1986)
Sulfadiazine	17/34	1gm q6h	I	q8–12h	q24h	q48–72h or avoid	HEMO/CAPD: No data	
Sulfameth- oxazole	10/20–50	1gm q8h	I	q12h	q18h Same dose for CAVH‡	q24h	HEMO: 1gm AD† CAPD: 1gm q24h	
Trimethoprim	11/20–49	100–200mg q12h	I	q12h	q18h Same dose for CAVH‡	q24h	HEMO: Dose AD† CAPD: q24h	CAVH‡: q18h
TMP/SMX-DS Treatment	As above	5mg/kg IV q8h	D	100%	50%	Not recommended		
Prophylaxis	As above	tab 1 q24h or 3x/wk po	No change	100%	100%	100%		
Vancomycin²	6/200–250	1gm q12h	D&I	1gm q12h	1gm q24–96h	1gm q4–7 days	HEMO/CAPD: Dose for CrCl <10	CAVH‡: 500mg q24–48h. New dialysis membranes ↑ clearance; **check levels.**
ANTIFUNGAL ANTIBIOTICS								
Amphotericin B & ampho B lipid complexes	24/unchanged	Non-lipid: 0.4-1.0mg/ kg/day; ABCD¹ 3-6mg/kg/day; ABLC:³ 5mg/kg/day; LAB:³ 3-5mg/kg/day	I	q24h	q24h Same dose for CAVH‡	q24–48h	HEMO: None CAPD: Dose for CrCl <10	Toxicity lessened by saline loading; risk amplified by concomitant cyclosporine A, aminoglycosides, or pentamidine

² Vancomycin serum levels may be overestimated in renal failure if measured by either fluorescence polarization immunoassay or radioimmunoassay; vanco breakdown products interfere. EMIT method OK.

¹ **ABCC** = ampho B cholesteryl complex; **ABLC** = ampho B lipid complex; **LAB** = liposomal ampho B

¹ **CAVH** = continuous arteriovenous hemofiltration (*NEJM* 336:1303, 1997) usually results in CrCl of approx. 30 ml/min.; **CVVH** = Continuous Venovenous Hemofiltration (*CID* 41:1159, 2005, & 42:435, 2006). Clearance dependent on ultrafiltration rate (L/hr). * **AD** = after dialysis. "**Dose AD**" refers only to timing of dose. **Supplement is to replace drug lost via dialysis;** "**extra drug**" **in addition to regimen used for CrCl <10 ml/min.**

TABLE 15A (4)

ANTIMICROBIAL	HALF-LIFE (NORMAL/ESRD) hr	DOSE FOR NORMAL RENAL FUNCTION	METHOD* (see footnote)	ADJUSTMENT FOR RENAL FAILURE Estimated creatinine clearance (CrCl), ml/min			SUPPLEMENT FOR HEMODIALYSIS, CAPD* (see footnote)	COMMENTS ± DOSAGE FOR CAVH/CVVH*
				>50-90	10-50	<10		
ANTIFUNGAL ANTIBIOTICS *(continued)*								
Fluconazole	37/100	200-400mg q24h	D	200-400 mg q24h	100-200 mg q24h **Same dose for CAVH**	100-200mg q24h	HEMO: 100% of normal renal function dose AD*; CAPD: Dose for CrCl <10	
Flucytosine[4]	3-6/75-200	25mg/kg q6h	I	q12h	q16h **Same dose for CAVH**	q24h	HEMO: Dose AD*; CAPD: 0.5-1 gm q24h	
Itraconazole solution, po	35/--	100-200mg q12h	--	100%	100%	100%	HEMO/CAPD/CAVH*: No adjustment	
Itraconazole, IV	35/--	200mg IV q12h	--	200 mg IV q12h Do not use if CrCl <30 due to accumulation of cyclodextrin carrier				
Voriconazole, IV	Non-linear kinetics	6mg/kg IV q12h x2, then 4mg/kg q12h	No change	No change	If CrCl <50 ml/min, accumulation of IV vehicle (cyclodextrin); switch to po or dc			
ANTIPARASITIC ANTIBIOTICS								
Atovaquone	No data	750mg po q12h		No data in patients with renal or hepatic impairment				
Dapsone	No data	100mg po/day		No data in patients with renal or hepatic impairment				
Pentamidine	29/118	4Mg/kg/day	I	q24h	q24h-36h	q48h	HEMO/CAPD/CAVH: None	
Pyrimethamine	96/96	50-75mg/day	No change	100%	100%	100%	HEMO/CAPD/CAVH: None	
ANTITUBERCULOUS ANTIBIOTICS *(Excellent review: Nephron 64:169, 1993)*								
Ethambutol	4/7-15	15mg/kg q24h	D	q24h **Same dose for CAVH**	q24-36h	q48h	HEMO: Dose AD*; CAPD: Dose for CrCl <10	25mg/kg 4-6hr prior to dialysis for usual 3x/wk dialysis. Streptomycin recommended in lieu of ethambutol in renal failure.
Ethionamide	2.1/?	250-500mg q12h	D	100%	100%	50%	HEMO/CAPD/CAVH*: None	
Isoniazid	0.7-4/8-17	5mg/kg/day (max. 300mg)	D	100%	100%	100%	HEMO: Dose AD*; CAPD/CAVH*: Dose for CrCl <10	
Pyrazinamide	9/26	25mg/kg q24h (max. dose 2.5gm q24h)	D	25mg/kg q24h	25mg/kg q24h	12-25mg/kg q24h	HEMO: 40mg/kg 24 hrs prior to each 3x/wk dialysis; CAPD: No reduction	

* Concentrations <25 mcg/ml should be avoided to prevent development of resistance, while >100 mcg/ml avoided because of toxicity (JAC 35:241, 1995).
‡ **CAVH** = continuous arteriovenous hemofiltration (NEJM 336:1303, 1997) usually results in CrCl of approx. 30 ml/min. **CVVH** = Continuous Venovenous Hemofiltration (CID 41:1159, 2005, & 42:435, 2006). Clearance dependent on ultrafiltration rate (L/h). ⁺ **AD** = after dialysis. "**Dose AD**" refers only to timing of dose. **Supplement is to replace drug lost via dialysis; "extra drug" in addition to regimen used for CrCl <10 ml/min.**

TABLE 15A (5)

ANTIMICROBIAL	HALF-LIFE (NORMAL/ESRD) hr	DOSE FOR NORMAL RENAL FUNCTION[1]	METHOD* (see footnote)	ADJUSTMENT for renal failure Estimated creatinine clearance (CrCl), ml/min			SUPPLEMENT FOR HEMODIALYSIS, CAPD* (see footnote)	COMMENTS ± DOSAGE FOR CAVH/CVVH*
				>50-90	10-50	<10		
Rifabutin	No data	300mg/day po			No data available		CAVH*: No data	
Rifampin	1.5-5/1.8-11	600mg/day	D	600mg q24h	300-600mg q24h	300-600mg q24h	HEMO: None CAPD/CAVH*: Dose for CrCl <10	Biologically active metabolite
ANTIVIRAL AGENTS								
Acyclovir	2.5/20	5-12.4mg/kg q8h	D&I	5-12.4mg/kg q8h	5-12.4mg/kg q12-24h	2.5-12.4mg/kg q24h	HEMO: Dose AD* CAPD: Dose for CrCl <10	Rapid IV infusion can cause renal failure. CAVH*: 3.5mg/kg/day
Adefovir		10mg po q24h	I	10mg q24h	10mg q48-72h	10mg q7 days	HEMO: q7 days AD*	Major toxicity is renal. No data
Cidofovir: Complicated dosing—see package insert								No efficacy, safety, or pharmacokinetic data in pts with moderate/severe renal disease.
Induction	2.5/unknown	5mg/kg 1x/wk for 2 wks	—	5mg/kg 1x/wk	0.5-2mg/kg 1x/wk	0.5-2mg/kg q2wks	No data	
Maintenance	2.5/unknown	5mg/kg q2wks	—	5mg/kg q2wks	0.5-2mg/kg q2wks	0.5mg/kg q2wks	No data	
Didanosine tablets—>60kg	0.6-1.6/4.5	400mg q24h, enteric-coated	D	400mg q24h	125-200mg q24h	125mg q24h	HEMO/ CAPD: Dose for CrCl <10	Data are estimates. If CrCl <10 & If <60 kg, do not use EC tabs.
Emtricitabine	10/>10	200mg q24h	I	200mg q24h	200mg q48-72h	200mg q96h	HEMO: Dose for CrCl <10	
Entecavir	128-149/?	0.5mg q24h	D	0.5mg q24h	0.15-0.25mg q24h	0.05mg q24h	HEMO/ CAPD: 0.05 mg q24h	Give after dialysis on dialysis days
Famciclovir	2.3-3.0 /10-22	500mg q8h	D&I	500mg q8h	500mg q12-24h Same dose for CAVH	250mg q24h	HEMO: 250 mg AD* CAPD: No data	CAVH-F: Dose for CrCl 10-50

Foscarnet (CMV dosage) Dosage adjustment based on est. CrCl (ml/ min) div by pt's kg — Normal half-life (T½) 3hrs with terminal T½ very long with ESRD: 18-88hrs. Dose: Induction: 60mg/kg q8h x2-3wks IV; Maintenance: 90-120mg/kg/day IV. Method: —. See package insert for further details.

Ganciclovir — Half-life 2.9/30 IV. Dose: Induction 5mg/kg q12h IV. Method: D&I.

CrCl = ml/min/kg body weight—ONLY FOR FOSCARNET

	>1.4	>1.0-1.4	>0.8-1.0	>0.6-0.8	>0.5-0.6	>0.4-0.5	<0.4
Foscarnet Induction	60 q8h	45 q8h	50 q12h	40 q12h	60 q24h	50 q24h	Do not use
Foscarnet Maintenance	120 q24h	90 q24h	65 q24h	105 q48h	80 q48h	65 q48h	Do not use
Ganciclovir	5mg/kg q12h	5mg/kg q12h	2.5mg/kg q24h	1.25-2.5mg/kg q24h	1.25 mg/kg q24h	1.25 mg/kg 3x/wk	HEMO: Dose AD* CAPD: Dose for CrCl <10

[1] CAVH = continuous arteriovenous hemofiltration (NEJM 336:1303, 1997) usually results in CrCl of approx. 30 ml/min. CVVH = Continuous Venovenous Hemofiltration (CID 41:1159, 2005, & 42:435, 2006). Clearance dependent on ultrafiltration rate (L/hr). * AD = after dialysis. "Dose AD" refers only to timing of dose. Supplement is to replace drug lost via dialysis; "extra drug" in addition to regimen used for CrCl <10 ml/min.

TABLE 15A (6)

ANTIMICROBIAL	HALF-LIFE (NORMAL/ESRD) hr	DOSE FOR NORMAL RENAL FUNCTION†	METHOD* (see footnote)	ADJUSTMENT FOR RENAL FAILURE Estimated creatinine clearance (CrCl), ml/min			SUPPLEMENT FOR HEMODIALYSIS, CAPD (see footnote)	COMMENTS = DOSAGE FOR CAVH/CVVH†
				>50-90	10-50	<10		
Indinavir/ nelfinavir/ nevirapine	No data	No data with renal insufficiency. Less than 20% renal excretion. Probably no dose reduction.						
Lamivudine	5-7/15-35	300mg po q24h	D&I	300mg po q24h	50-150 mg q24h	25-50 mg q24h	HEMO: Dose AD*; CAPD/CAVH†: No data	
Ritonavir & saquinavir		Negligible renal clearance. At present, no patient data						
Stavudine, po	1-1.4/5.5-8	30-40mg q12h	D/I	100%	50% q12-24h Same dose for CAVH†	≥60 kg: 20mg/day <60 kg: 15mg/day	HEMO: Dose as for CrCl <AD* 10; CAPD: No data	CAVH†: Dose for CrCl 10-50
Tenofovir	4-8/?	300mg po q24h	—	300mg q24h	CrCl 30-50: 300mg q48h; CrCl 10-30: 300mg 2 x wk	No data	Hemo: 300mg po after every 3rd dialysis	
Valganciclovir	4/67	900mg po q12h	D&I	900mg po q12h	450 mg q24h to 450 mg every other day	Do not use	Do not use	
Valacyclovir	2.5-3.3/14	1gm q8h (for H. zoster in healthy pts)	D&I	1gm q8h	1gm q12-24h Same dose for CAVH†	0.5 gm q24h	HEMO: Dose AD*; CAPD: Dose for CrCl <10	CAVH†: Dose for CrCl 10-50
Zalcitabine	2.0/>8	0.75mg q8h	D&I	0.75mg q8h	0.75 mg q12h Same dose for CAVH†	0.75 mg q24h	HEMO: Dose AD*; CAPD: No data	CAVH†: Dose for CrCl 10-50
Zidovudine	1.1-1.4/1.4-3	200mg q8h or 300mg q12h	D&I	200mg q8h or 300mg q12h	200 mg q8h or 300 mg q12h	100 mg q6-8h; if HEMO AD*	HEMO: Dose for CrCl <10; CAPD: Dose for CrCl <10	CAVH†: 100mg q8h

† Dosages are for life-threatening infections; * D = dosage reduction, I = interval extension; ** Per cent refers to % change from dose for normal renal function.
Abbreviations: HEMO = hemodialysis; CAPD = chronic ambulatory peritoneal dialysis; ESRD = endstage renal disease; NUS = not available in the U.S.

† CAVH = continuous arteriovenous hemofiltration (NEJM 336:1303, 1997) usually results in CrCl of approx. 30 ml/min., CVVH = Continuous Venovenous Hemofiltration (CID 41:1159, 2005, & 42:435, 2006). Clearance dependent on ultrafiltration rate (L/hr). † AD = after dialysis. "Dose AD" refers only to timing of dose. Supplement is to replace drug lost via dialysis; "extra drug" in addition to regimen used for CrCl <10 ml/min.

TABLE 15B: NO DOSAGE ADJUSTMENT WITH RENAL INSUFFICIENCY, BY CATEGORY:

Antibacterials		Antifungals	Anti-TBc	Antivirals
Azithromycin	Linezolid	Amphotericin B	Rifabutin	Abacavir
Ceftriaxone	Minocycline	Caspofungin	Rifapentine	Atazanavir
Chloramphenicol	Moxifloxacin	Itraconazole oral solution		Delvirdine
Ciprofloxacin XL	Nafcillin	Voriconazole, po only		Efavirenz
Clindamycin	Pyrimethamine	Micafungin		Fosamprenavir
Dirithromycin	Rifaximin	Anidulafungin		Indinavir
Doxycycline	Tigecycline			Lopinavir
				Nelfinavir
				Nevirapine
				Ribavirin
				Saquinavir
				Tipranavir

TABLE 15C: DOSAGE OF ANTIRETROVIRAL DRUGS IN PATIENTS WITH IMPAIRED HEPATIC FUNCTION
(See CID 40:174, 2005)

DRUG GENERIC (TRADE)	STANDARD DOSE	DOSING IF HEPATIC IMPAIRMENT CHILD-PUGH SCORE*	ADJUSTED DOSE	COMMENTS
Protease inhibitors				
Amprenavir (Agenerase)	1200mg q24h	5–8	450mg q12h	
		9–12	300mg q12h	
Atazanavir (Reyataz)	300–400mg po q24h	7–9	300mg q24h	
		>9	Do not use	
Fosamprenavir (Lexiva)	1400mg po q12h	5–8	700mg q12h	No ritonavir boosting
		9–12	Not recommended	if hepatic impairment
Indinavir (Crixivan)	800mg po q8h	Mild to moderate hepatic insufficiency	600mg q8h	
Lopinavir/ritonavir (Kaletra)	400mg/100 mg po q12h	No dosage recommendations; use with caution if hepatic impairment		
Nelfinavir (Viracept)	1250mg po q12h	No dosage recommendations; use with caution if hepatic impairment		
Ritonavir (Norvir)	600mg po q12h	No dosage recommendations; use with caution if hepatic impairment		
Saquinavir (Invirase)	1000mg po + 100 mg ritonavir b.i.d.	No dosage recommendations; use with caution if hepatic impairment		
Tipranavir	500mg + 200 mg ritonavir po b.i.d.	5-9	No dosage adjustment	
		>9	No data	
Fusion inhibitor				
Enfuvirtide (Fuzeon)	90mg subQ q12h	No dosage adjustment recommendations		

*CALCULATION OF CHILD-PUGH SCORE—Classification below

CLINICAL FEATURE	SCORE GIVEN		
	1	2	3
Encephalopathy *(see below)***	None	Grade 1–2	Grade 3–4
Albumin	>3.5 gm/dl	2.8–3.5 gm/dl	<2.8 gm/dl
Total bilirubin	<2 mg/dl	2–3 mg/dl	>3 mg/dl
If taking indinavir or if Gilbert's syndrome	<4 mg/dl	4–7 mg/dl	>7 mg/dl
Prothrombin time	<4	4–6	>6
or			
INR	<1.7	1.7–2.3	>2.3

CLASSIFICATION

Score	Class
5–6	A
7–9	B
>9	C

**GRADE OF ENCEPHALOPATHY

Grade	Clinical Criteria
1	Mild confusion, anxiety, restlessness, fine tremor, slow coordination
2	Drowsiness, asterixis
3	Somnolent but arousable, marked confusion, speech incomprehensible, incontinent, hyperventilation
4	Coma, decerebrate posturing, flaccidity

**TABLE 16A: DRUG/DRUG INTERACTIONS: ANTIRETROVIRAL DRUGS &
DRUGS USED IN TREATMENT OF HIV-ASSOCIATED INFECTIONS & MALIGNANCIES**
This is a selected list. For drug-drug interactions of other antimicrobials, please refer to Table 22 of the
2005 SANFORD GUIDE TO ANTIMICROBIAL THERAPY & NEJM 344:985, 2001.
Significance/Certainty: ± = theory/anecdotal; + = of probable clinical import; ++ = of definite clinical import

ANTI-INFECTIVE AGENT (A)	OTHER DRUG (B)	EFFECT	SIGNIFICANCE/ CERTAINTY
Aminoglycosides— parenteral (amikacin, gentamicin, kana- mycin, netilmicin, sisomicin, strep- tomycin, tobramycin) NOTE: *Capreomycin is an aminoglycoside, used as alternative drug to treat mycobacterial infections.*	Amphotericin B	↑ nephrotoxicity	++
	Cis platinum (Platinol)	↑ nephro & ototoxicity	+
	Cyclosporine	↑ nephrotoxicity	+
	Neuromuscular blocking agents	↑ apnea or respiratory paralysis	+
	Loop diuretics (e.g., furosemide)	↑ ototoxicity	++
	NSAIDs	↑ nephrotoxicity	+
	Non-polarizing muscle relaxants	↑ apnea	+
	Radiographic contrast	↑ nephrotoxicity	+
	Vancomycin	↑ nephrotoxicity	+
Aminoglycosides— oral (kanamycin, neo- mycin)	Oral anticoagulants (dicumarol, phenindione, warfarin)	↑ prothrombin time	+
Amphotericin B & ampho B lipid formulations	Antineoplastic drugs	↑ nephrotoxicity risk	+
	Digitalis	↑ toxicity of B if hypokalemia	+
	Nephrotoxic drugs: aminoglyco- sides, cidofovir, cyclosporin, fos- carnet, pentamidine	↑ nephrotoxicity of A	++
Amprenavir & fosamprenavir	Antiretrovirals—*see Table 16B & C*		
	Contraceptives, oral	↓ levels of A; use other contraception	++
	Lovastatin/simvastatin	↑ levels of B—**avoid**	++
	Methadone	↓ levels of A & B	++
	Rifabutin	↑ levels of B (↓ dose by 50–75%)	++
	Rifampin	↓ levels of A—**avoid**	++
Atazanavir	**See Protease inhibitors & Table 16B & C**		
Atovaquone	Rifampin (perhaps rifabutin)	↓ serum levels of A; ↑ levels of B	+
	Metoclopramide	↓ levels of A	+
	Tetracycline	↓ levels of A	+

Azole Antifungal Agents[1] [**Flu** = fluconazole, **Itr** = itraconazole, **Ket** = ketoconazole, **Vor** = voriconazole, + = occurs, **blank space** = either studied & no interaction OR no data found (may be in pharm. co. databases)]

Flu	Itr	Ket	Vor		OTHER DRUG (B)	EFFECT	SIGNIFICANCE/ CERTAINTY
+	+	+	+		Amitriptyline	↑ levels of B	+
+	+	+	+		Calcium channel blockers	↑ levels of B	+ +
	+		+		Carbamazepine (vori contraindicated)	↓ levels of A	+ +
+	+	+	+		Cyclosporine	↑ levels of B, ↑ risk of nephrotoxicity	+
	+	+			Didanosine	↓ absorption of A	+
+	+	+			Efavirenz	↓ levels of A, ↑ levels of B	+ + (avoid)
	+	+			H₂ blockers, antacids, sucralfate	↓ absorption of A	+
+	+	+	+		Hydantoins (phenytoin, Dilantin)	↑ levels of B, ↓ levels of A	+ +
	+	+			Isoniazid	↓ levels of A	+
	+	+			Lovastatin/simvastatin	Rhabdomyolysis reported; ↑ levels of B	+ +
+	+	+	+		Midazolam/triazolam, po	↑ levels of B	+ +
+	+	+	+		Oral anticoagulants	↑ effect of B	+ +
+	+	+	+		Oral hypoglycemics	↑ levels of B	+ +
	+	+			Pimozide	↑ levels of B	+ +
	+	+	+		Protease inhibitors	↑ levels of B	++
	+	+	+		Proton pump inhibitors	↓ levels of A, ↑ levels of B	++
+	+	+	+		Rifampin/rifabutin (vori contraindicated)	↑ levels of B, ↓ serum levels of A	++
	+		+		Sirolimus (vori contraindicated)	↑ levels of B	+ +
+		+			Tacrolimus	↑ levels of B with toxicity	+ +
+		+			Theophyllines	↑ levels of B	+
		+			Trazodone	↑ levels of B	+ +
+					Zidovudine	↑ levels of B	+
Caspofungin					Cyclosporine	↑ levels of A	++
					Tacrolimus	↓ levels of B	++
					Carbamazepine, dexamethasone, efavirenz, nelfinavir, nevirapine, phenytoin, rifampin	↓ levels of A; ↑ dose of caspofungin to 70 mg/day	++

---

[1] Major interactions given; unusual or minor interactions manifest as toxicity of non-azole drug due to ↑ serum levels: Caffeine (Flu), digoxin (Itr), felodipine (Itr), fluoxetine (Itr), indinavir (Ket), lovastatin/simvastatin, quinidine (Ket), tricyclics (Flu), vincristine (Itr), & ↓ effectiveness of oral contraceptives.

TABLE 16A (2)

ANTI-INFECTIVE AGENT (A)	OTHER DRUG (B)	EFFECT	SIGNIFICANCE/CERTAINTY
Clindamycin (Cleocin)	Kaolin	↓ absorption of A	+
	Muscle relaxants, e.g., atracurium, baclofen, diazepam	↑ frequency/duration of respiratory paralysis	+
Cycloserine	Ethanol	↑ frequency of seizures	+
	INH, ethionamide	↑ frequency of drowsiness/dizziness	+
Dapsone	Didanosine	↓ absorption of A	+
	Oral contraceptives	↓ effectiveness of B	+
	Pyrimethamine	↑ in marrow toxicity	+
	Rifampin/Rifabutin	↓ serum levels of A	+
	Trimethoprim	↑ levels of A & B (methemoglobinemia)	+
	Zidovudine	May ↑ marrow toxicity	+
Delavirdine (Rescriptor)	See Non-nucleoside reverse transcriptase inhibitors (NNRTIs) & Table 16C		
Didanosine (ddl) (Videx) NOTE: ddl & tenofovir can ↓ CD4 count without increase in viral "load"	Allopurinol	↑ level of A – AVOID	++
	Cisplatin, dapsone, INH, metronidazole, nitrofurantoin, stavudine, vincristine, zalcitabine	↑ risk of peripheral neuropathy	+
	Ethanol, lamivudine, pentamidine	↑ risk of pancreatitis	+
	Fluoroquinolones	↓ absorption 2° to chelation	+
	Ganciclovir	↑ levels of A	+
	Drugs that need low pH for absorption: dapsone, indinavir, itra/ketoconazole, pyrimethamine, rifampin, trimethoprim	↓ absorption	+
	Methadone	↓ levels of A	++
	Ribavirin	↑ levels of ddl metabolite—**avoid**	++
	Tenofovir	↑ levels of A (reduce dose of A)	++
Efavirenz (Sustiva)	See Non-nucleoside reverse transcriptase inhibitors (NNRTIs) & Table 16C		
Ethambutol (Myambutol)	Aluminum salts (includes didanosine buffer)	↓ absorption of A & B	+

Fluoroquinolones (*Cipro* = ciprofloxacin; *Gati* = gatifloxacin; *Gemi* = gemifloxacin; **Levo** = levofloxacin; **Lome** = lomefloxacin; **Moxi** = moxifloxacin; **Oflox** = ofloxacin)

NOTE: Blank space = either studied & no interaction OR no data found (pharmaceutical company may have data)

Cipro	Gati²	Gemi²	Levo	Lome	Moxi²	Oflox	OTHER DRUG (B)	EFFECT	SIGNIFICANCE/CERTAINTY
	+		+		+	+	**Antiarrhythmics (procainamide, amiodarone)**	↑ Q-T interval (torsade)	++
+	+		+	+	+	+	Insulin, oral hypoglycemics	↑ & ↓ blood sugar	++
+							Caffeine	↑ levels of B	+
+				+			Cimetidine	↑ levels of A	+
+						+	Cyclosporine	↑ levels of B	±
+	+		+	+	+	+	Didanosine	↓ absorption of A	++
+	+	+	+	+	+	+	**Cations: Al⁺⁺⁺, Ca⁺⁺, Fe⁺⁺, Mg⁺⁺, Zn⁺⁺ (antacids, vitamins, dairy products), citrate/citric acid**	↓ absorption of A (some variability between drugs)	++
+							Foscarnet	↑ risk of seizures	+
	+						Methadone	↑ levels of B	++
+					+	+	**NSAIDs**	↑ risk CNS stimulation/seizures	++
+							Phenytoin	↑ or ↓ levels of B	+
+	+	+					Probenecid	↓ renal clearance of A	+
+	+	+	+	+		+	Sucralfate	↓ absorption of A	++
+							Theophylline	↑ levels of B	++
+				+		+	Warfarin	↑ prothrombin time	+

ANTI-INFECTIVE AGENT (A)	OTHER DRUG (B)	EFFECT	SIGNIFICANCE/CERTAINTY
Foscarnet (Foscavir)	Ciprofloxacin	↑ risk of seizures	+
	Nephrotoxic drugs: aminoglycosides, ampho B, cis-platinum, cyclosporine	↑ risk of nephrotoxicity	+
	Pentamidine IV	↑ risk of severe hypocalcemia	++
Ganciclovir (Cytovene) & **Valganciclovir**	Imipenem	↑ risk of seizures reported	+
	Probenecid	↑ levels of A	+
	Zidovudine	↓ levels of A, ↑ levels of B	+
Gentamicin	See Aminoglycosides—parenteral		
Indinavir	See Protease Inhibitors & Table 16B & C		
Isoniazid	Alcohol, rifampin	↑ risk of hepatic injury	++
	Aluminum salts	↓ absorption (take fasting)	++
	Carbamazepine, phenytoin	↑ levels of B with nausea, vomiting, nystagmus, ataxia	++

---

² Neither Gati, Gemi, nor Moxi interacts with calcium but may interact with other multi-valent cations.

TABLE 16A (3)

ANTI-INFECTIVE AGENT (A)	OTHER DRUG (B)	EFFECT	SIGNIFICANCE/ CERTAINTY
Isoniazid *(continued)*	Itraconazole, ketoconazole	↓ levels of B	+
	Oral hypoglycemics	↓ effects of B	+
Lamivudine	Zalcitabine	Mutual interference—do not combine	++
Linezolid (Zyvox)	Adrenergic agents	Risk of hypertension	++
	Aged, fermented, pickled or smoked foods— ↑ tyramine	Risk of hypertension	+
	Serotonergic drugs (SSRIs)	Risk of serotonin syndrome	+
Lopinavir	*See Protease inhibitors*		

Macrolides (Ery = erythromycin, **Dir** = dirithromycin, **Azi** = azithromycin, **Clr** = clarithromycin; **+** = occurs, **blank space** = either studied & no interaction OR no data (pharmaceutical company may have data)

Ery	Dir	Azi	Clr			
+	+		+	Carbamazepine	↑ serum levels of B, nystagmus, nausea, vomiting, ataxia	++ (avoid with erythro)
+			+	Cimetidine, **ritonavir**	↑ levels of B	+
+			+	Clozapine	↑ serum levels of B, CNS toxicity	+
				Colchicine	↑ levels of B(Potent. Fatal)	++ (avoid)
+				Corticosteroids	↑ effects of B	+
+	+	+	+	Cyclosporine	↑ serum levels of B with toxicity	+
+	+	+	+	Digoxin, digitoxin	↑ serum levels of B (10% of cases)	+
			+	Efavirenz	↓ levels of A	++
+	+		+	Ergot alkaloids	↑ levels of B	++
+			+	Lovastatin/simvastatin	↑ levels of B, rhabdomyolysis	++
+				Midazolam, triazolam	↑ levels of B, ↑ sedative effects	+
+	+		+	Phenytoin	↑ levels of B	+
+	+	+	+	Pimozide	↑ Q-T interval	++
+			+	Rifampin, rifabutin	↓ levels of A	+
+			+	Tacrolimus	↑ levels of B	++
+			+	Theophyllines	↑ serum levels of B with nausea, vomiting, seizures, apnea	++
+	+	+	+	Valproic acid	↑ levels of B	+
+	+		+	Warfarin	May ↑ prothrombin time	+
			+	Zidovudine	↓ levels of B	+
Metronidazole				Alcohol	Disulfiram-like reaction	+
				Cyclosporin	↑ levels of B	++
				Disulfiram (Antabuse)	Acute toxic psychosis	+
				Lithium	↑ levels of B	++
				Oral anticoagulants	↑ anticoagulant effect	++
				Phenobarbital, hydantoins	↑ levels of B	++

Nelfinavir	*See Protease inhibitors & Table 16B & C*
Nevirapine (Viramune)	*See Non-nucleoside reverse transcriptase inhibitors (NNRTIs) & Table 16C*

Non-nucleoside reverse transcriptase inhibitors (NNRTIs): For interactions with protease inhibitors, *see Table 16C.* **Del** = delavirdine, **Efa** = efavirenz, **Nev** = nevirapine

Del	Efa	Nev	Co-administration contraindicated:		
+			Anticonvulsants: carbamazepine, phenobarbital, phenytoin		++
+			Antimycobacterials: rifabutin, rifampin		++
+			Antipsychotics: pimozide		++
+			Benzodiazepines: alprazolam, midazolam, triazolam		++
+	+		Ergotamine		++
+	+		HMG-CoA inhibitors (statins): lovastatin, simvastatin		++
+			St. John's wort		++
			Dose change needed:		
+			Amphetamines	↑ levels of B—caution	++
+		+	Antiarrhythmics: amiodarone, lidocaine, others	↓ or ↑ levels of B—caution	++
+	+	+	Anticonvulsants: carbamazepine, phenobarbital, phenytoin	↓ levels of A &/or B	++
+	+	+	Antifungals: itraconazole, ketoconazole	Potential ↓ levels of B	+
+	+	+	Antipsychotic: Pimozide	↑ levels of B	++ (avoid)
+	+	+	Antirejection drugs: cyclosporine, rapamycin, sirolimus, tacrolimus	↑ levels of B	++
		+	Benzodiazepines: *as above*	↑ levels of B	++
+		+	Calcium channel blockers	↑ levels of B	++
+		+	Clarithromycin	↑ levels of B metabolite	++
+		+	Cyclosporine	↑ levels of B	++
+			Dexamethasone	↓ levels of A	++
+	+	+	Sildenafil, vardenafil, tadalafil	↑ levels of B	++

TABLE 16A (4)

ANTI-INFECTIVE AGENT (A)			OTHER DRUG (B)	EFFECT	SIGNIFICANCE/CERTAINTY

Non-nucleoside reverse transcriptase inhibitors (NNRTIs): For interactions with protease inhibitors, *see Table 16C*. Del = delavirdine, Efa = efavirenz, Nev = nevirapine

Del	Efa	Nev	Co-administration contraindicated:		
+		+	Fentanyl, methadone	↑ levels of B	++
+			Gastric acid suppression: antacids, H-2 blockers, proton pump inhibitors	↓ levels of A	++
	+	+	Methadone, fentanyl	↓ levels of B	++
	+	+	Oral contraceptives	↑ or ↓ levels of B	++
+	+	+	Protease inhibitors—see Table 16B & C		
+	+	+	Rifabutin, rifampin	↑ or ↓ levels of rifabutin; ↓ levels of A—**caution**	++
	+	+	St. John's wort	↓ levels of A	
+	+	+	Warfarin	↑ levels of B	++

Pentamidine, IV	Amphotericin B	↑ risk of nephrotoxicity	+
	Foscarnet	↑ risk of hypocalcemia	+
	Pancreatitis-associated drugs, e.g., alcohol, valproic acid	↑ risk of pancreatitis	

ANTI-INFECTIVE AGENT (A)	OTHER DRUG (B)	EFFECT	SIGNIFICANCE CERTAINTY

Protease Inhibitors – Anti-HIV Drugs (**Atazan** = atazanavir; **Fosampren** = fosamprenavir; **Indin** = indinavir; **Lopin** = lopinavir; **Nelfin** = nelfinavir; **Riton** = ritonavir; Saquin = saquinavir; **Tipran** = tipranavir). For interactions with antiretrovirals, see Table 22B & C.

Atazan	Fosampren	Indin	Lopin	Nelfin	Riton	Saquin	Tipran	Also see http://aidsinfo.nih.gov	EFFECT	
								Analgesics		
					+		+	1. Alfentanil, fentanyl, hydrocodone, tramadol	↑ levels of B	+
			+		+		+	2. Codeine, hydromorphone, morphine, methadone	↓ levels of B	+
+	+	+	+	+	+	+		**Anti-arrhythmics: amiodarone, lidocaine, mexiletine, flecainide**	↑ levels of B; **do not co-administer**	++
	+	+	+	+	+	+		**Anticonvulsants: carbamazepine, clonazepam, phenytoin, phenobarbital**	↑ levels of A, ↑ levels of B	++
+	+				+	+		Antidepressants, all tricyclic	↑ levels of B	++
				+	+			Antidepressants, all other	↓ levels of B; **no pimozide**	++
		+		+				**Antihistamine:** Loratadine	↓ levels of B	+
			+					Atovaquone	↓ levels of B	
+	+	+	+	+	+	+	+	**Benzodiazepines, e.g., diazepam, midazolam, triazolam**	↑ **levels of B—do not use**	++
					+			Beta blockers: metoprolol, indolol, propranolol, timolol	↑ levels of B	+
+	+	+	+	+	+	+	+	Calcium channel blockers (all)	↑ levels of B	++
+								Clarithro, erythro	↑ levels of B if renal impairment	+
	+		+	+	+		+	Contraceptives, oral	↓ levels of B	++
	+		+		+	+		Corticosteroids: prednisone, dexamethasone	↓ levels of A, ↑ levels of B	+
+	+	+	+	+	+	+	+	Cyclosporine	↑ levels of B, monitor levels	+
+	+	+	+	+	+	+	+	Ergot derivatives	↑ **levels of B—do not use**	++
	+	+			+	+	+	Erythromycin, clarithromycin	↑ levels of A & B	+
		+				+		Grapefruit juice (>200ml/day)	↓ indinavir & ↑ saquinavir levels	
+	+	+	+	+	+	+	+	H2 receptor antagonists	↓ levels of A	++
+	+	+	+	+	+	+	+	HMG-CoA reductase inhibitors (statins): lovastatin, simvastatin	↑ **levels of B—do not use**	++
+								Irinotecan	↑ **levels of B—do not use**	++
	+	+	+	+	+	+	+	Ketoconazole, itraconazole, ?vori	↑ levels of A, ↑ levels of B	+

TABLE 16A (5)

ANTI-INFECTIVE AGENT (A)	OTHER DRUG (B)	EFFECT	SIGNIFICANCE CERTAINTY
+ + + +	Metronidazole	Poss disulfiram reaction, alcohol	+
+ + + + + + +	Pimozide	↑ levels of B—do not use	++
+ + + + + + +	Proton pump inhibitors	↓ levels of A	++

Protease Inhibitors – Anti-HIV Drugs (**Atazan** = atazanavir; **Fosampren** = fosamprenavir; **Indin** = indinavir; **Lopin** = lopinavir; **Nelfin** = nelfinavir; **Riton** = ritonavir; **Saquin** = saquinavir; **Tipran** = tipranavir). For interactions with antiretrovirals, see *Table 22B & C.*

Atazan	Fosampren	Indin	Lopin	Nelfin	Riton	Saquin	Tipran	OTHER DRUG (B)	EFFECT	SIGNIFICANCE CERTAINTY
								Also see http://aidsinfo.nih.gov		
+	+	+	+	+	+	+	+	Rifampin, rifabutin	↓levels of A, ↑levels of B (avoid)	++ (avoid)
+	+	+	+	+	+	+		Sildenafil (Viagra), tadalafil, vardenafil	Varies, some ↑ & some ↓ levels of B	++
+	+	+	+	+	+	+	+	St. John's wort	↓ levels of A—do not use	++
+								Tenofovir	↓ levels of B – add ritonavir	++
		+	+		+			Theophylline	↓ levels of B	+
+	+				+		+	Warfarin	↑ levels of B	+
Pyrazinamide								INH, rifampin	May ↑ risk of hepatotoxicity	±
Pyrimethamine								Lorazepam	↑ risk of hepatotoxicity	+
								Sulfonamides, TMP/SMX	↑ risk of marrow suppression	+
								Zidovudine	↑ risk of marrow suppression	+
Quinine								Digoxin	↑ digoxin levels; ↑ toxicity	++
								Mefloquine	↑ arrhythmias	+
								Oral anticoagulants	↑ prothrombin time	++
Quinupristin/ dalfopristin (Synercid)								Anti-HIV drugs: NNRTIs & PIs	↑ levels of B	++
								Antineoplastic: vincristine, docetaxel, paclitaxel	↑ levels of B	++
								Calcium channel blockers	↑ levels of B	++
								Carbamazepine	↑ levels of B	++
								Cyclosporine, tacrolimus	↑ levels of B	++
								Lidocaine	↑ levels of B	++
								Methylprednisolone	↑ levels of B	++
								Midazolam, diazepam	↑ levels of B	++
								Statins	↑ levels of B	++
Ribavirin								Didanosine	↑ levels of B → toxicity—avoid	++
								Stavudine	↓ levels of B	++
								Zidovudine	↓ levels of B	++
Rifamycins (rifampin, rifabutin) *Ref.: ArIM 162:985, 2002* **The following is a partial list of drugs with rifampin-induced ↑ metabolism & hence lower than anticipated serum levels: ACE inhibitors, dapsone, diazepam, digoxin, diltiazem, doxy-cycline, fluconazole, fluvastatin, haloperidol, nifedipine, progestins, triazolam, tricyclics, voriconazole, zidovudine**								Al OH, ketoconazole, PZA	↓ levels of A	+
								Atovaquone	↑ levels of A, ↓ levels of B	+
								β adrenergic blockers (metoprolol, propranolol)	↓ effect of B	+
								Caspofungin	↓ levels of B—increase dose	++
								Clarithromycin	↑ levels of A, ↓ levels of B	++
								Corticosteroids	↑ replacement requirement of B	++
								Cyclosporine	↓ effect of B	++
								Delavirdine	↑ levels of A, ↓ levels of B—avoid	++
								Digoxin	↓ levels of B	++
								Disopyramide	↓ levels of B	++
								Fluconazole	↑ levels of A[3]	+
								Amprenavir, indinavir, nelfinavir, ritonavir	↑ levels of A (↓ dose of A), ↓ levels of B	++
								INH	Converts INH to toxic hydrazine	++
								Itraconazole[3], ketoconazole	↓ levels of B, ↑ levels of A[3]	++
								Methadone	↓ serum levels (withdrawal)	+
								Nevirapine	↓ levels of B—avoid	++
								Oral anticoagulants	Suboptimal anticoagulation	++
								Oral contraceptives	↓ effectiveness; spotting, pregnancy	+
								Phenytoin	↓ levels of B	+
								Protease inhibitors	↑ levels of A, ↓ levels of B—Caution	++
								Quinidine	↓ effect of B	+

---

[3] Up to 4wks may be required after RIF discontinued to achieve detectable serum itra levels; ↑ levels associated. with uveitis or polymyolysis

TABLE 16A (6)

ANTI-INFECTIVE AGENT (A)	OTHER DRUG (B)	EFFECT	SIGNIFICANCE/CERTAINTY
	Sulfonylureas	↓ hypoglycemic effect	+
	Tacrolimus	↓ levels of B	++
	Theophylline	↓ levels of B	+
	TMP/SMX	↑ levels of A	+
	Tocainide	↑ effect of B	+
Ritonavir	*See Protease inhibitors & Table 16B & C*		
Saquinavir	*See Protease inhibitors & Table 16B & C*		
Stavudine	Dapsone, INH	May ↑ risk of peripheral neuropathy	±
	Ribavirin	↓ levels of A—**avoid**	++
	Zidovudine	Mutual interference—do not combine	++
Sulfonamides	Cyclosporine	↓ cyclosporine levels	+
	Methotrexate	↑ antifolate activity	+
	Oral anticoagulants	↑ prothrombin time; bleeding	+
	Phenobarbital, rifampin	↓ levels of A	+
	Phenytoin	↑ levels of B; nystagmus, ataxia	+
	Sulfonylureas	↑ hypoglycemic effect	+
Telithromycin (Ketek)	Carbamazine	↓ levels of A	++
	Digoxin	↑ levels of B—do digoxin levels	++
	Ergot alkaloids	↑ **levels of B—avoid**	++
	Itraconazole; ketoconazole	↑ levels of A; no dose change	+
	Metoprolol	↑ levels of B	+ +
	Midazolam	↑ levels of B	+ +
	Phenobarbital, phenytoin	↓ levels of A	++
	Pimozide	↑ **levels of B; QT prolongation—avoid**	++
	Rifampin	↓ **levels of A—avoid**	+ +
	Simvastatin & other "statins"	↑ levels of B	+ +
	Sotalol	↓ levels of B	+ +
	Theophylline	↑ levels of B	+ +
Tenofovir (Viread))	Atazanavir	↓ levels of B—add ritonavir	++
	Didanosine (ddI)	↑ **levels of B (reduce dose)**	++
Tigecycline	Oral contraceptives	↓ levels of B	++
Trimethoprim	Amantadine, dapsone, digoxin, methotrexate, procainamide, zidovudine	↑ serum levels of B	++
	Potassium-sparing diuretics	↑ serum K$^+$	++
	Thiazide diuretics	↓ serum Na$^+$	+
Trimethoprim/ Sulfamethoxazole	Azathioprine	Reports of leucopenia	+
	Cyclosporine	↓ levels of B, ↑ serum creatinine	+
	Loperamide	↑ levels of B	+
	Methotrexate	Enhanced marrow suppression	++
	Oral contraceptives, pimozide, & 6-mercaptopurine	↓ effect of B	+
	Phenytoin	↑ levels of B	+
	Rifampin	↑ levels of B	+
	Warfarin	↑ activity of B	+
Vancomycin	Aminoglycosides	↑ frequency of nephrotoxicity	++
Zalcitabine (ddC) (HIVID)	Valproic acid, pentamidine (IV), alcohol, lamivudine	↑ pancreatitis risk	+
	Cisplatin, INH, metronidazole, vincristine, nitrofurantoun, d4T, dapsone	↑ risk of peripheral neuropathy	+
Zidovudine (ZDV)	Atovaquone, fluconazole, methadone	↑ levels of A	+
	Clarithromycin	↓ levels of A	±
	Indomethacin	↑ levels ZDV toxic metabolite	+
	Nelfinavir	↓ levels of A	++
	Probenecid, TMP/SMX	↑ levels of A	+
	Ribavirin	↓ **levels of A—avoid**	++
	Rifampin/rifabutin	↓ levels of A	++
	Stavudine	Interference – do not combine	++

TABLE 16B: DRUG-DRUG INTERACTIONS BETWEEN PROTEASE INHIBITORS

(Adapted from Guidelines for the Use of Antiretroviral Agents in HIV-Infected Adults & Adolescents; see www.aidsinfo.nih.gov)

NAME (Abbreviation, Trade Name)	Amprenavir (APV, Agenerase)	Atazanavir (ATV, Reyataz)	Fosamprenavir (FOS-APV, Lexiva)	Indinavir (IDV, Crixivan)	Lopinavir/Ritonavir (LP/R, Kaletra)	Nelfinavir (NFV, Viracept)	Saquinavir (SQV), (Invirase)	Tipranavir (TPV)
Amprenavir (APV, Agenerase)				Levels: APV AUC[1]↑ 33%. Doses: standard	Dose: APV 750mg q12h, LP/R either standard or to 533/133 mg q12h	Levels: APV AUC[1]↑ 1.5X. Inadequate data	Levels: APV AUC[1]↑ 32%. Dose: Insufficient data	No data
Atazanavir (ATV, Reyataz)				Do not co-administer; risk of additive ↑ in indirect bilirubin	RTV 100mg ↑ ATV AUC[1]238%		SQV (Invirase) 1600mg + ATV 300mg + RTV 100mg, all q24h	
Fosamprenavir (FOS-APV, Lexiva)				↑ serum conc. both drugs; do not co-administer			Insufficient data	Fos APV levels ↓. **Do not co-administer**
Indinavir (IDV, Crixivan)	Levels: APV AUC[1]↑ 33%. Doses: not established	Do not co-administer; risk of additive ↑ in bilirubin	↑ serum conc. both drugs; **do not co-administer**		IDV AUC[1]↑, IDV dose 600mg q12h	↑ IDV & NFV levels. Dose: IDV 1200mg q12h, NFV 1250mg q12h	SQV levels ↑ 4-7 fold. Dose: Insufficient data	No data
Lopinavir/Ritonavir (LP/R, Kaletra)	Dose: APV 750 mg q12h; LP/R either standard or ↑ to 533/133mg q12h	RTV 100mg ↑ ATV AUC[1]238%	↓ serum conc. both drugs; **do not co-administer**	IDV AUC[1]↑; IDV dose 600mg q12h		LP levels ↓; NFV levels ↑. Dose: LP/R 533/133mg q12h; NFV 1000mg q12h	SQV levels ↑. Dose: SQV 1000mg b.i.d., LP/R-standard	LPV levels ↓. **Do not co-administer**
Nelfinavir (NFV, Viracept)	Levels: APV AUC[1]↑ 1.5X. Dose: Inadequate data			↑ IDV & NFV levels. Dose: IDV 1200mg q12h; NFV 1250mg q12h	Dose: LP/R 533/133mg q12h; NFV 1000mg q12h		SQV levels ↑. Dose: SQV 1200mg b.i.d., NFV 1250mg b.i.d.	No data
Saquinavir (SQV, Fortovase/Invirase)	Levels: APV AUC[1]↑ 32%. Dose: Insufficient data	SQV (Invirase) 1600mg + ATV 300mg + RTV 100mg, all q24h	SQV (Invirase) 1000mg q12h + RTV 100-200mg q12h + FOS-APV 700mg q12h	IDV AUC[1]↑; Dose: Insufficient data	SQV levels ↑. Dose: SQV 1000mg b.i.d., LP/R-standard	SQV levels ↑ 1.5X. Dose: SQV 1200mg b.i.d., NFV 1250mg b.i.d.		SQV ↓. **Do not co-administer**
Tipranavir (TPV)	No data		Fos-APV levels ↓. **Do not co-administer**	No data	LPV levels ↓. **Do not co-administer**	No data	SQV ↓. **Do not co-administer**	

[1] AUC = area under the curve

TABLE 16C: DRUG–DRUG INTERACTIONS BETWEEN NON-NUCLEOSIDE REVERSE TRANSCRIPTASE INHIBITORS (NNRTIs) & PROTEASE INHIBITORS.
(Adapted from Guidelines for the Use of Antiretroviral Agents in HIV-Infected Adults & Adolescents; see www.aidsinfo.nih.gov)

NAME (Abbreviation, Trade Name)	Amprenavir (APV, Agenerase)	Atazanavir (ATV, Reyataz)	Fosamprenavir (FOS-APV, Lexiva)	Indinavir (IDV, Crixivan)	Lopinavir/Ritonavir (LP/R, Kaletra)	Nelfinavir (NFV, Viracept)	Saquinavir—softgel (SQV, Invirase)	Tipranavir (TPR)
Delavirdine (DLV, Rescriptor)	APV AUC↑ 130%. DLV AUC↓ 61%. **Do not co-administer**	No data	**Co-administration not recommended**	IDV levels ↑ 40%. Dose: IDV 600mg q8h, DLV standard	Expect LP levels to ↑. No dose data	NFV levels ↑ 2X; DLV levels ↓ 50%. Dose: No data	SQV levels ↑ 5X. Dose: SQV 800mg q8h, DLV standard	No data
Efavirenz (EFZ, Sustiva)	APV AUC↓ 36%. Dose: EFZ standard—add RTV 200mg to standard APV	ATV AUC↓ 74%. Dose: EFZ standard; ATA/RTV 300/100mg q24h with food	FOS-APV levels ↓. Dose: EFZ standard; FOS-APV 1400mg + RTV 300mg q4h or 700mg FOS-APV + 100mg RTV q12h	Levels: IDV ↓ 31%. Dose: IDV 1000mg q8h; EFZ standard	Level of LP ↓ 40%. Dose: LP/R 533/133 mg q12h; EFZ standard	Standard doses	Level: SQV ↓ 62%. Dose: SQV softgel 400mg + RTV 400mg q12h	No dose change necessary
Nevirapine (NVP, Viramune)	No data	No data	No data	IDV levels ↓ 28%. Dose: IDV 1000mg q8h or combine with RTV, NVP standard	LP levels ↓ 53%. Dose: LP/R 533/133 mg q12h; NVP standard	Standard doses	Dose: SQV softgel + RTV 400/400mg, both q12h	No data

TABLE 17: ANTIMICROBICS IN PREGNANCY

Drug	FDA Pregnancy Categories*	Placental Transfer (%)	Breastfeeding	Adverse Effects: Fetus, Mother
Antibacterial Agents				
Beta Lactams				
Imipenem/cilastatin	C	ND	OK	None
Clindamycin	B	6–46	OK	None
Fluoroquinolones	C	80–90	No	Potential arthropathy
Linezolid	C	ND	ND	
Macrolides:				
Azithromycin	B	ND	ND	None
Clarithromycin	C	ND	OK	Fetal toxicity in primates
Erythromycin	B	5–20	OK	None
Metronidazole	B	+	No	None: do not use in 1st trimester
Telithromycin	C	ND	ND	
Antifungal Agents:				
Amphotericin B	B	+	OK	None
Caspofungin	C		?	
Fluconazole, itraconazole	C	ND	ND	NHS
Voriconazole	D		?	**Risk of birth defects**
Antiparasitic Agents:				
Nitazoxanide	B	ND	ND	ND
Pentamidine	C	+	No	NHS
Pyrimethamine	C	+	No	None: do not use in 1st trimester
Sulfonamides	C	70–90	No	Potential kernicterus & hem-G6PD
Trimethoprim	C	30–100	OK	None
Antimycobacterial Agents:				
Dapsone	C	+	OK	Hem-G6PD
Ethambutol	ND	30	OK	None
Isoniazid	C	100	OK	None
Pyrazinamide	C	ND	OK	None
Rifabutin	B	ND	ND	
Rifampin	C	33	OK	Postnatal bleeding in infant
Streptomycin	C	10–40	OK	Ototoxicity (16% deafness)
Thalidomide	**X**	Presumably	ND	**Major risk birth defects**
Antiviral Agents:				
Abacavir	C	Yes (%?)	No	Teratogen: 35x human exposure
Acyclovir, valacyclovir	B	70	OK., ?	None. No data with vala—administer with caution to breast-feeding .
Adefovir	C	ND	No	
Amprenavir, fosamprenavir	C	ND	No	Teratogen in rodents
Atazanavir	B	ND	No	
Cidofovir	C	ND	No	–
Delavirdine	C	ND	No	Teratogenic in rats; rodent tumors
Didanosine	B	50	No	None
Efavirenz	D	ND	No	**High risk of birth defects**
Emtricitabine	B	ND	No	
Enfuvirtide	B	ND	No	
Entecavir	C	ND	?	
Famciclovir	B	ND	?	–
Foscarnet	C	ND	ND	
Ganciclovir, valganciclovir	C	No	No	Carcinogenic in animals, NHS
Indinavir	C	ND	No	
Interferons	C	ND	?	
Lamivudine	C	100	No	–
Lopinavir	C	ND	No	
Nelfinavir	B	ND	No	–
Nevirapine	C	100	No	
Ribavirin	**X**	ND	No	**Major risk of birth defects**
Ritonavir	B	15–100	No	Rodent tumors
Saquinavir	B	Minimal	No	–
Stavudine	C	76	No	Tumors in rodents
Tenofovir	B	ND	No	
Tipranavir	C	ND	?	
Zalcitabine	C	30–50	No	Tumors in rodents
Zidovudine	C	85	No	None
Anabolic Agents:				
Megestrol acetate (oral)	**X**	ND	No	Use contraindicated

* **FDA Pregnancy Categories: A**—adequate studies in pregnant women, no risk; **B**—animal studies no risk, but human studies not adequate or animal toxicity but human studies no risk; **C**—animal studies show toxicity, human studies inadequate but benefit of use may exceed risk; **D**—evidence of human risk, but benefits may outweigh; **X**—fetal abnormalities in humans, risk > benefit; **ND** = no data
***Abbreviations: Hem-G6PD** = hemolysis in individuals with G6PD deficiency; **NHS** = no controlled human studies

TABLE 18: SPECTRUM & TREATMENT OF HIV/AIDS-ASSOCIATED MALIGNANCIES*
(Treatment Review: *Oncologist* 10:412, 2005)

I. **Spectrum of associated malignancies: AIDS-defining neoplasms**
  A. **Kaposi's sarcoma** & other KSHV/HHV8 related neoplasms:
    1. Primary body cavity lymphoma (primary effusion lymphoma)
    2. Multicentric Castleman disease
  B. **HIV-associated lymphoma**
    1. Primary CNS lymphoma (EBV)
    2. Non-Hodgkin's lymphoma (EBV)
    3. Body cavity lymphoma; primary effusion lymphoma (HHV8/EBV)
  C. **Cervical carcinoma** (human papillomavirus)
  D. **Other neoplasms with increased incidence in AIDS patients**
    1. Anogenital neoplasia & squamous cell carcinoma of the anus (human papillomavirus)
    2. Basal cell carcinoma of the skin
    3. Hodgkin's disease
    4. Seminoma
    5. Pediatric leiomyosarcoma
II. **Kaposi's sarcoma (KS)—Selected issues: *CID 37:82, 2003***
  A. **Etiology & pathogenesis**
    1. Human herpesvirus type 8 (HHV8); also called Kaposi's sarcoma-associated herpesvirus (KSHV)
    2. HHV8/KSHV
      a. Viral DNA found in all KS tumors
      b. Infection precedes KS
      c. Seropositivity rate predicts KS rate
      d. Virus latent in most cells; lytic in <5% of cells
      e. Targets spindle cells
  B. **Diagnosis**
    1. Clinical appearance & then biopsy
    2. HHV8/KSHV serology; can now quantitate HHV8 in plasma by PCR
  C. **Treatment** (*Lancet Oncology 4:576, 2003; Crit Rev Onco; Hematol 53:253, 2005*)
    1. **Immune reconstitution** (improvement) with effective antiretroviral therapy of HIV infection leads to:
      a. Reports of clearance of HHV8 from circulating cells; 60–80% response rate
      b. Protease inhibitors have anti-tumor activity in mice & patients: *Nature Med 8:225, 2002*
    2. **Local therapy**—often used for cosmetic purposes

Therapy	Drug/Dose	Comment
Radiation	Single dose: 8–12 Gy	For single/grouped lesions. Relieves facial edema.
Intralesional therapy & other treatment of localized disease	Vinblastine 0.01 mg in 0.1 ml sterile water Liquid nitrogen Laser therapy	
Topical alitretinoin (9-cis retinoic acid)*	Apply 0.1% gel q12h	18% response

* *Arch Derm 139:178, 2003*

    3. **Systemic therapy**—see next section for doses

Stage of KS	Recommended Treatment
a. All stages, if possible	Observe response to combination antiretroviral rx & concomitant improvement in immune status of the patient
b. If progression despite combination antiretroviral rx or failure of antiretrovirals to substantially ↓ HIV viral burden or ↑ CD4 count:	
(1) Slowly progressive KS	(a) Observe or (b) Add antiretrovirals or (c) Investigational therapy: Thalidomide (*CID 23:501, 1996*)
(2) Rapidly progressive widespread/symptomatic KS	Liposomal doxorubicin or liposomal daunorubicin
(3) KS disease non-responding to liposomal doxorubicin or daunorubicin	Paclitaxel (Taxol) or [liposomal doxorubicin + vincristine + bleomycin]

    4. Doses, reported responses, & toxicity of drugs used for systemic therapy** of Kaposi's sarcoma*.

Drug(s)	Dose	Reported Response, %	Toxicity/Comment
Bleomycin (with doxorubicin & vincristine)	10 mg/M² q14 days	25	**Doxorubicin: marrow suppression; G-CSF 5 mcg/kg/day (usually 300 mcg) may be required.**
Doxorubicin (with bleo & vincristine)	10–20 mg/M²	50–88 (includes partial response)	Bleomycin: myocardial toxicity & heart failure with total dose of 550 mg/M² Vincristine: peripheral neuropathy (sensory loss, paresthesias)
Liposomal doxorubicin-polyethylene glycol conjugated	20 mg/M² q2–3 wks	59	Neutropenia (15–25%), alopecia, nausea, back pain, flushing, chest tightness
Liposomal daunorubicin	40 mg/M² q2–3 wks	30–95	

TABLE 18 (2)

Drug(s)	Dose	Reported Response, %	Toxicity/Comment
Paclitaxel (Taxol)	135 mg/M² q3 wks	49–71	Severe hypersensitivity reaction in 2% pts; premedicate with steroids, diphenhydramine & H₂ antagonist; pancytopenia; many others

* For drugs, review package insert regarding dosage, precautions in administration & toxicities. For details, see Kaplan, LD, Northfelt, DW: Malignancies associated with AIDS, in *Medical Management of AIDS*, 6th Ed., Eds.: M.A. Sande, P.A. Volberding, W.B. Saunders & Co., 1999, pg467–496, & *NEJM 342:1027, 2000.*

** With systemic disease, chemotherapy is palliative only, does not alter survival.

III. **Primary body cavity lymphoma; primary effusion lymphoma**
   A. Etiology: HHV8/KSHV; some cells also positive for EBV
   B. Diagnosis: Biopsy of tumor masses in pleural space, pericardial space, intraabdominal cavity
   C. Treatment: Chemotherapy—*see non-Hodgkin's lymphoma (V.C.)*; complete remission reported with antiretroviral therapy.
   D. Concomitant HAART prolongs survival *(AIDS 17:1787, 2003)*.
IV. **Multicentric Castleman disease**
   A. Rare lymphoproliferative disorder
   B. Etiology: HHV8/KSHV
   C. Clinical: Fever, lymphadenopathy, splenomegaly
   D. Treatment: Very effective—Either vinblastine 6–10 mg q2 wks or etoposide 150–200 mg for 2 consecutive days q2 wks. Also reports of success with foscarnet *(CID 26:527, 1998)* & interferon alfa *(CID 31:602, 2000)*.
V. **HIV-associated lymphoma** *(AIDS Reader 14:605, 2005; Blood 107:13, 2006)*
   A. **General**
      1. Compared to immunocompetent pts, present in advanced stage; median survival only 6 months
      2. HIV-associated non-Hodgkin's lymphomas virtually all of B-cell origin
      3. Viral association
         a. Systemic lymphomas—no viral association
         b. CNS lymphoma—EBV DNA present in 100% but predictive value low *(CID 38:1629, 2004)*
         c. Body-cavity lymphomas—HHV8 genome present in virtually all
      4. Prognosis improving coincident with effective antiretroviral therapy
   B. **Primary CNS lymphoma**
      1. Usually in patients with very low CD4 counts
      2. Detection of EBV DNA by PCR in CSF in >90% pts but predictive value low *(CID 38:1629, 2004)*
      3. Treatment
         a. Whole brain irradiation; prolongs survival 1–3 months; longer survival with concomitant HAART *(AIDS 15:2119, 2001)*
         b. Responses to combination of ZDV, ganciclovir, & IL-2 in a few patients *(CID 34:1660, 2002)*
   C. **Non-Hodgkin's lymphoma** *(AIDS Reader 14:605, 2004)*
      1. **Continuous infusion EPOCH** (etoposide, prednisone, vincristine, cyclophosphamide, doxorubicin) leads to 92% probability of remission at 53 months *(Blood 101:4853, 2003)*. **No HAART during chemo**—controversial.
      2. Another option: Rituximab (anti-CD20 antibody) plus HAART plus chemotherapy
         a. U.S.—negative results: data in Abst. S17 of International Conference on Malignancies in AIDS, 2003.
         b. Two European trials—definite benefit *(Blood 100:470a, Abst 1824, 2002; AIDS 17:137, 2003)*.
VI. **Cervical carcinoma:** *JID 188:555, 2003; MMWR 53(RR-15):46, 2004*
   A. Epidemiology
      1. More frequent, more severe
         a. As CD4 count falls
         b. If co-infection with human papillomavirus (co-infection in 66% of HIV-infected women)
      2. 25–40% Pap smears abnormal in HIV-infected women
   B. Terminology of pre-invasive cervical disease
      Following terms more or less synonymous: cervical dysplasia, cervical intraepithelial neoplasia (CIN), & squamous intraepithelial lesions (SIL)
   C. **Recommendations**
      1. Pap smears x2 in year one & then annually if normal initially; every 3 yrs if CD4 >500/mm³ *(JAMA 293:1471, 2005)*.
      2. More frequent Pap smears if:
         a. Previous abnormal Pap smear
         b. History of papilloma (wart) virus infection
         c. Post-treatment for CIN (SIL)
         d. Symptomatic AIDS or CD4 count <200/mm³
      3. If Pap smear shows SIL or evidence of papillomavirus, refer for colposcopy &/or biopsy.
      4. Low-grade lesions, follow closely
      5. High-grade lesions, treat by ablation (e.g., radiotherapy) or excision. Avoid cryosurgery due to high recurrence rates.
VII. **Anal neoplasia:** *MMWR 53(RR-15):46, 2004*
   A. Epidemiology
      1. HIV-infected immunodeficient patients at increased risk of human papillomavirus (HPV)-related anal neoplasia.
      2. HPV DNA found in roughly 50% of anal cytology specimens from HIV-infected men.
   B. Recommendations for HIV-infected pts with history of anal intercourse
      1. Anal Pap smear
      2. Routine anoscopy with biopsy as indicated
      3. Wide surgical resection for established neoplasia

TABLE 19: RECOMMENDATIONS FOR ROUTINE IMMUNIZATION OF HIV+ CHILDREN (ASYMPTOMATIC & SYMPTOMATIC)
[Modified from USPHS/IDSA Guidelines (MMWR 49:RR-9, Oct. 6, 2000; MMWR 51:32, 2002; AnIM 137, Nov. 5 [Suppl.]:468, 2002; MMWR 54:Q1, 2006)]

Vaccine	Age												
	Birth	1 mo.	2 mos.	4 mos.	6 mos.	12 mos.	15 mos.	18 mos.	24 mos.	4–6 yrs.	11–12 yrs.	14–16 yrs.	
↓ Recommendations for these vaccines are the same as those for immunocompetent children ↓													
Hepatitis B¹	Hep B #1												
		Hep B #2				Hep B #3				Hep B			
Diphtheria & Tetanus toxoids, Pertussis²			DTaP	DTaP	DTaP		DTaP			DTap	Tdap		
Hemophilus influenzae type b⁴			Hib	Hib	Hib	Hib					Hib		
Inactivated Polio⁴			IPV	IPV	IPV					IPV	IPV		
Hepatitis A³						Hep A series				Hep A series			
Meningococcal⁵									MPSV 4	MPSV 4	MCV4	MCV4	
↓ Recommendations for these vaccines differ from those for immunocompetent children ↓													
Pneumococcus⁶			PCV	PCV	PCV	PCV			PPV23	PPV23 (age 5–7yrs)			
Measles, Mumps, Rubella⁷	Do not give to severely immuno-suppressed (Category 3) children				MMR				MMR	MMR			
Varicella⁸	Give only to asymptomatic non-immunosuppressed (Category 1) children. Contraindicated in all other HIV-infected children			Var	Var	Var			Var				
Influenza⁹	A dose is recommended every year												

☐ Range of recommended ages for vaccination

▨ Vaccines to be given if previously recommended doses were missed or were given earlier than the recommended minimum age

This schedule indicates the recommended ages for routine administration of licensed childhood vaccines as of Jan. 1, 2006, for children aged birth–18yrs. Additional vaccines might be licensed & recommended during the year. Licensed combination vaccines might be used whenever any components of the combination are indicated & a vaccine's other components are not contraindicated. Providers should consult the manufacturer's package inserts for detailed recommendations.

¹ **Hepatitis B vaccine (HepB). AT BIRTH:** All newborns should receive monovalent HepB soon after birth & before hospital discharge. **Infants born to mothers who are hepatitis B surface antigen (HBsAg)-positive** should receive HepB & 0.5mL of hepatitis B immune globulin (HBIG) within 12hrs of birth. **Infants born to mothers whose HBsAg status is unknown** should receive HepB within 12hrs of birth. The mother should have blood drawn as soon as possible to determine her HBsAg status; if HBsAg-positive, the infant should receive HBIG as soon as possible (no later than age 1wk). **For infants born to HBsAg-negative mothers,** the birth dose can be delayed in rare circumstances but only if a physician's order to withhold the vaccine & a copy of the mother's original HBsAg-negative laboratory report are documented in the infant's medical record. **FOLLOWING THE BIRTH DOSE:** The HepB series should be completed with either monovalent HepB or a combination vaccine containing HepB. The second dose should be administered at age 1–2mos. The final dose should be administered at age 24wks. Administering four doses of HepB is permissible (e.g., when combination vaccines are administered after the birth dose); however, if monovalent HepB is used, a dose at age 4mos is not needed. **Infants born to HBsAg-positive mothers** should be tested for HBsAg & antibody to HBsAg after completion of the HepB series at age 9–18mos (generally at the next well-child visit after completion of the vaccine series).

² **Diphtheria & tetanus toxoids & acellular pertussis vaccine (DTaP).** The fourth dose of DTaP may be administered as early as age 12mos, provided 6mos have elapsed since the third dose & the child is unlikely to return at age 15–18mos. The final dose in the series should be administered at age 4yrs. **Tetanus toxoid, reduced diphtheria toxoid, & acellular pertussis vaccine (Tdap adolescent preparation)** is recommended at age 11–12yrs for those who have completed the recommended childhood DTP/DTaP vaccination series & have not received a tetanus & diphtheria toxoids (Td) booster dose. Adolescents aged 13–18yrs who missed the 11–12yr Td/Tdap booster dose should also receive a single dose of Tdap if they have completed the recommended childhood DTP/DTaP vaccination series. **Subsequent Td** boosters are recommended every 10yrs.

³ Three **Hemophilus influenzae type b (Hib) conjugate vaccines** are licensed for infant use. If Hib conjugate vaccine (polyribosylribitol phosphate-meningococcal outer membrane protein [PRP-OMP]) (PedvaxHIB® or ComVax™ [Merck & Company, Inc., Whitehouse Station, NJ]) is administered at ages 2 & 4mos, a dose at age 6mos is not required. Because clinical studies among infants have demonstrated that certain combination products might induce a lower immune response to the Hib vaccine component, DTaP/Hib combination products should not be used for primary immunization among infants at ages 2, 4, or 6mos, unless approved by the FDA for these ages.

⁴ An all-inactivated poliovirus vaccine (IPV) schedule is recommended for routine childhood polio vaccination in the U.S. All children should receive 4 doses of IPV at age 2mos, age 4mos, ages 6–18mos, & ages 4–6yrs. Oral poliovirus vaccine should not be administered to HIV-infected persons or their household contacts.

TABLE 19 (2)

⁵ **Hepatitis A vaccine (Hep A).** HepA is recommended for all children at age 1yr (i.e., 12–23mos). The 2 doses in the series should be administered at least 6mos apart. States, counties, & communities with existing HepA vaccination programs for children aged 2–18yrs are encouraged to maintain these programs. In these areas, new efforts focused on routine vaccination of children aged 1yr should enhance, not replace, ongoing programs directed at a broader population of children. HepA is also recommended for certain high risk groups (see MMWR 1999;48[No. RR-12]).

⁶ **Heptavalent pneumococcal conjugate vaccine (PCV).** PCV is recommended for all children aged 2–59mos. Children aged ≥2yrs should also receive the **23-valent pneumococcal polysaccharide vaccine (PPV23);** a single revaccination with the 23-valent vaccine should be offered to children after 3–5yrs. Refer to the Advisory Committee on Immunization Practices recommendations (see CDC. Preventing pneumococcal disease among infants & young children: recommendations of the Advisory Committee on Immunization Practices [ACIP], MMWR 49(RR-9):1–38, 2000) for dosing intervals for children starting the vaccination schedule after age 2mos.

⁷ **Measles, mumps, & rubella (MMR)** should not be administered to severely immunocompromised (Category C) children. HIV-infected children without severe immunosuppression would routinely receive their 1st dose of MMR as soon as possible after reaching their 1st birthdays. Consideration should be given to administering the 2nd dose of MMR at 1mo (i.e., a minimum of 28 days) after the 1st dose rather than waiting until school entry.

⁸ **Varicella-zoster virus vaccine** should be administered only to asymptomatic, non-immunosuppressed children. Eligible children should receive 2 doses of vaccine with a ≥3mo interval between doses. The 1st dose can be administered at age 12mos.

⁹ **Inactivated split influenza virus vaccine** should be administered to all HIV-infected children aged ≥6mos each year. For children aged 6mos–<9yrs who are receiving influenza vaccine for the first time, 2 doses administered 1mo apart are recommended. For specific recommendations, see CDC. Prevention & control of influenza: recommendations of the Advisory Committee on Immunization Practices (ACIP), MMWR 51(RR-4):1–32, 2002.

¹⁰ **Meningococcal vaccine (MCV4).** Meningococcal conjugate vaccine (MCV4) should be administered to all children at age 11–12yrs as well as to unvaccinated adolescents at high school entry (age 15yrs). Other adolescents who wish to decrease their risk for meningococcal disease may also be vaccinated. All college freshmen living in dormitories should be vaccinated, preferably with MCV4, although **meningococcal polysaccharide vaccine (MPSV4)** is an acceptable alternative. Vaccination against invasive meningococcal disease is recommended for children & adolescents aged 2yrs with terminal complement deficiencies or anatomic or functional asplenia & for certain other high risk groups (see MMWR 2005;54[No. RR-7]); use MPSV4 for children aged 2–10yrs & MCV4 for older children, although MPSV4 is an acceptable alternative.
For further information, see www.cdc.gov.

TABLE 20: IMMUNIZATION OF HIV+ ADULTS (ASYMPTOMATIC & SYMPTOMATIC)

General Principles/Guidelines:

• In HIV+ individuals, there are activated T-cells (CD25+) & quiescent T-cells (CD25-). Only activated T-cells produce virus & spread infection. In HIV+ adults, significant (2-36 fold) transient (≤6wks) ↑ in plasma viral RNA after pneumococcal, influenzal & tetanus immunization (NEJM 334:1222, 1996). A similar phenomenon occurs with acute infections, i.e., influenza. At present, there are no data suggesting that this is clinically relevant (AnIM 131:430, 1999; CID 28:548, 1999). Concurrently, antibody responses are ↓ in HIV+ individuals. Our recommendations are presented in the following table.

• **Administration of live attenuated vaccines is contraindicated in individuals with advanced HIV infection (AIDS) (MMR is an exception).**

• Immunization (when indicated) with killed whole cell vaccines &/or purified antigens should be done as soon as reasonable after HIV infection diagnosed, before CD4 cells ↓ further (JID 171:1217, 1995).

• Extended primary series &/or more frequent boosters often indicated.

• When specifically indicated, immune globulin (IG) & specific immune globulins can be administered.

• For general reference on licensed vaccine use in immunocompromised hosts, see Clin Microbiol Rev 11:1, 1998.

RECOMMENDATIONS FOR ROUTINE IMMUNIZATION OF HIV+ ADULTS (United States)

(From Update on Adult Immunization, Centers for Disease Control, MMWR 51:904, 2002, MMWR 54:Q1, 2006)

VACCINE/TOXOID	STAGE OF HIV INFECTION		BOOSTER DOSE	AUTHORS' RECOMMENDATIONS³ (AIDS Clin Care 8:11, 1996)
	ASYMPTOMATIC HIV+*	SYMPTOMATIC (AIDS)*		
Td (tetanus/ diphtheria)	Yes	Yes	10 yrs	0
HbCV (Haemophilus influenzae type b conjugate vaccine)	Yes	Yes	None	+ (if IDU)
Pneumococcal	Yes	Yes	6yrs	+
influenza	Yes	Yes	Annual	+
Hepatitis A	Yes	Yes	None	+
HBV (Hepatitis B)	Yes	Yes	None	+
eIPV (polio)	(Yes)**	(Yes)**	(None)	0
MMR (Measles, mumps, rubella)	Yes	(Yes)**	**	NA
Meningococcal	Yes**	Yes**	None	NA

Abbreviations: Td = tetanus & diphtheria toxoids, adsorbed (for adult use); **MMR** = measles, mumps & rubella vaccine; **HbCV** = Haemophilus influenzae type b conjugate vaccine; **Pneumococcal** = pneumococcal polysaccharide (23 component) vaccine; **HBV** = Hepatitis B vaccine; **eIPV** = enhanced-potency inactivated polio vaccine; **IDU** = injection drug user.

* Asymptomatic-CDC category A1, A2; Symptomatic-CDC A3, B1-3, C1-3; ** See Comments; ³ + = benefit > risk, 0 = benefit probably < risk. For further information, see www.cdc.gov.

TABLE 20 (2)
COMMENTS ON "ROUTINE" VACCINES/TOXOIDS*

VACCINE/TOXOID	COMMENTS
Td	"Injection" drug users at ↑ risk of tetanus
HbCV	Is of unproven benefit & immune responses ↓; although the risk of H. influenzae type b disease is ↑ & adverse reactions are minimal, it is no longer recommended.
Pneumococcal	Risk of bacteremia is ↑ [as high as 9.4/1000/yr (*J Inf Dis 162:1012, 1990*)]. Revaccination 6yrs after 1st dose is recommended. Benefit appears > risk.
Hepatitis A	In the past several years hep A has ↑ in frequency in homosexual men in the U.S., Canada & Australia (*MMWR 45:155, 1992*). Outbreaks also reported in injection drug users (IDU) (*Am J Pub Health 79:463, 1989*). <10% U.S.-born young adults have antibody (*Mil Med 157:579, 1992*). 2 hep A vaccines, inactivated, are licensed in U.S. FDA-approved indications include: persons engaged in high-risk sexual activity (homosexually active men), IDU (*MMWR 47:708, 1998; MMWR 48:RR-12, 1999*).
Hepatitis B	If lifestyle or occupation was risk factor for HIV it is also a risk factor for hepatitis B. Series of 3 IM injections in deltoid, using 12-in needle (not into the buttocks), should be given. Test for antibody to HBs Ag 1-6 months after completing series. If anti-HBs is <10 milli-international units, revaccinate with 1 or more doses.
Influenza	Annual immunization with the current vaccine is recommended regardless of age. Benefit appears > risk (*AnIM 131:430, 1999*). Poor immune response in pts with CD4 count <200. Some recommend amantadine, rimantadine or neuraminidase inhibitors instead of immunization in this group (*CID 28:548, 1999*).
eIPV (enhanced-potency inactivated polio vaccine)	In adults ≥18yrs, use only if specifically indicated: travel to developing countries (not Central or South America), prior to (~8wks, time for initial 2 doses) household exposure to individuals given oral polio vaccine.
OPV (oral polio vaccine)	Contraindicated
Specific immunoglobulins: Hepatitis B (HBIG), human rabies (HRIG), tetanus (TIG), vaccinia (VIG), varicella-zoster (VZIG)	Can be used for same indications, same dosage as in non-HIV infected individuals
MMR	Withhold MMR or other measles-containing vaccines from HIV-infected persons with severe immunosuppression
Meningococcal	*Medical indications:* adults with anatomic or functional asplenia or terminal complement component deficiencies. *Other indications:* 1styr college students living in dormitories; microbiologists who are routinely exposed to isolates of *Neisseria meningitides*; military recruits; & persons who travel to or reside in countries in which meningococcal disease is hyperendemic or epidemic (e.g., the "meningitis belt" of sub-Saharan Africa during the dry season [Dec–June]), particularly if contact with local populations will be prolonged. Vaccination required by the government of Saudi Arabia for all travelers to Mecca during the annual Hajj. Meningococcal conjugate vaccine is preferred for adults meeting any of the above indications who are aged <55yrs, although meningococcal polysaccharide vaccine MPSV4) is an acceptable alternative. Revaccination after 5yrs might be indicated for adults (previously vaccinated with MPSV4) who remain at high risk for infection (e.g., persons residing in areas in which disease is epidemic). See also Table 21B.

* For further details, see Wilson, et al., *AnIM* 114:582, 1991

TABLE 21A: MEASURES TO BE TAKEN BY PHYSICIANS IN PREPARING HIV+ PATIENTS & INDIVIDUALS LIKELY TO HAVE "RISKY" BEHAVIOR FOR OVERSEAS TRAVEL*[1]

The likelihood of developing an illness during a 3-wk vacation in a tropical area is about 50% (*J Travel Med 6:71, 1999*). Since illnesses are likely to be more serious &/or become chronic in the HIV+ patient, there is advice to be given & measures to be taken to minimize risks. These include:

• If the traveler is likely to engage in risky behavior during travel, ascertain the HIV antibody status before travel, especially if travel is planned to a developing country.
• If the traveler is known to be HIV+, take account of legal restrictions on travel for persons with HIV infection[2]. Assess the immune status (CD4 cell count) in infected persons.
• Review planned itinerary & activities in light of the patient's immune status & review the added risks for travel, especially to developing or tropical countries. In some instances, it may be prudent to recommend a change in itinerary or activities because of serious risks that cannot be eliminated or reduced.
• Recommend the following measures to reduce exposure to pathogens:
 Assiduously avoid food & beverages that may be contaminated, especially raw or undercooked shellfish, fish, meat, or eggs; raw, unpeeled fruits & vegetables; tap water & ice; as well as unpasteurized milk & milk products (cheese). Insist on eating only well-cooked foods & on drinking only very hot or bottled beverages.
 Reduce contact with vectors, for example, by using insect repellent & avoiding outdoor exposure at dusk or other times & places of increased insect activity.
• Urge the patient to obtain prompt evaluation of symptoms of illness & early treatment of infection. Where possible, identify a physician knowledgeable about HIV infection at the destination[3]. Arrange for continuation of medical management during travel (for example, prophylaxis for Pneumocystis carinii pneumonia).
• Use vaccine & prophylactic therapy as indicated by the planned itinerary & activities. Prescribe antimicrobial agents (with or without antimotility drugs) & counsel the patient on their use for early treatment of diarrheal disease.[4]

[1] The most up-to-date source is: Health Information for the International Traveler, 1995. HHS Public Health (CDC) No. 93-8280. Available from U.S. Government Printing Office, Washington, DC 20402. See also www.travmed.com; www.fitfortravel.scot.nhs.uk.
[2] Duckett M, Orkin AJ: AIDS-related migration & travel policies & restrictions: a global survey. AIDS 3:(Suppl 1) S231-252, 1989.
[3] For a list of English-speaking doctors abroad & health information: International Association for Medical Assistance to Travelers (IAMAT), 417 Center St., Lewiston, NY 14092.
[4] For suggestions regarding a medical kit & advice (for all travelers): Sanford JP: Self-help for the traveler who becomes ill. Inf Dis Clin NA 6:405, 1992.
* Reproduced with permission from Wilson ME, von Reyn CF, Fineberg HV: Infections in HIV-infected travelers: risks & prevention (Table 2). AnIM 114:582, 1991. USPHS/IDSA Guidelines CID 21(Suppl. 1):520, 199

TABLE 21B: IMMUNIZATION OF HIV+ ADULTS TRAVELING TO DEVELOPING COUNTRIES*

| VACCINE/TOXOID | STAGE OF HIV INFECTION | | COMMENTS |
	ASYMPTOMATIC HIV+*	SYMPTOMATIC (AIDS)*	
"Routine" for All Developing Countries			
eIPV	Yes	Yes	See Tables 19 & 20. OPV contraindicated
Hepatitis A	Yes	Yes	See Table 20 (2).
Typhoid Vi polysaccharide vaccine (Connaught)	Yes	Yes	Boosters recommended q2yrs. Live attenuated oral typhoid vaccine contraindicated
Immune globulin (IG)	Yes	Yes	For 2–3mos travel, 0.02ml/kg IM single dose
"Special" Depending on Itinerary: Country & Activity			
Cholera (inactivated vaccine)	See Comments	See Comments	Vaccine does not prevent infection, efficacy ~50%, risk to U.S. travelers very low. WHO does not recommend, but some countries require (check with Health Dept.). If required, have vaccination completed, signed, dated & validated to avoid risk of revaccination & quarantine.
Rabies (pre-exposure) (inactivated vaccine)	Yes, if indicated (Animal handlers, travelers spending 1mo or more in country where rabies is a constant threat)	Yes, if indicated	Course: Three 1ml of HDCV or RVA IM on days 0, 7, 28. Test serum for antibodies 2wks after 3rd dose.
Meningococcal (polysaccharide vaccine)(Menomune) or polysaccharide-protein conjugate (Menactra)	Yes, if traveling to area where meningococcal disease is epidemic or endemic (sub Sahara Africa)		Note recent CDC advisory: 5 cases of Guillain-Barre syndrome reported after Menactra vaccination. Causal relationship NOT clear (www.phppo.cdc.gov)
Yellow Fever (live attenuated)	Yes (±); offer choice if potential exposure unavoidable	No (contra-indicated)	
Japanese Encephalitis	Yes, if indicated: travel to Asia, in monsoon (summer) months, staying in rural areas		Requires 3 injections: day 0, 7, & 30. An abbreviated schedule on days 0, 7, 14 can be used but less effective (MMWR 42:RR-1, 1993).
Plague (inactivated)	Yes, if indicated: to areas of endemic plague, esp. if staying in rural areas, not in tourist hotels		
BCG (Bacillus Calmette-Guerin) vaccine	No	No	Is live attenuated vaccine

* All travelers should have current routine immunizations, Table 20
** Asymptomatic-CDC categories A1, A2; Symptomatic-CDC A3, B1-3, C1-3 (Table 4A).
For further information, see www.travmed.com; www.fitfortravel.scot.nhs.uk.

TABLE 22: BIOLOGICS IN TREATMENT OF HEMATOCYTOPENIAS*

DRUG NAME, GENERIC (TRADE) COST	COMMENTS ON USE, ADVERSE EFFECTS
Erythropoietin (Epogen, Procrit) 4000 units $54.00–$57.00 Ref.: NEJM 352:1011, 2005 **Darbepoetin** (Aranesp, Nesp) = long-acting erythropoietin. 0.025mg/kg $128	Indicated if erythropoietin (EPO) level ≤500mU/ml. **Dose:** 100units/kg IV or subQ 3x/wk for 8wks. If no response, can increase dose 50–100units/kg increments to a max. dose of 300units/kg 3x/wk. Follow retic. count & replace iron if necessary. No significant adverse effects. 40,000–60,000units subQ once weekly may equal efficacy of 3x/wk. q (J AIDS 34:368, 2003). **Dose of darbepoetin:** 0.45mcg/kg IV or subQ **q wk.**
Granulocyte-CSF or G-CSF, Filgrastim (Neupogen), 300mcg $215; Pegfilgrastim (Neulasta), 6mg $3,062; & **Granulocyte-monocyte-CSF or GM-CSF,** Sargramostim (Leukine), 250mcg $153	**G-CSF:** Standard dose 5mcg/kg/day subQ; lower doses may work in HIV pts, i.e., 1mcg/kg/day subQ until ANC >1000 cells/dl, then 1–2x/wk. No effect on HIV replication. Pegylated G-CSF—pegfilgrastim: 6mg subQ once per chemotherapy cycle. **GM-CSF:** Dose 5mcg/kg/day subQ → ↑ PMNs, monocytes, eosinophils assoc. with ↑ in viral load; also ↑ efficacy of ZDV. Adverse effects: fever, myalgia, fatigue, malaise, headache, bone pain.
Intravenous immune serum globulin (IVIG) (Gamimune N, Gammar, & others). $900 for 100 ml of 10% prep of Gamimune General dosage: (1) Adults: 200–400mg/kg q21 days; (2) Children: 400mg/kg/ month	Example uses: (1) **Parvovirus B-19** infection. Effective. Dose: 400mg/kg/day x10 days. (NEJM 321:519, 1989.) (2) **Immune thrombocytopenia.** Use IVIG only if pt bleeding &/or immediate invasive procedure. Rapid effects but transient. Dose: 1–2gm/kg over 2 days. Anti-Rh immune globulin (see below) more cost effective. (3) **Autoimmune neutropenia.** 1–2mo. benefit in pts who failed G-CSF. Dose: 20–25gm/day x 4–6 days.
Rho (D) Immune Globulin (Anti-Rh immunoglobulin, human) (WinRho). 1500 intl units $324.50 1500 intl units = 300mcg	Treatment for **HIV-induced ITP** in non-splenectomized Rh+ pts. Coats Rh+ RBC with antibody; competes with antibody-coated platelets for binding sites on splenic macrophages. Some RBC hemolysis. Effective AIDS pts. Dose: 25–50mcg/kg/day x7 days, then q3wks.

* **NOTE:** Majority of hematologic problems resolve, or substantively improve, with control of HIV replication. In general, treat HIV first before using drugs outlined above.

TABLE 23: AIDS INFORMATION & REFERRAL SERVICES

- AIDS/HIV Clinical Trials conducted by National Institutes of Health & FDA-approved efficacy trials: 1-800-874-2572
- For a wide variety of AIDS/HIV information, resources, publications, call the National AIDS Clearinghouse: 1-800-458-5231
- To find out about AIDS resources in your area, call the National AIDS Hotline: 1-800-342-2437
- The AIDS/HIV Treatment Directory is published by the American Federation for AIDS Research (AmFAR) & is updated semi-annually; 733 Third Ave., 12th Floor, New York, NY 10017-3204. Telephone: 1-800-392-6327
- The HIV/AIDS Treatment Information Service (Public Health Coordinating Group): 1-800-HIV-0440
- Travel information for patients: www.travmed.com & www.fitfortravel.scot.nhs.uk

Helpful Websites for Questions About HIV/AIDS:

CDC National Information Prevention Network: www.cdcnpin.org
amFAR (American Foundation for AIDS Research): www.amfar.org
The HIV/AIDS Treatment Information Service (ATIS): www.hivatis.org
San Francisco General Hospital: http://hivinsite.ucsf.edu
Johns Hopkins AIDS Service: www.hopkins-aids.edu
WHO Treatment Guidelines: www.who.org

TABLE 24: LIST OF GENERIC & COMMON TRADE NAMES

GENERIC NAME: TRADE NAMES	GENERIC NAME: TRADE NAMES	GENERIC NAME: TRADE NAMES
Abacavir: Ziagen	Ethambutol: Myambutol	**Pegylated interferon alfa-2b: PEG Intron**
Acyclovir: Zovirax	Ethionamide: Trecator	Pentamidine: Pentam 300
Adefovir: Hepsera	Etoposide: VePesid	Pentamidine aerosol: NebuPent
Amikacin: Amikin	Famciclovir: Famvir	Primaquine: Primachine
Amphotericin B: Fungizone	Filgrastim (G-CSF): Neupogen	Pyrazinamide: Pyrazinamide
Ampho B cholesteryl complex: Amphotec	Fluconazole: Diflucan	Pyrimethamine: Daraprim
Ampho B lipid complex: Abelcet	Flucytosine: Ancobon	Quinupristin/dalfopristin: Synercid
Ampho B liposomal: AmBisome	Fomivirsen: Vitravene	Ribavirin: Virazole, Rebetol
Amprenavir: Agenerase	Fosamprenavir: Lexiva	Rifabutin: Mycobutin
Atazanavir: Reyataz	Foscarnet: Foscavir	Rifampin: Rifadin, Rimactane
Atovaquone: Mepron	Ganciclovir: Cytovene	Ritonavir: Norvir
Azithromycin: Zithromax	Human growth hormone (rHGH): Serostim	Saquinavir: Invirase (hard cap)
Bleomycin: Blenoxane	Imipenem: Primaxin	Fortovase (softgel)
Capreomycin: Capastat	Indinavir: Crixivan	Sargramostim (GM-CSF): Leukine, Prokine
Caspofungin: Cancidas	Interferon alfa: Roferon-A, Intron A	Stavudine (d4T): Zerit
Cidofovir: Vistide	Iodoquinol: Yodoxin	Tenofovir: Viread
Ciprofloxacin: Cipro	Isoniazid: INH, Laniazid, Tubizid	Thiacetazone: Tibione
Clarithromycin: Biaxin, Biaxin XL	Itraconazole: Sporanox	Tipranavir: Texega
Clindamycin: Cleocin	Ketoconazole: Nizoral	Trimethoprim: Proloprim, Trimpex
Clofazimine: Lamprene	Lamivudine (3TC): Epivir, Epivir-HBV	Trimethoprim/Sulfamethoxazole: Bactrim, Septra
Cycloserine: Seromycin	Linezolid: Zyvox	Trimetrexate: Neutrexin
Daunorubicin-liposome: DaunoXome	Megestrol: Megace	Valacyclovir: Valtrex
Delavirdine: Rescriptor	Nelfinavir: Viracept	Valganciclovir: Valcyte
Didanosine (ddl): Videx	Nevirapine: Viramune	Vidarabine: Vira-A
Doxorubicin: Adriamycin	Norfloxacin: Noroxin	Vinblastine: Velban
Doxorubicin-liposome: Doxil	Ofloxacin: Floxin	Vincristine: Oncovin
Dronabinol: Marinol	Paclitaxel: Taxol	Voriconazole: Vfend
Efavirenz: Sustiva	Palivizumab: Synagis	VP16: VePesid
Emtricitabine: Emtriva	Paromomycin: Humatin	Zalcitabine (ddC): HIVID
Enfuvirtide: Fuzeon	PAS: Paser	Zidovudine (ZDV): Retrovir
Erythropoietin: Epogen, Procrit	**Pegylated interferon alfa-2a: Pegasys**	

TRADE NAME: GENERIC NAME	TRADE NAME: GENERIC NAME	TRADE NAME: GENERIC NAME
Abelcet: Ampho B lipid emulsion	Intron A: Interferon alfa	Seromycin: Cycloserine
Adriamycin: Doxorubicin	Invirase: Saquinavir hard cap	Serostim: Human growth hormone [HGH(m)]
Agenerase: Amprenavir	Kaletra: Lopinavir + ritonavir	Sporanox: Itraconazole
AmBisome: Ampho B liposomal	Lamprene: Clofazimine	Sustiva: Efavirenz
Amikin: Amikacin	Leukine: Sargramostim (GM-CSF)	Synagis: Palivizumab
Amphotec: Ampho B cholesteryl complex	Lexiva: Fosamprenavir	Synercid: Quinupristin/ dalfopristin
Ancobon: Flucytosine	Marinol: Dronabinol	Taxol: Paclitaxel
Bactrim: TMP/SMX	Megace: Megestrol	Texega: Tipranavir
Biaxin, Biaxin XL: Clarithromycin	Mepron: Atovaquone	Tibione: Thiacetazone
Blenoxane: Bleomycin	Myambutol: Ethambutol	Trecator: Ethionamide
Cancidas: Caspofungin	Mycobutin: Rifabutin	Trimpex: Trimethoprim
Capastat: Capreomycin	NebuPent: Pentamidine aerosol	Trizivir: Abacavir + zidovudine + lamivudine
Cleocin: Clindamycin	Neupogen: Filgrastim (CSF)	Truvada: Tenofovir + emtricitabine
Cipro: Ciprofloxacin	Neutrexin: Trimetrexate	Valcyte: Valganciclovir
Combivir: Zidovudine + lamivudine	Noroxin: Norfloxacin	Valtrex: Valacyclovir
Crixivan: Indinavir	Norvir: Ritonavir	Velban: Vinblastine
Cytovene: Ganciclovir	Oncovin: Vincristine	VePesid: Etoposide (VP16)
Daraprim: Pyrimethamine	Paser: PAS	Vfend: Voriconazole
DaunoXome: Daunorubicin-liposome	PEG Intron: Pegylated interferon alfa-2b	Videx: Didanosine (ddl)
Diflucan: Fluconazole	Pegasys: Pegylated interferon alfa-2a	Viracept: Nelfinavir
Doxil: Doxorubicin- liposome	Pentam 300: Pentamidine	Viramune: Nevirapine
Emtriva: Emtricitabine	Primachine: Primaquine	Virazole: Ribavirin
Epivir, Epivir-HBV: Lamivudine	Primaxin: Imipenem + cilastatin	Viread: Tenofovir
Epogen: Erythropoietin	Procrit: Erythropoietin	Vistide: Cidofovir
Famvir: Famciclovir	Prokine: Sargramostim (GM-CSF)	Vitravene: Fomivirsen
Floxin: Ofloxacin	Proloprim: Trimethoprim	Yodoxin: Iodoquinol
Fortovase: Saquinavir softgel	Rebetol: Ribavirin + interferon alfa-2b	Zerit: Stavudine (d4T)
Foscavir: Foscarnet	Rescriptor: Delavirdine	Ziagen: Abacavir
Fungizone: Amphotericin B	Retrovir: Zidovudine	Zithromax: Azithromycin
Fuzeon: Enfuvirtide	Reyataz: Atazanavir	Zovirax: Acyclovir
Hepsera: Adefovir	Rifadin: Rifampin	Zyvox: Linezolid
HIVID: Zalcitabine (ddC)	Rimactane: Rifampin	
Humatin: Paromomycin	Roferon-A: Interferon alfa	
	Septra: TMP/SMX	

INDEX TO MAJOR ENTRIES

Bold numbers indicate: Major description OR Drug dosage, side-effects, & modification in renal/hepatic insufficiency

Abacavir   10–12, 14, 19–**22**, **28**, 30, 31, 39,
                                   43, 44,84, 148, 155,164,172
Abscess, lung   93, **94**
Acalculous cholecystitis   85
Acanthamoeba   69
Acute retroviral syndrome   **55**, **64**, 71, 74, 99
Acyclovir   48, 72–74, 78, 79, 86, 90, 129
                             133–135, **145**, 147, **153**, 164, 172
Addison's disease   **67**, 101, 139
Adenovirus   42, 73, 76, 78, 82, 87, **90**, **98**
Adrenal   66, **67**, 138
AIDP (acute inflammatory demyelinating
    polyradiculopathy)   64
AIDS cholangiopathy   42, **85**
AIDS dementia complex (ADC)   41, **56**–58, 61, 63, 89
Amikacin   110, 111, 113, 122, 135,
                                   140, **149**, 150, 156, 172
Amphotericin B   43, 66, 83, 98, **116–123**,
                                   136, 137, 144, 147, 151,
                                   155, 156, 159, 164, 172
Amprenavir   21, 23, 25, **29**, 32, 39, 40, 45, 46,
                             109, 148, 155, **156**, 160, 162–164, 172
Anabolic agents   2, **164**
Analgesics   66, 159
Anemia   4, 28, 29, 31, 35, 71, **82**, **83**, 93, 94,
                   104, 131, 134, 136, 137, 140, 142–144, 146
Anergy   108
Antiretroviral drugs   21**–24, 28–30, 38**, 39, 51,
                             52, 65, 66, 74, 75, 78, 148,
                             155, 156, **158–161**, 163
Anxiety   58, 76, 146, 155
Aphthous ulcers   65, **73**, 135
Arthritis   95, **96**, 101, 106
Ascites   88, **97**, 140
Aseptic meningitis   62, **63**, 73, 142
Aspergillosis   60, **94**, 95, **116**, 136
Atazanavir   4, 10, 12, 19, 21, 23, **24**, **29**, 31–33, 39
                   40, 45, 52, 148, 155, 156, 161–164, 172
Atovaquone   38, 48, 49, 53, 124, 125, **142**, 147,
                   148, 152, 156, 159, 160, 161, 172
Attachment Inhibitor   33
Azithromycin   40, 47, 49, 54, 86, 104, 135, **142**,
                             150, 155, 158, 164, 172
AZT   See Zidovudine, ZDV

Bacillary angiomatosis 15, 42, 60, 72, 75, **86**, 100, 106
Bacterial vaginosis   1, 81, **126**
Bartonella   3, 70, 86, **98**, 100, 106
BCG   3, 107, 170
Blastocystis hominis   123
Blastomycosis   **93**, 94, **117**, 122
Bleach, household   2
Bleomycin   165, 172
Blindness   59, 62, **69**, 128
Bowel perforation   **75**
Branched DNA assay   15
Breastfeeding   35, 37, **55**, 164
Bronchiectasis   88
Bronchitis   15, **88**
"Buffalo hump"   **32**

Calymmatobacterium
    granulomatis   *See Granuloma Inguinale*
Campylobacteriosis   41, 75, 78, **106**
Candidiasis   3, 15, 35, 37, 43, 54, 69, **71**, **73**, **80**, **81**
                   89, 92, **99**, 104, **117**, **118**, 119, 126, 137
Capreomycin   108, 111, 135, **140**, 156, 172
Carcinoma   15, **72**, 74, 78, 79, 83, 87, 95,
                             131, 165, **166**
Cardiomyopathy   41, **82**, 105
Caspofungin   **43**, **116–120**, **137**, 147, 155,
                             156, 160, 164, 172
Cauda equina syndrome   64, 66
CCR5 Chemokine Inhibitors   33

CD4 cell count   1, 4, **5**, **8**, **9**, 11, 13, **15**, **18**, 20, 22
                   24, 27, 29, 30, 25, 36–40, 42, 45, 49, 51,
                   53–56, 58, 59, 61–65, 67–77, 79, 80, 82,
                   84, 86–95, 98–101, 103–111, 115, 119,
                   121, 122, 125–129, 131–134, 157, 165
                                   166, 168, 169
Central nervous system disease   41, **55–65**, 100
Cervical carcinoma   15, 165, **166**
Cervical dysplasia   15, **79**, 166
Cervicitis   1, **79**, **80**, 96, **106**, **112**
Chagas' disease   61, 82
Chancroid   **79**, 80, **106**
Chickenpox (varicella)   49, 90, **135**
Child-Pugh Score   26, **155**
Chlamydia   3, 4, 35, 78, 80, 81, 89,
                   90, 96, **106**, 112, 113
Cholangiopathy   *See AIDS Cholangiopathy*
Cholecystitis   *See Acalculous Cholecystitis*
Chorioretinitis (CMV Retinitis)   15, 41, 58, 69, **70**,
                   105, **128**, 133, 145
Cidofovir   48, 61, 69, 72, **128–129**, 133,
                   134, **144**, **153**, 156, 164, 172
CIDP (chronic inflammatory demyelinating
    polyradiculopathy)   64
CIN (cervical intraepithelial neoplasm) **35**, **79**, 134, 166
Ciprofloxacin   79, 99, 135, **141**, 150, 155, 157, 172
Clades of HIV   5
Clarithromycin   40, 47, 49, 54, 86, 106, 109–112,
                   114, 135, 141, **142**, **150**, 158, 159,
                   161, 164, 172
Clindamycin   72, 75, 78, 113, 114, 124–126,
                   135, **142**, 155, 157, 164, 172
Clofazimine   48, 70, 101, 110–112, 122, **141**, 172
Clostridium difficile   **78**, 106
Cocaine, crack   1–3, 59, 82
Coccidioidomycosis   15, 84, **92**, 94, 95, **119**, **120**
Combination antiretroviral
    therapy   18–27, 38–40, 134, 165
Combivir   **18–20**, 22, 44, 172
Condoms   1–3, 35, 79
Condyloma acuminatum   **79**, 100, **134**
Congestive heart failure   42, **97**
Contraception   1, 3, 21, 23, 29, 35, 80,
                   139, 156, 157, 159–161
Cotton wool spots   41, **69**, 70
Crabs   *See Pediculosis pubis*
Cryptococcosis   15, 16, 42, 43, 54–56, 58–**62**,
                   63, 64, 67–**69**, 70, 72, **92**, 94, 99, 100,
                   102, 103, 113, 119, **120**, **121**, 122, 134
Cryptosporidium   15, 54, 75, **76**, 84, 85, 98,
                   102, 103, **123**, 143
Cunnilingus   1
CVA (cerebral vascular accident)   59
Cycloserine   108, 109, 111, 140, 157, 172
Cyclospora   75, **76**, 85, **123**
Cytomegalovirus (CMV)   4, 15, 41, 54, 55, **58**,
                   60, 67–**69**, 70, **72–74**, 75, **77**,
                   78, 82–92, 84, 85, 87, **94**, 95, 97, 98,
                   103, 105, **127**, **128**, 129, 133, 144, 145, 153

D4t   See Stavudine
Dapsone   36, 38, 48, 49, 53, 66, 67, 83, 84,
                   95, 112, 124, **125**, 142, 147, **152**, 157,
                   160, 161, 164
ddC   See Zalcitabine
ddI   See Didanosine
Delavirdine   10, 12, **23**, **28**, 31, 44, 148,
                   157–160, 163, 164, 172
Delirium   58, 138, 145
Dementia complex (ADC) See AIDS dementia complex
Depression   4, 29, **57**, 58, 63, 68, 141, 146
Desensitization, pencillin See Penicillin desensitization
Desensitization, TMP/SMX   16

Diarrhea 15, 16, 19, 21, 22, 25, 26, 28–33, 37, 40, 41, 46, 47, 51, 54, 56, 66, 71, **75**, **78**, 90, 93, 98, 102–107, 111, 124, 137, 138, 141–146, 169
Didanosine (ddI) 9–12, 14, 19, 21, **22**, **28**, 30–32, 34, 36, 43, 67, 70, 73–75, 86, 148, **149**, 156, **157**, 160, 164, 172
Disulfiram 21, 29, 138, 139, 143, 158, 159
Donovanosis 106
DOT (directly observed therapy) 88, **107–109**, 135
Doxorubicin 165, 167, 172
Drug dosage & adjustments (renal & hepatic dysfunction) **149–155**
Drug-drug interactions **156–163**
Drug pharmacokinetics **147–148**
Dysphagia 41, **73–75**

EB virus (Epstein Barr 42, 55, 60, 72, 82, 87, virus, EBV) 95, **129**, 165, 166
Efavirenz 10, 12, **18–21**, **23–25**, 29, 31, 32, 34–36, 39, 43, 45, 46, 52, 68, 109, **148**, 155–159, **163**, 164, 172
Ehrlichiosis 90
ELISA (Enzyme-linked Immuno-Sorbent Assay) 7, 15, 37
Emphysema 88
Emtricitabine 10, 11, 19, 21, **22**, 27, 28, 30, 39, 40, **43**, 44, 130, 148, **153**, 164, 172
Encephalitis **55–59**, 60, 62, 104, 106, 125, 127, 133, 170
Encephalitozoon helium 68, 124
Endocarditis **84**, 89, **106**, 114, 122
Endophthalmitis **68–69**
Enfuvirtide 10, 13, **26**, **30**, 39, 40, 47, **148**, 155, 164, 172
Entamoeba histolytica 76, **77**, 78, **123**
Enteroadherent E. coli 76
Enterocytozoon bieneusi/hellum 77, 85, **124**
Entry Inhibitors 13, 33
Eosinophilia 26, 29, **84**, 95, 101, 122, 140, 142
Eosinophilic folliculitis 99, 101
Epoetin alfa (erthropoietin) 28, 82, 83
Esophagitis **74**, 119, 127
Ethambutol 47, **107–112**, 135, **139**, 147, **152**, 157, 164, 172
Ethionamide 108, 109, **140**, **152**, 157, 172
Etoposide 166, 172

Famciclovir **133**, **134**, 135, 145, **147**, **153**, 164
Filgrastim (G-CSF) 31, 83, 144, 165, **170**, 172
Fingernail changes 28, 101
Fluconazole 43, 54, 62, 67, 73, 74, 86, 99, 100, 117, **118–121**, 122, **123**, **126**, 137–139, 147, **152**, 156, 160, 161, 164
Flucytosine (5-FC) 83, **120**, **137**, 147, **152**, 172
Fluoroquinolones 106, 109, 111–113, 114, **141–142**, **150**, 157, 164
Fosamprenavir 10, 12, 19, **21**, 24, 25, **29**, 39, 40, **46**, 52, 148, 155, 156, **162–163**, 164, 172
Foscarnet 48, 66, 69, 74, 80, 83, 86, 90, 98, 127–**129**, 133, **134**, **144**, 147, **153**, 156, 157, 159, 164, 166, 167, 172
FUO (Fever of unknown origin) **70–71**
Fusariosis 121

Gamma globulin **40**, 42, 129
Ganciclovir 48, 54, 64, 66, 67, 69, 74, 77, 78, 83, 84, 86, 90, 94, **127**, **128**, 129, 133, **144**, **145**, 147, **153**, 157, 164, 166, 172
Gastritis 74, 75
G-CSF See Filgrastim
Genotype resistance testing 10, 11, 13, 14, 27, 131
Giardia lamblia 77, 84, 88, **124**, 143
Giemsa stain 77, 80, 91
Gingivitis 71, **72**, 135
Glomerulosclerosis 97, 98
GM-CSF See Sargramostim
Gonads 68

Gonorrhea (GC) 3, 4, **79**, **112**
Granulocytopenia 28, **83**, 144
Granuloma inguinale **80**, **106**
Guillain-Barre syndrome 28, 31, **61**, 66, 106, 170

HAART (Highly Active 2, 4, **18–27**, 36, 37, 39, 41, Antiretroviral Therapy) 53–62, 64–73, 75–79, 81–87, 89, 91–100, 102, **103–105**, 107, 110, 112, 119–121, 127–134, 166
Haemophilus influenzae pneumonia 63, 89, 98, 168
Haemophilus influenzae vaccine 168
Hairy leukoplakia 3, 4, 71, **72**, **129**
Headache 18, **50**, **52**, 88, **101**
Health care worker, exposure 18, **50**, **52**, 88, **101**
Heart failure 42, 81, 82, 95, 97, 165
Hematemesis 74, 75
Hepatic steatosis See Steatosis
Hepatitis 2–4, 6, 25–31, 36, 45, **50–52**, 53, 55, 81, 85, **86–87**, 97, 103, 104, 107, 109, **131–135**, 137–140, **145–146**, 167–170
Herpes simplex 1, 3, 4, 15, 48, **58**, 60, 64, 68, **69**, **73**, **74**, **78**, 79, 80, 87, 100, 104, 128, **133**, **145**
Herpes zoster 3, 16, 48, 49, 60, 64, 68, **69**, **100**, 104, 105, 128, **134**, **135**, 154, 168, 169
Heterosexual transmission 2, 35, 37
HHV-6 (human herpes virus-6) 61, 90
HHV-8 See Kaposi's syndrome
Hilar lymphadenopathy 42, 94
Histoplasmosis 15, 70, 72, 74, 92, **93**–95, 98, **99**, 100, **121**, 122, 134
HIV-1 antibody tests 6, 7
HIV-1 subtypes 5, 6, 11, 14
HIV-2 5, 6, 8, 9, 98
HIV testing, recommendations 1, 4, 5–9, 35, 36
HPV (human paillomavirus) 35, 72, **79**, **134**, 166
HTLV-1 (human T-lymphocytic virus) 5, 7, 9, 64, 101
HTLV-2 (human T-lymphocytic virus) 5, 7
Hydroxyurea 28, 32, 86
Hyperkalemia 58, **66**, 67, 143
Hypocalcemia **66**, 143, 157, 159
Hypoglycemia **67**, 147, 143
Hyponatremia 58, **66**, 67

IDU (IVDU) See Injection drug use
IL-2 (interleukin-2) 84, 102, 166
Imidazoles 135, 138
Imipenem cilastatin (IMP) 111, 113, 122, 135
Immune reconstitution syndrome 27, 38, 39, 55, 59, 61, 62, 64, 66, 67, 70, 75, 78, 86, 89, 91, 94, 95, **98**–100, **103–105**, 130, 133, 165
Immunization 3, 4, 6, 9, 40, 89, 90, **167–170**
Impetigo 42, 100
Indinavir 4, 10, 12, 14, **20**, **21**, **25**, **29**, 31, 32, 36, 46, 52, 57, 83, 84, 90, 103, 109, 148, 154, 155, 157, 159, 160, **162**, **163**, 164, 172
Infection control 88
Influenza 4, 6, 7, 9, 63, 80, 87–**90**, 98, 167–169
Integrase Inhibitors 33
Injection drug use (IDU, IVDU) 1–3, 7, 27, 35, 37, 50, 52, 80, 82, 86, 89, 102, 129, 132, 133, 135, 168, 169
Interferon alfa 70, 83, 84, 87, 134, **146**, 166, 172
Iodoquinol 123, 124, **142**, 172
Isolation practices 15, 77, 80, 87, **88**, 92, 93, 108
Isoniazid (INH) 47, 49, 139, 147, 156–158, 164, 172
Isospora belli 75–**77**, 84, 85, 124
Itraconazole 43, 54, 99, 116, 117, **119–124**, 126, 135, **138**, 147, 152, 155, 156, **158**–161, 164, 172
Ivermectin 121, 126, 127, **143**, 147

Kaletra **25**, **30**, **46**, 155, **162**, **163**, 172
Kaposi's sarcoma 15, 41, 67, 68, **72**–74, 78, 81–83, 85, **92**, 94, 95, **100**, 102, 104, **133**, 165
Karnofsky scale 16

Ketoconazole 66, 68, 74, 86, 121, **122**, 135, 156–161, 172

Lactic acidosis 21–23, 27, **28**, 30, **31**, 35, 36, 39, 44, 66, 85, 96, 103, 145
Lamivudine (3TC) 12, 18, **19–22**, **28**, 31, 34, 43, 44, 52, 65, 67, 75, 83, 86, 97, 129, 130, 146, 164, 172
Legionella 89, 90
Leiomyosarcoma 42, 165
Leishmaniasis 3, 70, 72, **75**, 81, 83, 101, 104
Leprosy 99
"Lightning pain" syndrome 96
Lipodystrophy **66**, 87, 103
Lipomatosis **32**, 87
Listeriosis 63, 81, 106
Loeffler's syndrome 95
Lopinavir 10, 12, 14, **19**, 23, **25**, 30, 32, 35, 36, 39, 40, 43, 46, 52, 84, 109, 148, **155**, 158–160, **162**, **163**, 164, 172
Lung abscess See Abscess, lung
Lupus anticoagulant 84
Lymphogranuloma venereum (LGV) 78, 79, **80**, **107**
Lymphoid interstitial pneumonia (LIP) 42, **92**
Lymphoma 7, 15, 56, 58, 59, **60**–62, 64, 66, 67, 70, 72–75, 78, 81–83, 85, **92**, 94, 95, 97, 100, 102, 104, 165, 166

MAC or MAI (Mycobacterium avium complex or intracellulare) 15, 40, 47–49, 54, 56, 66–68, 70, 71, 73, 75, 77, 83, 85, 88, 90, **94**, 95, 97, 98–**100**, 102–105, **110**–112, 139, 141, 142
Malignancies 3, 4, 37, 40, 82–85, 97, 116, 117, 122, 133, 136, 156, **165–166**
Maturation Inhibitor 33
Measles **90**, 168, 169
Megestrol acetate 67, 96, 164, 172
Meningitis 16, 37, 43, 54–56, 59, **62**, **63**, 68, 69, 73, 84, 89, 103, 106, **115**, 119–123, 137, 138, 144, 169
Menstrual dysfunction 35, 67, 68, 140, 145
Metronidazole 21, 29, 72, 99, **106**, 123, 124, 126, 135, **143**, 147, 151, 157–159, 161, 164
Microsporidia 68, 75–77, **85**, 98, 103, **124**
Molluscum contagiosum 62, 68, **99**, 104, 122, **134**
Mononeuritis multiplex **64–66**, 127
Myalgia 26, 28, 51, 55, **65**, **66**, 74, 87, 96, 136, 140, 143, 144, 146, 170
Mycobacteria, atypical 70, 75, 81, 95, 98, 100, 111, 112, 142, 156
Mycobacterium avium complex or intracellulare See MAC or MAI
Mycobacterium kansasii 15, **93**–95, 99, 111
Mycobacterium tuberculosis (TB) 3, 4, 9, 37, 53, 62, 63, 69, 71, 75, 78, 81, 85, 88, 89, 90, 93–95, 98, 103, **107–109**
Myelopathy 7, 64
Myocarditis 82
Myopathy 4, 23, 28, **65**, **96**

Natural history, HIV **17**, 37
Neisseria gonorrhoeae 4, 78, **112**, 113
Nelfinavir 10, 12, **19**, **20**, **25**, 30, 40, 46, 109, 148, 155, 158, 161, **162–163**, 164, 172
Nephropathy 42, **97–98**, 104
Neuropathy 21–23, 26, 28, 31, **32**, 55, 64–**66**, 74, 106, 139, 140, 142–144, 146, 157, 161, 165
Neuropsychiatric syndromes 27, 29, 56, 57, 132
Nevirapine 10, 12, **20**, **24**, 25, 27, **29**–31, 34–36, 39, 45, 46, 52, 83, 86, 99, 148, 154–156, 158–160, **163**, 164, 172
NMDA 56
Nocardiosis 61, 68, 81, 92, 94, 95, 97, **122**
Non-Nucleoside Reverse Transcriptase Inhibitors 4, 10, 12, 23, 24, 27, **28–29**, (NNRTI) 31, 33, 38–40, 44, 45, 48, 157–160, 163
Nonoxynol 1, 2, 35

Norwegian scabies 80, **84**, **101**, 127
Nucleoside Reverse Transcriptase Inhibitors (NRTI) 4, 10, 21, 23, 27, **28**, 36, 39, 65, 86, 97, 99
Numbness, foot 65

Occupational exposure **2–3**, 7, 18, **50–52**
Odynophagia 41, 73, **74**, 75
Ofloxacin 106, 108, 135, **141**, **157**, 172
Organ transplantation 122, 128, 136–138, 145

P. carinii pneumonia (PCP) 6, 15, **38–39**, 42, 48, 53, 59, 66, 67, 69, 70, 73, 75, 88, 89, **91**–95, 99, 102, 105, 125, 142, 144, 169
p24 antigen 2, 5, 6, **7**, 15, 37, 55, 75
Paclitaxel 160, 165, 166, 172
Pancreatitis 19, 21–23, 25, 28, 30, **31**, 55, **67**, **75**, 96, **97**, 131, 143, 157, 159, 161
Pap smear 4, 35, 73, 134, 166
Papillitis, CMV 68, **69**, 128
Papillomavirus (HPV) See HPV
Paromomycin 123, 124, 143, 172
Parotid enlargement 42, **73**, 104
Parvovirus B-19 83, 104, **134**, 170
PCP See P. carinii pneumonia
PCR (polymerase chain reaction) 5, 7, 8, 11, 15, 37, 38, 42, 54, 58–61, 69, 70, 72, 79, 82, 84, 91, 102, 106, 124, 131, 134, 165, 166
Pediatric AIDS 36–49
Pediculosis pubis 80, 126
Pegylated interferon 70, **146**, 164, 172
Peliosis hepatis 42, **86**, 106
Pelvic inflammatory disease (PID) 35, **80**, **113**
Penicillin desensitization 34
Penicillium marneffei 70, **72**, 85, 93, 99, **122**
Pentamidine 36, 38, 48, 49, 53, 58, 66, 67, 69, 75, 83, 91, 95, 97–99, **125**, **143**, 144, 151, 152, 156, 157, 159, 161, 164, 172
Performance status 16
Pericarditis 81, 105
Perinatal infection 2, 20, **37**, **38**, 42, 87, 131, 133
Peritonitis **75**, 80, 97, 113, 119, 137
Pets 3, 68, 90
Pharmacokinetics See Drug pharmacokinetics
Phenotype resistance testing 4, 11, 13, 14, 27
Pituitary 67
Plasma viremia 2, 4, 6, 9, 11, 14, 15, 18, 27, 33, 35–39, 41, 51, 54, 55, 57, 61–63, 66, 79, 84, 86, 87, 89, 97, 100, 103–105, 170
Pleural effusion 50, 88, 91–**95**
PML See Progressive multifocal leukoencephalopathy
Pneumococcal pneumonia 9, 89, **98**
Pneumococcal vaccine 3, 4, 9, 89, **167–169**
Pneumocystis carinii (PCP) See p. carinii pneumonia
Pneumonia 4, 9, 15, 26, 30, 37, 42, 62, 63, 66, 69, 70, 73, 81, 87, 88, 91–**94**, 95, 98, 102, 103, 105, **114**, 116, 116, **125**, **128**, 135, 169
Pneumothorax 91, **95**, 143
Podophyllin 72, 79, 129, 134
Polymyositis 96
Porphyria cutanea tarda 101
Post-exposure prophylaxis (PEP) 1, 18, 50–52, 133
Prednisone 29, 74, 96, 97, 107, **125**, 159, 166
Pregnancy, HIV 2–4, 6, 10, 18–24, 27–30, **35–37**, 38, 45, 51, 52, 80, 83, 106, 124, 126, 127, 132, 134, 135, 137–139, 142, 143, 145, 146, 160, **164**
Primaquine 83, 125, **143**, 172
Proctitis **78**, 80, 112
Progressive multifocal leukoencephalopathy (PML) 41, 55, 57–**61**, 104, 134
Prophylaxis (OIs) 53, 54
Prostatitis 113
Protease inhibitors (PI) 4, 10–13, 19–21, 23, **24–26**, 27, **29**, 30–32, 33, 36, 38–40, **45–47**, 48, 67, 70, 102, 103, 104, 109–111, **155**–158, **159–163**, 165

Protein S 42
Proteinuria 97–98, 144
Psoriasis 96, 101, 127, 135
Psychoses 139, 140, 158
Pulmonary hypertension, primary 82
Pyomyositis 95
Pyrazinamide (PZA) 47, 53, 108, 109, 11, 112,
135, 140, 141, 160, 164, 172
Pyrimethamine 53, 83, 124, 125, 143, 147,
152, 155, 157, 160, 164, 172

Quinacrine 124

RAU (Recurrent aphthous ulcers) 73, 135
Reiter's syndrome 80, 96
Resistance, antiviral drug 10–14, 18–21, 27, 36, 39, 40
Retinitis 15, 41, 58, 68–70, 80, 103, 105,
106, 127, 128, 129, 133, 145
Rheumatoid arthritis 96
Rho immune globulin 42
Rhodococcus 68, 70, 81, 93, 94, 98, 113
Rifabutin 40, 47–49, 53, 54, 70, 107–112, 135,
141, 153, 155–161, 164, 172
Rifampin 26, 47, 49, 53, 67, 75, 86, 106–115,
121, 135, 138, 139–141, 147, 153,
156–161, 164, 172
Rifater (INH, RIF, PZA) 140
Risk assessment 1
Ritonavir 10, 12, 14, 19–21, 23–27, 30–33, 35, 36,
39, 40, 43, 45–47, 52, 84, 86, 87, 103, 109,
148, 154, 155, 158–161, 162, 163, 164, 172
Rotavirus 41

'Safe' sex 1–3
Salivary gland anti-HIV antibody test 3
Salivary gland enlargement 73, 123
Salmonella 15, 41, 63, 70, 76, 88, 98, 113
Salpingitis 80, 113
Saquinavir 10, 12, 20, 21, 26, 30, 32, 40, 47, 52,
75, 109, 148, 154, 155, 159, 160, 162,
163, 164, 172
Sargramostim (GM-CSF) 83, 144, 170, 172
Scabies 80, 84, 99, 100, 101, 127, 143
Scedosporium 122–123
Seborrhea 50, 101, 135
Seizures 4, 59–64, 141, 142, 144, 145, 157, 158
Sepsis 42, 58, 98
Septata intestinalis 77, 124
Sexual transmission of HIV 1, 2, 105, 131
Shigellosis 76, 78, 113
Shingles (varicella zoster) See Herpes zoster
Sinusitis 70, 98
Sjögren's syndrome 73
Skin 3, 16, 19, 22, 24, 28–31, 36, 42, 51, 54, 60,
62, 80, 81, 83, 86, 93, 99–101, 104, 111,
114, 115, 119, 121–123, 127, 133, 135,
137–144, 165
Skin/nail discoloration 22, 28, 100, 101, 141
Sporotrichosis 100, 123
Staphylococcus aureus 42, 81, 89, 94, 95, 98, 114
Stavudine (d4T) 10–12, 14, 21, 22, 28, 30, 34–36,
39, 40, 43, 44, 52, 62, 65, 67, 75, 83, 96,
97, 148, 154, 157, 160, 161, 164, 172
Steatosis 21, 22, 27, 28, 30, 66, 85
Stevens-Johnson syndrome 24, 28–31, 34, 45, 99,
100, 139, 143, 144
Stomach 74–75
Stomatitis 23, 72, 119, 135, 140
Streptococcus pneumoniae 63, 89, 114, 116
Streptomycin 47, 108, 109, 135, 140, 147,
149, 150, 152, 164
Sulfadiazine 122, 125, 143, 151
Syphilis 2–4, 55, 56, 58, 59, 63, 64, 68, 70,
72, 78–80, 81, 95, 99, 115, 135

T
3TC See Lamivudine

Tenofovir 4, 9, 10–12, 14, 18, 19, 21, 22, 23, 24,
27, 28, 30, 31, 39, 40, 43, 44, 45, 97, 98,
130, 148, 154, 157, 160, 161, 164, 172
Terbinafine 122, 138
Testes 68
Testosterone 4, 68, 139
Tests for HIV (viral load, viral burden) 5–14, 16
Thalidomide 65, 73, 74, 78, 135, 164, 165
Thiacetazone (amithiozone) 141, 172
Thrombocytopenia 40, 42, 55, 71, 84, 90, 137,
138, 143–145, 170
Thrush (oral candidiasis) 4, 16, 50, 71, 73, 104
Thyroid 41, 67, 142, 146
TIA (transient ischemic attack) 159
Tinidazole 124, 126, 147
TMP/SMX desensitization See Desensitization,
TMP/SMX
Torsade de pointes 141, 143
Toxoplasma gondii 3, 4, 15, 16, 41, 53, 55, 56,
58–62, 64, 67, 68, 70, 75, 82,
88, 93, 95, 101, 105, 125, 142
Transfusion (blood products) 2, 83, 87, 124, 133, 140
Transmission of HIV 1–3, 8, 18, 20, 35–37, 50–52,
79, 83, 87, 91, 105, 131
Travel, advice & immunization 3, 77, 85, 169–170, 171
Trichomonas vaginalis 80, 126
Tricyclic antidepressants 32, 66, 159, 160
Trimethoprim (TMP) See TMP/SMX
Trimethoprim/sulfamethoxazole 16, 31, 36, 38, 48, 49,
(TMP/SMX) 53, 59, 66, 67, 74–76, 83, 84,
86, 89–91, 97, 99 111–114, 122–125,
135, 142, 144, 151, 157, 160, 161, 164, 172
Trimetrexate 83, 172
Trizivir 20, 21, 43, 44, 172
Trovafloxacin 150
TTP (thrombotic thrombocytopenic purpura) 84, 145
Tuberculin test (PPD) 3, 4, 54, 88, 89, 107
Tuberculosis See Mycobacterium tuberculosis
Typhlitis 75, 78

Urethritis 2, 79, 80, 96, 106, 112
Uveitis 68–70, 80, 103, 110, 141

Vacuolar myelopathy 64
Vaginitis 1, 81, 119, 126
Valacyclovir 79, 84, 133, 134, 135, 145,
148, 154, 164, 172
Valganciclovir 54, 66, 83, 127–129, 145,
148, 154, 157, 164, 172
Varicella zoster virus (VZV) See Herpes zoster
Vascular line sepsis 42
Ventricular tachycardia 139, 143
Vinblastine 165, 166, 172
Vincristine 65, 157, 160, 161, 165, 166, 172
Viral load See Plasma viremia
Voriconazole 116–119, 121–123, 139, 147,
152, 155, 156, 160, 164, 172
vRNA (viral load) 8, 15, 18, 37, 55, 105, 168
VZIG (varicella zoster immunoglobin) 49, 169
VZV (varicella zoster virus) See Herpes zoster

Warts 72, 79, 81, 100, 104, 134, 146
Wasting syndrome 4, 15, 41, 50, 66, 68,
75–77, 102, 104
Weakness 28, 31, 60, 61, 64, 65, 66, 96, 116
Western blot 3, 5–7, 15, 37

Xerostomia 73, 143
Xerotic eczema 101

Zalcitabine (ddC) 23, 28, 32, 39, 44, 62, 65, 67, 73, 74,
83, 84, 86, 96, 97, 107, 135, 161, 172
Zidovudine (ZDV, AZT) 3, 4, 12, 18–21, 22, 24, 27,
28, 30–32, 34, 36, 39–41, 43,
44, 50, 52, 62, 65, 74, 75, 83,
84, 86, 87, 96, 101, 102, 110,
135, 144, 161, 166, 170, 172